The Cult of Remembrance and the Black Death

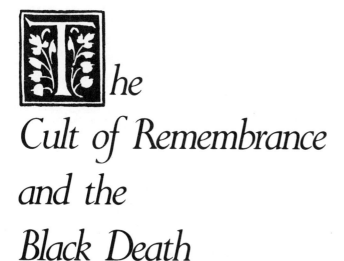

The
Cult of Remembrance
and the
Black Death

SIX RENAISSANCE CITIES
IN CENTRAL ITALY

SAMUEL K. COHN, Jr.

The Johns Hopkins University Press   Baltimore and London

This book was originally brought to publication with the generous assistance
of the National Endowment for the Humanities.

Johns Hopkins Paperbacks edition, 1997
06 05 04 03 02 01 00 99 98 97   5 4 3 2 1

The Johns Hopkins University Press
2715 North Charles Street
Baltimore, Maryland 21218-4319
The Johns Hopkins Press Ltd., London

The Library of Congress has cataloged the hardcover edition as follows:
Cohn, Samuel Kline.
    The cult of remembrance and the Black Death : six Renaissance cities in central
Italy / Samuel K. Cohn, Jr.
        p.   cm.
    Includes bibliographical references and index.
    ISBN 0-8018-4303-0
    1. Italy — Social conditions — 1268–1559.   2. Life style — Italy — History.
    3. Black death — Social aspects — Italy — History.   4. Charitable bequests — Italy
    — History.   5. Art and society — Italy — History.   6. Renaissance — Italy.   I. Title.
    HN475.C59   1992
    306′.0945 — dc20   91-45267

ISBN 0-8018-5606-X (pbk.)

Pages xiv — xv:
Abraham Ortelius, "Tusciae antique typus" (Antwerp, 1584).

Contents

Tables and Illustrations

Acknowledgments

This study began neither in Florence nor with testaments. Instead, while surveying materials in the Marche for a study of comparative city-state development in the Middle Ages, I heard that the Florentine state archives were about to close. Despite the official pronouncement of nine months, many predicted that they would remain shut for decades. The perverse thought then crossed my mind: why not return for one last Florentine topic? *Veluti canis ad vomitum* (as medieval chroniclers sometimes expressed the lure of sin), I rushed back to Florence in the summer of 1987. Places in the *sala di consultazione* were then becoming hard to come by. But the atmosphere became more charged by late fall 1987, when I was able to return again to Florence, this time funded by a half-year sabbatical from Brandeis University. To secure a seat when the archives opened (9 a.m.), the *studioso* had to line up under Vasari's arches at 7 and once inside had to remain zealously reading the documents or else face forfeiting the valiantly won place to hungry researchers waiting in the corridor. Tensions ran high, and work was periodically punctuated by shouting matches between overworked archival personnel and overstressed *studiosi*. Nonetheless, the common predicament gave rise to a community of good will and an intellectual camaraderie that I have rarely experienced in academic life. I fondly remember intellectual exchanges, complaints, and gossip over quick lunches *al banco* and after-archive beers with Deborah Krohn, Gianni Cappelli, Chris Wickham, Robert Black, John Nadis, Adrienne Atwell, Amanda Lillie, Daniela Lamberini, and others.

After the archives had closed, I was able to return to Italy to continue research in Pisa, Arezzo, Perugia, Siena, and Assisi through a generous project grant awarded by the Getty Center for the Humanities. To the archivists, researchers, and photographers in these towns, I owe a special thanks, especially to Don Costanzo Tabarelli, O.S.B., who left the doors to the rich collections of the convent of San Pietro open until 8 p.m. and sometimes later, and to Maria Immacolata Bossi, who introduced me to the rich *pergamene* collections housed in the Sacro Convento of Assisi.

I spent the academic year 1988-89 as a Guest Fellow at the Villa I Tatti (Harvard University). In this unique center for Renaissance studies I was able to discuss my ideas about the Renaissance and cycling in Tuscany with art historians, musicologists, historians, and students of Italian literature. I am indebted to the staff and the scholars then in residence, Amanda George, Nelda Feracci, Fortunato Pratesi, Walter Kaiser, Eve Borsook, Margaret Haines, Eileen Reeves, Peter Urquhart, Chris Reynolds, Erling Skaug, and especially Salvatore Camporeale. Back in Cambridge, I benefited from conversations with John Shearman.

Many friends and scholars have read versions of the manuscript at various moments in its development. My colleagues Philip Ethington, Alice Kelikian, and David Fischer read the Introduction, as did Anthony Molho. Deborah Krohn, Stephen Campbell, John Paoletti, Megan Holmes, William Hood, Jane Bestor, and Julia Sheehan read the sections on art and painting; and, at different stages, Salvatore Camporeale, Rudolph Binion, Genevieve Warwick, William Bowsky, and the manuscript editor at the Johns Hopkins University Press, Carol Ehrlich, read through the entire manuscript. Beyond exposing errors and infelicities in style, these scholars forced me to state assumptions, rethink arguments, and draw out more boldly conclusions blanketed by mounds of empirical findings. They may be disappointed with what resulted from their careful readings and comments; nonetheless, without their encouragement, criticism, and intellectual exchange, I can safely say my research would have produced a different book—a weaker one.

My research assistant during the summer of 1990, Megan Holmes, took special pains beyond my meager sums, reading drafts on testamentary commissions, directing me to relevant secondary research, instructing me in late medieval Italian art history, and following her own leads searching for the survival of testamentary commissions through documents, churches, and museums. Finally, I wish to thank Genevieve Warwick, my friends at Vincigliata, and the ragazzi del Gruppo Sportivo di Maiano, who made research on this book more than an academic endeavor.

Like small plaques or the coats of arms that late Trecento testators ordered to be embossed on candlestick holders, this book is dedicated to the memories of earthly endeavors—that of two of my teachers.

A Note on Names and Dates

Names

In this text, names and citations from archival sources have been rendered according to the orthography found in the originals.

Dates

The city-states in this study used various calendars. Florence and Siena began the year on 25 March, the feast of the Annunciation (*stile dell'Incarnazione*). Thus, a testament dated February 1348 would have been redacted in 1349 according to the modern Gregorian calendar. For Arezzo, Assisi, and Perugia, the new year began with Christmas (*stile della Natività*). Finally, Pisa had its own style (*stile pisano*). The new year began on the feast of the Annunciation but was one year ahead of the Florentine calendar. Thus, a testament dated 25 June 1349 would have been redacted in the year of the Black Death (1348), and one dated 6 February 1349 would have been issued in 1349 according to our calendar. Although Adriano Cappelli (*Cronologia, cronografia, e calendario perpetuo*, 14) maintains that this Pisan style persisted until 1749, the testaments found in my samples changed their dating to the Florentine calendar with the Pisan subjection to the Florentines in 1406. For my statistics and for the text of this book, dates have been rendered in the modern style of the Gregorian calendar. In the Notes, I have left the dates as they appeared in the original documents.

Apennini montes.

Annetanum

Apua.

CLVS ENTI

AP VA NI
LIGVR ES.

LIGVRIAE PARS.

E T R V

Segesta Tigu
liorum.

Marcalla flu.

Pistorium, vel
ad Pistores.

Florentia co
lonia, quae, et Flu
entia, forte

T

Fossa Pa
phriana.

Massa

STELLATES

Phocensis lacus.

R

Luna, quae et
ad Carrari.

Carrea, a siue
et Potentia.

Phocenses.

I

Fluentini, qui et
Arnien ses.

A

Ericis
portus.

Montes Feroniani.

Luca co
lonia

Sena colonia

ETR

Arnus flui.

Volaterrani, cognomi
ne Etrusci.

Pisae colonia, Aeneas
cognominat Virgilius.

VRI.

Volaterra
colonia

MARE

TYRRHENVM, SI

Volaterranus ager.

OCCIDENS.

Arni ostium,
et Pisanus
portus.

Lamellum.

Ligurnus portus. Videsurg
ad Herculem. Antonin.

Cecinna flu.

Volaterra
na Vada.

GORGON

Inter Pisanum Cyrna
cumq lacus.

Cecinna fl.

Rusellae Ptol.

Vetulonienses.

R

A

Vetulonium
Suderetum.

M

IM

Squalet lucifugis insula plena
viris. Rutil. lib. 1.

Capraria

Statona.

Prilis
lacus.

Salebro
portus.

Pandataria Agrippinae
Aug. exilio celebr's

CORSI
CAE in
sulae
pars

ILNA, quae
et AE THA
LIA.

Anpus portus.

VE TVSCVM

Insula inexhaustis talibum
generosa metallis. Virg.

M

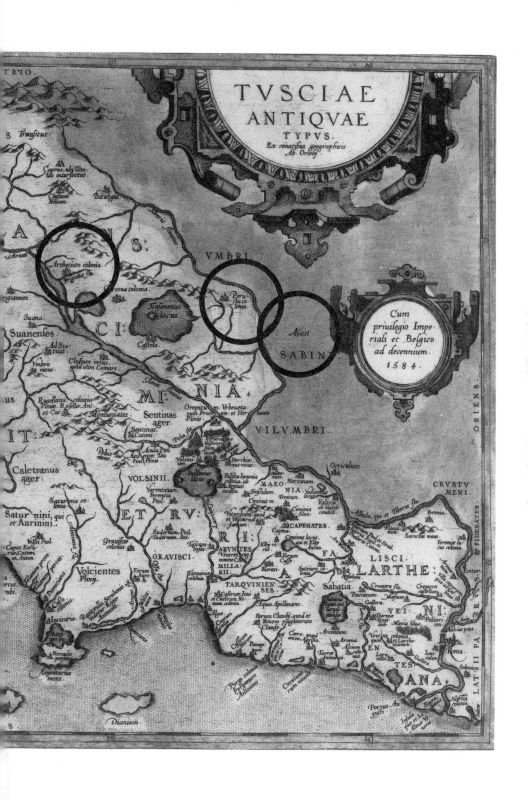

1

Introduction

While the proper realm of religions is the afterlife, they have their foundations on earth. They lead the faithful towards the everlasting and infinite, but then live in time and space. Each has its history and its geography.
—Gabriel Le Bras, "Un programme: La géographie religieuse"

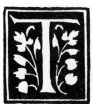his book began as an exercise in comparative history. A single practice—the writing of a testament and its bequests, to friends, to kin, to pious and charitable causes—serves as the key for comparing six societies of late medieval and early Renaissance Tuscany and Umbria. Changes in Arezzo, Assisi, Florence, Perugia, Pisa, and Siena are measured against one another through the quantitative analysis of 3,389 wills from some of the earliest notarized specimens of the twelfth and thirteenth centuries through the Black Death of 1348 and its recurrent attacks until 1425. While the social ambit of those redacting wills tended to expand over the period investigated in this book, testators possessing little or no landed property can be found in these samples from the outset. Only the *miserabili,* those without substantial property of any sort, landed or movables, are seriously underrepresented.

My concentration on testaments means that this study focuses on intentions more than eventualities. While last wills and testaments and codicils may have constituted the major source of income for charitable institutions (at least by the middle of the thirteenth century),[1] they tell us little about the actual ebb and flow of properties to particular charitable organizations or whether particular bequests indeed ended up in the coffers of the desired beneficiaries. An institutional approach—from the perspective of a hospital, a monastery, or a cathedral—would better enable the researcher to answer such questions about contested testaments, incomes, and expenditures of charitable organizations. However, this more traditional approach to charity can only follow a few institutions or concentrate on big donors, which (as we will discover in Chapter 2) may be misleading and seriously limits the study of broader changes in mentalities.

The Comparative Approach

A recent anthology dedicated to questions of "life and death" in Renaissance Florence begins by "celebrating" the interdisciplinary success achieved by historians of the Florentine Renaissance over the past twenty years.[2] Indeed, the meticulous record keeping of the late medieval and early modern city-states of Italy has provided "laboratories"[3] for quantitative and interdisciplinary history unmatched by many other cultures before the rise of modern nation-state bureaucracies in the eighteenth century. Armed with computers, anthropological models, and economic theories, scholars have made impressive headway in uncovering everyday experience across social classes for late medieval and Renaissance Tuscany.[4] Subjects completely beyond the purview of the great nineteenth-century Swiss historian Jacob Burckhardt[5] now provoke lively debate and stimulate new research in areas such as the structure and texture of peasant life, the importance of the mezzadria,[6] the church and political patronage,[7] the political organization of the laboring classes,[8] family structure, ideology, and demography. Yet, social and economic historians of the late medieval and early modern Italian city-state have failed to observe one of the first and most elemental requirements of social science inquiry since Marx, Weber, and Durkheim—a comparative approach.[9] We now know, for instance, that patrician families in Quattrocento Florence remained clustered in their traditional neighborhoods, where they continued to exert local power and influence.[10] Yet we have no idea to what extent these patterns of residence and patronage characterized other Renaissance city-states. Did the Florentine patriciate hold on to their traditional bonds of neighborhood longer than elites in other cities? Were the bonds of family lineage stronger in Florence than elsewhere? Was the neighborhood ward here a more significant power base than elsewhere?[11] Similarly, questions as diverse as confraternal religiosity and the power of women in their households and over property now cry out for comparative analysis.

Two tendencies have characterized Florentine historiography. Historians with political orientations as diverse as Hans Baron[12] and Eugenio Garin[13] have redefined humanist culture and Italian politics in the early Renaissance roughly along those lines, which in the sixteenth century Medicean publicist and painter Giorgio Vasari sketched for Italian art history.[14] They have stressed Florence's peculiarity—its precocious and exceptional character, its centrality for understanding a rebirth in politics, economy, letters, and art. More recently, historians who have borrowed models and categories from anthropology have gone to the opposite extreme, seeing Florence as a "Mediterranean society" characterized by modes of comportment, notions of "honor" and "shame,"[15] and systems of patronage largely without temporal or other spatial delineations.[16] At least in one regard, the broad conclusions of these historians are more suspect than those drawn by the previous generation of scholars. While Baron compared Florentine humanists with those in Milan and Venice, and Myron Gilmore and Eugenio Garin placed their thinkers in larger geographical contexts than the single city-state, these recent historians of an anthropological bent have yet to compare Florence concretely with other localities to determine just how exceptional or unexceptional Renaissance Florence happened to be.

Quantitative and social science research on Italy has been curiously entrenched in a spirit of localism that once characterized more traditional narrative and political histories of Italy.[17] It is difficult to know why the study of the individual city-state in isolation has persisted for so long especially among French and Anglophone historians of the Renaissance in Italy, who have had no immediate stake in a city-state's local traditions. Perhaps it has resulted from the Promethean task that these post–World War II historians have assumed—"total history"—daunting enough for a single locality and nearly inconceivable for the comparison of numbers of territories.[18] While my study goes beyond the margins of individual testaments and their aggregation, I have made no attempt to reconstruct other areas of social, economic, and public life, since this would require an attention to archival sources equal to that given here to the analysis of thousands of testaments. Nonetheless, the conclusions that I have reached from comparisons of piety, inheritance, and property relations should serve other scholars now mining the rich archival collections in these towns on other themes and for different purposes.

The city-states of Italy from the appearance of Europe's earliest communal charters in the late eleventh century until political unification in 1871 supply the historian with an ideal "laboratory" for comparative studies. Unlike the difficulties presented for historians of northern Europe, where in moving from one culture to another, especially across national or language boundaries, the scholar must regard so many institutional differences, a nearly uniform notarial culture tied large zones and various regions of the Italian peninsula together, at least with regard to certain legal, institutional, and administrative practices. Institutions such as the *podestà*, the Captain of the People, and the antimagnate legislation exemplified by the Florentine Ordinances of Justice (1293) structured a civil and criminal legal system with deeply ingrained characteristics. Often the same state dignitaries (Podestà and Captains of the People with their bevies of notaries and police) carried and implemented these legal and administrative practices from one town to the next. This was certainly the case in the six cities examined in this study.[19] We shall see, however, that within these broad administrative and legal structures much room was left for profound differences in custom and practice.

The Six City-States

The city-states[20] chosen for this study were selected not arbitrarily but largely for the available documentation—large numbers of testaments that survived before and after the Black Death of 1348.[21] Several other towns in central Italy also possess archives with numerous last wills stretching back well before 1348 and qualify as interesting candidates. I avoided Bologna, Orvieto, and Borgo San Sepolcro, because other scholars are now engaged in systematic research of testaments in these towns.[22] To the west of Florence, Lucca would have been an obvious choice. I picked Pisa instead so as to include a maritime city. Similarly, the rich municipal archives in Umbria offer opportunities other than Perugia and Assisi. In addition to Orvieto, Todi, Gubbio, Foligno, and Spoleto could provide adequate numbers of testaments through the Trecento. I preferred Perugia for the obvious reasons that, like Florence in Tuscany, it became a regional center after the Black Death, crossing the terrains of earlier medieval city-states.[23] Moreover, today it possesses the richest notarial and parchment archives of any city in Umbria.[24] I

finally selected Assisi because of its extraordinary collection of early
testaments and because, as the birthplace of the Franciscan movement,
it might be isolated as an early center of mendicant values. I wanted to
know how long these values may have characterized this town and its
countryside, whether it resisted the changes I had uncovered in Siena
and was then finding across Tuscany, or whether it would fit what I then
thought (and still think) forms a general pattern of change in the late
Trecento.

POPULATION   All of these towns were major European cities before
the Black Death. Florence was the most populous, numbering at its
height (circa 1300) as many as 120,000. Depending on whose estimates
the historian believes, Siena comes next in size (about 52,000 at its
apex),[25] then Pisa (40,000 in the late thirteenth century[26] and perhaps
as many as 50,000 in 1315),[27] Perugia (28,505 according to estimates
derived from the estimo of 1285),[28] Arezzo (as large as 20,000),[29] and
last Assisi (approximately 12,397 according to a hearth tax initiated in
1232).[30] After the Black Death, and increasingly through the late fourteenth and early fifteenth centuries, the rank ordering as well as the
spacing between them changed. While waves of pestilence (in 1348,
1362–63, 1373–74, 1375, 1383–84, 1389, 1390, and 1399–1400) devastated towns and villages throughout Tuscany and Umbria, the ensuing
demographic histories were not everywhere the same. Pisa, Arezzo, and
Assisi shrunk to mere shadows of their former size. But despite their
losses, Florence, Perugia, and to some extent Siena grew relative to their
territories and in particular to the towns within their economic, political,
and administrative ambits.[31] If the early fifteenth-century population of
Florence (36,909, according to the Catasto of 1427)[32] was between half
and one-third of what it had been one hundred years earlier, Pisa—
the second largest city within the Florentine "district"—was less than
one-fifth of its late thirteenth-century size: according to the Catasto of
1427, its urban population stood at 7,106.[33] Arezzo's decline was not
quite as steep; in 1384, it numbered no more than 6,000[34] and in 1427
only 3,992.[35] Siena, on the other hand, was four times the size of these
provincial centers after the Black Death,[36] and Perugia had become the
second regional center of the six cities here investigated (at least by
1495, when its population can again be estimated); it was the only city
in this study to recoup its pre-plague head count before the late nineteenth century. Its population in 1495 stood at 28,455,[37] a population
size that Siena did not regain before the modern period.[38] For Assisi,

the population figures are more fragmentary than elsewhere. By a census of 1533, after more than a century of general upturn in European population, Assisi had reached only Arezzo's population at its low-water mark in the early fifteenth century (800 households).[39]

ECONOMY   All six cities were centers for textiles, banking, and commerce. The mix and extent of these activities, however, varied significantly from place to place. As an industrial center—particularly for wool production—Florence towered over the rest by the beginning of the Trecento.[40] The Florentine testaments witness this city's international climate as a center of banking and long-distance trade, corroborating those career scenarios which we know well from numerous merchant diaries and the lives of merchant-writers such as Giovanni Boccaccio and the chronicler Giovanni Villani. They also give insights into the situations of those international men of the merchant elite during the late Middle Ages who divided their lives and ultimately their property between their place of birth and their place of work. For instance, the international merchant Iacobus Juochi filius quondam[41] Geraldi Juochis, of Florence, "merchant in the city of Paris," devoted a large portion of his will to arranging the precise privileges and property settlements for an illegitimate daughter whom he had sired and left behind in Paris.[42] The will of the Florentine merchant Martinus f.q. Bizzi provided in comparable detail for the division of his properties *tam in denariis quam in mercantiis* that he held in his *fondaco* in Avignon as well as his businesses in Florence.[43]

But the testaments from the smaller and less wealthy maritime city of Pisa lend a more international aura than those of the other five cities.[44] Pisan merchants such as Palmerius f.q. Vicini,[45] Angelus Spina f.q. Ruggeri Spine,[46] and the citizen Romenus Ruberis,[47] divided their pious gifts between Pisa and foreign places—a village in the district of Marseilles, the territory of Messina in Sicily, or the city of Genoa. Even those without mercantile occupations stretched interregional relations through their wills: thus, the Pisan widow Guida f.q. Bonuiani, from the village of Vico, provided her son's illegitimate daughter with a dowry on condition that she return from Sardinia.[48]

Furthermore, slaves appear more often in pious bequests in Pisa than in any other city; indeed, Florence is the only other city where slaves appear in these records as objects of charitable manumissions.[49] All came from distant lands.[50] When the slaves were identified beyond a Christian name, almost invariably they were referred to as "Tartars."[51] In only one case was a slave identified more specifically. Panchuccius f.q. Iacobi Pilati, from the Pisan parish[52] of San Lorenzo, "liberated" his domestic slave (*schiava mea*)—"Maria, the Greek, from Romania in the lands of Constantinople"—as well as her children "both feminine and masculine according to the customs of the city of Rome."[53]

In line with the demographic trends, after the Black Death Florence and Perugia experienced less economic decline than did their provincial cities, which increasingly became incorporated into the larger regional economies of Tuscany and Umbria.[54] Florentine historians over the past two decades have seriously questioned the notions of "Renaissance depression"[55] and have pushed beyond the aggregate trade and production estimates to investigate more closely changes in the character of economy and society from the Black Death through the fifteenth century. Despite repeated regional waves of famine, pestilence, and bankruptcies in 1369–71, 1374–75,[56] and the 1390s,[57] David Herlihy has argued that Tuscany formed a "rational" and integrated regional economy by the early Quattrocento.[58] In a glowing assessment of Florentine urban economy, Richard Goldthwaite claimed it was more "dynamic" and prosperous during the fifteenth century than ever before and that rapid social mobility distinguished this center of art and culture from other mercantile towns of the Renaissance, whether in Italy or north of the Alps.[59]

In the same vein, scholars working independently of one another in the local histories of various provincial cities in central Italy have revised the earlier pictures of these towns as sliding relentlessly into corruption, decline, and decadence after their moments of glory in the late Duecento or early Trecento, becoming by the early Quattrocento little more than market towns servicing the agricultural production of their surrounding hinterlands.[60] David Hicks has stressed the revival of industry and commerce in early Quattrocento Siena.[61] Giuseppe Mira argues that the wool industry in Perugia developed capitalistic relations of production only in the second half of the Trecento;[62] Romano Pierotti has shown the vitality and prosperity of Perugian cobblers in the last decades of the Trecento;[63] and Alberto Grohmann claims that the economy of Perugia remained resilient through the fifteenth and early sixteenth centuries.[64] Marco Tangheroni[65] has argued that after a depression from the 1320s through the 1340s, Pisan trade improved. Although it may have lost its competitive edge in the Mediterranean as a whole after defeat by the Genoese at Meloria (1284),[66] Pisa continued to dominate traffic in the Tyrrhenian Sea through the fourteenth century, while traffic with Sicily actually increased. Federigo Melis,[67] Marco Tangheroni,[68] and Michael Mallett,[69] moreover, have revised the older thesis of Pietro Silva,[70] who saw Pisa's loss of independence and incorporation into the Florentine territory in 1406 as the maritime city's death knell.

The economy of Arezzo, unfortunately, lacks a recent book-length scholarly analysis,[71] and according to Giovanni Cherubini, Arezzo remains the least studied and least well-known city in Tuscany.[72] According to cultural and general histories, this town entered its decline in the first decades of the Trecento,[73] or even as early as the Ghibelline defeat at Campaldino (1289). But my statistics on the resources itemized in last wills and testaments suggest that this provincial city may have also experienced economic recovery and even growth in certain sectors after the Black Death, at least for the short run of the later Trecento.[74] Based on the business accounts of notable merchants, such as the powerful Francesco Datini of Prato and Lazzaro Bracci of Arezzo, Melis has argued that Florentine occupation opened Aretine commerce to a larger regional network of trade stretching from the coastal towns of the Marche to Pisa, thus making the trade routes and networks of communication with Florence, the new regional hub of commerce, more efficient.[75] Indeed, the population history of Arezzo to some degree lends credence to this optimistic view. Between the tax records of 1390 and 1427, Arezzo declined less severely than the other two Tuscan cities of comparable importance — Pisa and Pistoia.[76] Furthermore, in regard to Arezzo's wool industry, Bruno Dini finds that Florence's political incursion in 1384 made no difference whatsoever to the type or the levels of production.[77] The Aretine wool industry experienced "a stable vitality" through the Trecento and into the first decades of the Quattrocento.[78] Instead, the decline of this industry came later with the protectionist policies that the Florentines initiated at the end of the 1420s. By 1450, imports of wool had fallen to two-thirds of the figures at the turn of the century, and exports had almost disappeared. According to Dini, the "progressive ruralization" of the Aretine economy characterized the Quattrocento and not the Trecento, leading by midcentury to the city's "general impoverishment" and by the second half of the sixteenth century to the complete disappearance of its wool industry.[79]

Even Assisi, the smallest of these places and the one that faded fastest and most decisively from the limelight of history, may have developed economically and industrially after the Black Death. According to Giuseppe Mira, only at the end of the Trecento did this pilgrimage center create a wool industry of regional importance with "the possibility of external markets, even of international dimensions."[80] Further, Giuseppe Zaccaria and Antonio Cristofani claim that the statutes of the cotton, linen, and hemp guild indicate that the city was a regional entrepôt for these goods from 1351 onward.[81]

GOVERNMENT   Politically, these cities represent different traditions. For the late thirteenth and early fourteenth centuries, Florence and Perugia were the bulwarks of Guelph diplomacy in central Italy, while Pisa, Arezzo, and Siena were strongholds of the Ghibelline factions.[82] The interlocking networks of diplomacy created by these webs of alliance may have created a more unified cultural and political world (at least from the point of view of the nobility and the merchant elites) during the Duecento than during the communal development of the early Trecento when internecine conflict intensified. Because of the frequent treaties and alliances between Florence and Perugia, the cultural distance between these two bastions of the Guelph cause may have been shorter during the thirteenth century than at any other time before the advent of modern communications.[83] In a political sense, Perugia was drawn into a greater Tuscany. To combat the incursions of the Holy Roman Emperor, Henry VI, and, as Heywood and Tabacco suggest, to consolidate possession in their respective *contadi,* Perugia joined Florence, Siena, and other Tuscan cities at the end of the twelfth century in an alliance called the Tuscan League or the Lega di San Genesio.[84]

All of these places except Arezzo retained corporative and representative institutions through at least the early fourteenth century. With the "class struggle" of 1287 in Arezzo,[85] culminating in the rise of Guido Tarlatus, bishop of Arezzo, as despot in 1312,[86] and the much less violent rise of the Donoratico in Pisa (1316),[87] signorial families ruled these two communes through most of the first half of the century, and Assisi became a vassal of Perugia in 1322.[88] On the other hand, merchant oligarchies ruled Florence (except for several short intervals—the rule of Walter of Brienne, 1342–43, and that of the Ciompi, a coalition of workers and minor guildsmen, 1378–81), Siena (under the Nine, 1287–1355, and later under other competing factions, called *monti*), and Perugia (under the Raspanti) throughout the period under investigation.

Nonetheless, the political histories of all these places from the mid-thirteenth through the early fourteenth centuries were rife with conflict between forces that contemporaries distinguished as the magnates and the *popolo* ("bourgeois artisans, tradesmen and manufacturers organized into guilds and armed societies from which workers and wage-earners were excluded").[89] Each commune passed antimagnate legislation during the late Duecento or early Trecento—most importantly, the *Breve Pisani Communis*[90] in 1286 and 1288,[91] the Ordinances of Justice of Florence in 1293,[92] the Ordinamenti del Buon Stato of Siena in 1310,[93] and the *Libro Rosso* of Perugia in 1333.[94] The extent to which members of the old lineages were excluded from governmental participation, however, varied from city-state to city-state.[95] William Bowsky has argued that the old magnate lineages played a more significant role in the political culture of Siena under the Nine than in Florence during the Trecento.[96] Similarly, in Perugia, the merchant elites never effectively excluded the old magnates from political patronage.[97] In Pisa, under the guise of republican rule,[98] and in Arezzo, with fewer overtures to the *popolani,* feudal lineages dominated communal politics,[99] especially after the abortive and bloody revolt of the *popolo* against the Aretine bishop Guglielmo Ubertini in 1287 and more so after Bishop Guido Tarlati was elected by the General Council as *"signore a vita"* in 1321.[100]

At the other end of the political spectrum, popular protest in Florence was distinctive in the character of its ideology, organization, and forms of revolt.[101] And in Siena popular insurrections, which allied artisans and workers with middling levels of society, managed to topple more regimes than anywhere else.[102] In contrast, popular movements were considerably weaker in late Trecento Perugia[103] and, according to Tangheroni, nonexistent in Pisa throughout the fourteenth century, despite widespread social unrest, which he claims was characteristic throughout Europe.[104] The Pisan chroniclers, however, do not confirm this picture of total social quiescence, reporting instances of popular unrest in Pisa in 1356 and 1369. In 1392, moreover, forces described by an anonymous chronicler as "all the *populo di Pisa,* armed with naked swords," toppled the oligarchy of the Gambacorta family and brought the notary D'Appiano to power.[105]

Finally, three of these city-states lost their communal sovereignty during the period examined in this study. Perugia relegated Assisi to the status of vassalage from 1322 until 1369, when the city of Saint Francis freed itself from Perugian control only to be immediately incorporated into the Papal States, its allies. The Florentines acquired Arezzo for a brief moment, 1337–1343, but took definitive control in 1384[106] and subjugated Pisa by force in 1406.

In Chapter 8, "Conclusion," I consider the possible impact of these demographic, economic, and political factors on the patterns of piety uncovered in my statistical analyses. The statistics show that the political incorporations and the loss of communal independence of three of these city-states did not effect the broad changes in piety and mentality that can be gleaned from testamentary practice. In Arezzo and Pisa, cultural convergence was already well on its way before the Florentines, through purchase and war, redrew the political boundaries of Tuscany. Assisi, for its part, despite its proximity to Perugia, remained until sometime after the recurrence of pestilence in 1363 as different from Perugia as any two city-states here examined in their testamentary habits and in the devotional practices seen from these acts.

The Testament

Testament writing was not identical in these diverse societies.[107] First, the survival of testaments (perhaps reflecting the actual frequency of testament writing) differed among the six cities. From the numerous testaments surviving in the hospital chartularies of Pisa's principal hospital, testament writing appears to have been well entrenched in this civil culture by the late thirteenth century. Only two testaments used in this study come from the twelfth century; both were Pisan (one dated 1155, the other 1185). In Arezzo, sufficient numbers of testaments for statistical analysis appeared later. While Ubaldo Pasqui finds two testaments from the eleventh century in his four volumes of Aretine medieval documents, he records no other wills until the early fourteenth century.[108] In the notarial protocols and parchment collections, which I have surveyed, none surfaced before 1305. Nonetheless, the Aretine testaments appear early relative to other towns not included in this study, such as Cortona and Ancona, where significant numbers of testaments do not appear until well into the Quattrocento.

The surviving evidence from Assisi presents a more perplexing pattern. An unusually large number of testaments has survived from the thirteenth century (40), constituting more than a quarter of the documents found for this village-town before the beginning of the fifteenth century. But the numbers preserved in the archives of this community fall off sharply by the 1320s and 30s—at the very time when these acts became numerous in Arezzo and Florence. This decline did not result from a transfer of charters or archives to Perugia after its conquest of Assisi in 1322.[109] Furthermore, testaments all but disappear in the years after the Black Death until the recurrence of plague in 1374, when they once again mount in numerical importance with the earliest appearance of notarial protocols now housed in the city's Biblioteca Comunale.

The formulaic clauses that preface the testaments from the various regions reveal other differences that transcend facts of documentary survival. This rich variety cannot be simply pinned to the notarial formula books (at least, the famous published ones that derive mostly from the mid-thirteenth century)—the anonymous "summa" from Arezzo, Florence's *Formularium,* the "summa of Rolandus Rodulfi and the most important prototype for central Italy, the formularium of the Bolognese lawyer Raniero (Raynerius) da Perugia.[110] Differences from notary to notary and, more strikingly, from town to town abound in the introductory clichés such as the "Cum nihil sit quod magis hominibus debeatur quam quod supreme voluntatis" recommended by Raniero. Furthermore, beneath the rungs and rubrics common to the formula books, variations in testamentary practice from city to city are found in the structure of the wills, such as whether the notary regularly prompted the testator to estimate the funerary expenses or the choice of burial.

In addition, the commune made its appearance in testament writing in three of these cities by demanding canonical portions for certain pious causes (in effect, the fees appear fixed with few exceptions). By the mid-Trecento, Siena's citizens and other subjects were generally required to grant a portion of their estates to the hospital of Santa Maria della Scala, to the building of the cathedral (its *opera*), and to the archbishop. Except in the wills of nobles and rich merchants, the sums for each of these imposed charities rarely exceeded the meager sum of 20 soldi until well into the fifteenth century.[111] From the late thirteenth century until shortly after 1348, the Commune of Assisi imposed a "postulatio" (or obligatory charity) on testators, which customarily ranged from ten to forty soldi. By the second half of the Trecento, this spiritual imposition almost disappears from the pious ledgers, but in its place testators consistently gave five soldi to the city's communal hospital as their opening bequest.[112] Florence required testators to support the Opera del Duomo, the cathedral, and the building and maintenance of the city walls, each cause to receive a payment that varied from several soldi to several florins but usually equaled 20 soldi.[113]

Curiously, of the published communal statutes of these six city-states, only those from Arezzo (1327) ordered its citizens to leave sums in their testaments for a pious cause, in this case the episcopal *opera,* then under construction. If the notary failed to alert a testator to leave a gift to the *opera,* the commune's *podestà* would fine him 20 soldi and the testator's estates would be levied 40 soldi, which would go to the *opera.*[114] From the testamentary evidence, it appears that the construction of the *opera* was completed quickly, and, unlike in other cities, its maintenance charges were not collected by retaining the mandatory legacy, or else Aretines simply ignored the *podestà*'s punitive threats. In contrast to testaments from Florence, Siena, and Assisi, which true to formula began with the imposed charities to the archbishop, the *opera,* its central hospital, or the city walls, those from Arezzo only occasionally offered a canonical gift to their *opera*.

Although these canonical levies represented paltry sums for all but the most impoverished testators, such impositions may have had repercussions on pious giving. For instance, additional gifts beyond the customary five soldi to the archbishop of Siena nearly disappeared during the fourteenth century (though such gifts had never been common). The same cannot be said, however, for gifts to the major hospital of the city, Santa Maria della Scala, which through the next two centuries succeeded in dominating pious bequests to hospitals in the region. By contrast, after Assisi levied such a canonical tax on testators to support its communal hospital, additional bequests to it, though rare to begin with, all but disappeared.

Testators from Arezzo, Pisa, and Perugia appear to have been spared such customary and imposed charities for most of the period under analysis. Only for the brief period of the Opera del Duomo's construction in Arezzo and after the city became subject to Florentine rule in 1384 were Aretines subject to mandatory charities. Similarly, after 1406 Pisan testators were charged the Florentine customary payments to the cathedral, its *opera,* and the maintenance of the Florentine city walls. Since these canonical gifts were required by law and did not reflect the pious choices of testators, they have not been tallied in my statistics of pious bequests. As we shall see, these discrepancies in legislated charity from city to city do not account for the regional differences, which I discuss in Chapter 3.

Notarial formula and practice gave special importance to the funeral in Pisa and Perugia. As early as the 1270s, the testament customarily opened with the choice of burial and the expenses to be paid for wax, masses, and meals and clothing for the poor. Usually lumped together with these expenses were additional sums for the poor, either in money, clothing, or food, to be doled out on the seventh and thirtieth days after the burial and occasionally on the anniversary. By the last quarter of the fourteenth century, notarial formulas still structured the testament such that the first itemized bequests were payments for burial and the ensuing customary days; however, the costs for these last rites were increasingly left to the discretion of spouses, kin, and heirs.

In contrast, the records from Siena, Florence, and Arezzo throughout the period of this study seldom mentioned funeral preparations or allocated specific sums for these rites. Does this mean that ordinary Pisans or Perugians planned more elaborate funerals? Do these omissions from the documents tell us anything about the mentality of Aretines and Florentines? Or were these simply matters handled by oral arrangements, the apparent differences simply stemming from differences in notarial customs? Certainly, the Florentines showed little modesty in celebrating lavish state funerals for their war heroes and on occasion even for men of letters.[115] The chronicles often listed in detail the mammoth expenditures that these occasions drew. For the funerals of ordinary citizens and villagers we are, however, left largely in the dark, forced perhaps to read the obverse from what the sumptuary laws prohibited.[116]

Communal restrictions impinged on testamentary practice in ways that were less subtle than those imposed by the traditions of notarial formularies. From the earliest testaments,[117] Florentines forbade women to redact last wills without the consent of a male protector (mundualdus), who might be the testatrix's husband or the next male kin, but who might bear no obvious kinship to the woman.[118] This special requirement is consistent with other restrictions that Florentine men placed on women kin in the late Middle Ages. Indeed, in Chapter 5 we find that Florence, far from being the norm in relations between the sexes, was the least desirable place of these six city-states in the late Middle Ages or the early Renaissance to have grown up female, at least in regard to the control of property.[119] On the other hand, legal ordinances and communal restrictions cannot be read alone in assessing a problem as complex as women's property rights. By the beginning of the fifteenth century, the Commune of Assisi similarly required women testators to have the consent of their husbands or, when widowed, the nearest blood relative. If no male blood relatives survived, women in Assisi were required to say so at the start of these early Quattrocento wills. Yet, at least in their discretionary power over their principal source of property, the dowry, women in this Umbrian town appear to have been better served than in Arezzo or neighboring Perugia, where the commune imposed no such regulations restricting the testamentary prerogatives of women. I shall argue that the differences in notarial formulas and in the institutional practice of will writing, as important as they were for the form and frame of this set of property contracts, cannot begin to account for the broad differences or similarities among these communities, which the statistics on giving and their implications for piety reveal.

How well does the testament reflect individual or collective mentalities? Were there clear differences in local practice that reflect differences in belief or in charitable practice? First, the number of autographs and wills in the vernacular was minute in all six towns in the period under study.[120] The testamentary choices were wedged within the rungs of the notary's formularies that lend the documents their legal mystique and that varied only slightly from city to city. These differences were mostly confined to the beginning of the document: the preambles, such as in Siena and Florence, might divide "the nobler part" of the soul from the body and the supposed less weighty matters of property or, as in Pisa and Perugia, might delve right into the choice of the grave and its accouterments or, as in Arezzo, jump straight from the opening formula, phrases such as "there is nothing so certain as death and nothing so uncertain as the hour of death," into the itemized bequests. Notaries no doubt asked the testator leading questions about certain charitable causes. For instance, in Perugia the notary was to demand from each lay member of the confraternity of the Misericordia dying without male heirs to bequeath 10 libbre di denari piccoli or at least five, if they could not afford more.[121] In Arezzo, city notaries were supposed "to suggest to testators" that they make bequests to the Misericordia of Arezzo and that any legacies be reported to the rectors of this congregation within three days of the testament's redaction.[122] In Siena, the statutes of the Misericordia required all of its oblates to redact a notarized last will and testament.[123] But none of the notaries in these cities during the time span covered by this study were expected to practice anything approaching the bureaucratic heavy-handedness required of Venetian notaries, who, during the sixteenth century, "were furnished with an ever-lengthening list of approved charities, and were obliged by law to mention them to clients making their wills."[124]

Each itemized list of bequests reflects to some extent a distinct personality with its own sentiments, prejudices, hopes, and desires. If the formulaic casts appear invariable for a particular notary or group of notaries, the itemized lists could vary sharply from one testator to the next within the same notarial protocol. Like the notarial preambles, the phrases that prefaced the choice of grave were less flexible than the actual choices that followed not only from one testator to the next but from one notary to the next and even between notaries of these different regions. But even here the odd testator might begin the list of last decisions over property with words that were not always stamped in the notarial formularies. To what extent these notarized documents expressed the apprehensions of those societies here under inspection, and how they varied by place and across time, is a central focus of the first half of this book.

However individual the character of these documents, outside forces—the notary, the priest or monk (who may or may not have been present at the bedside), the testator's kin, and even the formulaic character of the documents themselves—channeled and confined the testator's choices.[125] Attilio Bartoli Langeli has considered the testament the production of a triangle of forces—testator, notary, and confessor[126]—and Martin Bertram has gone farther in emphasizing the pressures placed on the individual testator's "free will" by pointing to the unwritten practices imposed by pious corporations, notarial conventions, and "the very mode" by which testaments were drafted.[127] The extent of such influences and whether they affected the six cities differently is difficult to determine. Certainly, the range of women's choices, as with the law and local custom, varied from city to city. But even if the testamentary provisions themselves only reflected notarial convention, as they do not, the geographical differences over time in patterns of piety and decisions over property would merit attention. For even a view from the perspective of the notary would deepen our picture of late medieval and early Renaissance culture now drawn largely from the heights of humanist or religious tracts. By looking at changes in testamentary practice—choices over time and differences from place to place—I do not mean to endorse the romantic presumption that these testamentary decisions could somehow be purely the desires of "the individual" late medieval man or woman; rather, the very fact that these testaments were socially determined "products" makes them all the more valuable for interpreting societal change and difference.

Finally, one might even go beyond these influences and pressures which framed the individual's testamentary form and choices by considering who might or might not write a will: what were the rules of property succession *ab intestato?* Here, the communal statutes from these various city-states present a fairly uniform legal culture, that of customary law, in which male kin had rights of inheritance over female kin and in which property succeeded through the male line.[128]

The Model from Siena

My previous study of wills, *Death and Property in Siena, 1205–1800: Strategies for the Afterlife,* initially spurred the questions behind this present work. While the Sienese study looked at changes in mentality and decisions about property over the long haul of six centuries in a single place— the city and territory of Siena—the present work considers only one "historical block" demarcated by this earlier study but across a more vast geography. From the Sienese documents, the first major transformation (that can be observed statistically) in the patterns of piety and giving came not with the Black Death of 1348 but when pestilence returned in 1363.[129] While the massive mortality of 1348 caused drastic changes in church finances and the needs of the poor, the mentality of individual testators appears unchanged even while these cataclysmic events engulfed their very bodies and souls. They continued to give in the ways of the past, which harked back to the last decades of the thirteenth century. When facing the final arbitration over their worldly goods, hard-headed peasants, petty merchants, and craftsmen, as well as notables from the old patrician lines, practiced what the mendicants were then preaching, despite protocapitalist commercial habits.[130] By liquidating, splintering, and scattering their pious bequests over large numbers of ecclesiastical entities, they strove to break what Saint Catherine of Siena called "the earthly cell"—their mundane attachments to worldly gains.[131]

The testaments placed under the scrutiny of the computer show the Sienese striving to avoid earthly remembrance through works of art, chapel endowments, or even dowry funds. With 1363, testators lost confidence in the efficacy of this mendicant strategy of self-denial. The change, moreover, did not point in the directions argued recently by historians looking at charity and piety more globally for late medieval Europe.[132] Plague, economic and social dislocation, war, and famine did not provoke a new pessimism or rejection of this-worldly values.[133] Nor did testators' pious bequests to hospitals, monasteries, or religious confraternities change dramatically.[134] The one significant exception was poor relief. As opposed to the earlier indiscriminate handouts of pennies or bread to the "Poor of Christ," the Sienese henceforth predominantly supported dowry funds, which would be allocated to a few carefully chosen girls of "good character." This change, furthermore, pointed toward a more general transformation in piety, which I pointed to as the structure of giving. Beginning with the summer months of pestilence that struck Siena as well as other parts of central Italy in 1363, through the eighteenth century, testators would not return to the old mendicant habits of spreading their pious monies in paltry sums over the gamut of Sienese charities and religious entities. Instead, they sought to leave a mark in much the way that modern donors adorn classrooms, hospitals, or water fountains with plaques to memorialize themselves.

Sienese testators expressed similar obsessions with earthly memory through the allocation of their nonpious gifts to friends and kin. Increasingly, from the latter half of the fourteenth through the sixteenth century, they tried to manipulate from the grave the behavior of their heirs, the flow of properties through successive generations, and the pious obligations of those who received them.

At least for Siena over the long run, the change wrought by the renewed trauma felt in 1363 does not appear to have turned exactly in those directions described by contemporaries such as Giovanni Boccaccio, Matteo Villani, and the principal chronicler of Siena, Agnolo di Tura. They argued that pestilence divided the survivors into two groups— the few who saw the wrath of God and thereby attended to mending their ways, and those constituting the vast majority who turned away from religious practice to gaming, gambling, and feasting off the newborn wealth left in the wake of the high levels of mortality. On the contrary, the Sienese may have even given more in terms of value if not in number of bequests to pious entities, at least by the early Quattrocento. The value of these pious gifts, moreover, did not decline significantly in real terms or in relation to their other, nonpious bequests until the last decades of the Quattrocento.

Should the case of Siena be generalized? For other cities and regions, did 1348 fail to register deep shock waves in the plans ordinary citizens and villagers made for the afterlife and in their strategies over property? Was the plague's less lethal return of 1363 the more significant for the history of attitudes and the afterlife? Indeed, in *Death and Property in Siena* I suggested that the pattern did go beyond the borders of the Sienese territory. The one figure whose correspondence and everyday reflections on life, death, and salvation ran the gauntlet of the plague's first strike and recurrence did not come from Siena: the international scholar and early humanist Francesco Petrarch lived through the mortality of 1348 in Avignon and its recurrence (1361) in Milan. Like the patterns of bequests quantified from the testaments of peasants and artisans, Petrarch's letters on consolation, earthly endeavors, and glory signal an abrupt change in philosophy with the plague of 1361 looming in the suburbs around Milan. In 1348, Petrarch's views on earthly purpose and the self remained unshaken. Instead the mammoth mortality had a silver lining—it had, after all, liberated "the fortunate" from the corrupt, fleshly chains enslaving humanity in its present wretched state of earthly reality. In his letters of condolence he berated friends and dignitaries who, myopically, were mourning the recent losses of loved ones, unable to grasp that the deceased were the lucky ones.

Yet, in his opening letter to his second collection of epistles, the *Senilium Rerum Libri,* Petrarch did an about-face as he wept for the loss of his own loved ones struck down by the plague of 1361—his friend Socrates, to whom he dedicated the first collection of letters, the *Rerum Familiarum,* and his son Giovanni. Soon afterward, Petrarch fired off a letter to Giovanni Boccaccio ridiculing him for doing what Petrarch himself, before the onslaught of 1361, had recommended. A monk had momentarily convinced Boccaccio to give up his profligate worldly concerns with literature and antiquity and concentrate instead on preparing for death. Now Petrarch, who had previously characterized the mortal life as the "antechamber," a place of "exile," urged Boccaccio on the contrary not to "dwell on death" but to "learn to improve life" and in concrete terms to preserve his library as a fund for the perpetuation of letters for future generations. In a letter to Charles of Bohemia dated the same year, Petrarch exhorted the king to "seize the opportunity" to enter and bring order to Italy, "to use your life to acquire eternal glory."[135] While the other cities present discrepancies from the patterns drawn from Siena, I nevertheless argue that 1363 had broad consequences for changes in mentality across central Italy.

The Choice of Geography

At first, I planned to cast my net far afield, to search for fourteenth-century testaments in Lyons, Avignon, London, and other European cities that might have preserved substantial numbers of testaments before, during, and immediately after the Black Death of 1348. My initial forays into the early archival collections for Arezzo, however, convinced me that only fifty kilometers to the northeast I was already in a different world from that of the Sienese, at least for the period before the Black

Death. Charitable legacies found in testaments of certain early Trecento Aretines exemplified ideals that the Sienese records do not portray until well after the plague of 1363 and in some instances not even until the sixteenth century. Thus Dominus Symoneus of Arezzo, a notary[136] and son of a notary whose will dates from 1338, concentrated his last thoughts on the preservation of prized possessions and the connections between worldly things and earthly posterity. Unlike the long itemized lists of pious bequests of paltry sums to a myriad of ecclesiastical institutions characteristic of the pre-plague well-to-do in Siena, the major portion of Symoneus's long testament comprising extensive landed properties turned on only two bequests: one set aside property to finance the construction of his burial chapel and the future flow of its *ius patronatus* or rights of electing future generations of chaplains; the other carefully divided his private library holding 156 books bound in 66 volumes between the Dominican and Franciscan houses of Arezzo.[137] He then specified in systematic detail the friars' library privileges and the rules for preserving his collection ad infinitum, down to the locks and cages to secure these properties' physical preservation.[138] This gift, reminiscent of Petrarch's concern with Boccaccio's dispersing his library, is not paralleled in the Sienese documents until 1512.[139] Nor was Dominus Symoneus alone in these preoccupations with property and remembrance. Others in the middle-sized town of Arezzo, renowned for its university and especially for legal studies,[140] used their testaments to ensure that their libraries would remain intact after death. In the year of the Black Death, 1348, a testament of an Aretine surgeon even estimated the values of each of the volumes in his medical collection.[141] Letters and libraries did not, however, constitute the major avenue through which Aretine testators sought to leave an earthly imprint of their names and reputations. In marked contrast to the Sienese, from the earliest surviving testaments Aretines patronized works of art in their wills. While only one in one hundred from Siena before 1426 left instructions to build chapels or monumental graves, nearly one in ten from Arezzo left substantial properties for the purposes of memorializing their bones and those of their descendants. In Siena, not until the latter half of the fifteenth century did testators use their wills to attempt to regulate the succession of chaplains elected to skim off the *usufructus* of their landed properties to sponsor the singing of perpetual masses to commemorate their own and their predecessors' souls.

Testamentary patronage of other works of art, from altarpieces to painted candlestick holders, did not require financing from large inalienable landed properties. Here too the testamentary evidence reflects sharp differences in attitudes toward salvation between these two neighboring city-states. In a sample of 446 testaments constituting 3,088 pious bequests, the Sienese commissioned only six paintings. In Arezzo, by contrast, the desire to leave a concrete mark on one's parish church, neighborhood monastery, or cathedral peppered the early Trecento documents and increased in frequency after the recurrence of plague in the second half of the Trecento. Few of these paintings survive, whether on wood (*tabula*), walls, or cloth. If a large proportion of them were actually painted (as I suspect), then artworks must have crammed the walled spaces of these ecclesiastical houses to their rafters, giving an appearance very unlike the puritanical starkness that the poorer ones in particular now convey. According to Wackernagel, despite the antique-inspired changes in architectural aesthetics around the middle of the Quattrocento, paintings appeared here and there on exposed sections of wall, frequently on the front side of nave piers without association with an altar.[142] The testamentary commissions, moreover, descended the social ladder to the ranks of peasants and wage workers, as I show in Chapter 7.

On occasion these commissions explicitly evoked the desire for individual immortalization through their stipulated content and their hoped-for future maintenance in sacred spaces. In the year of the Black Death, for instance, the son of a blacksmith then living in the Casentine town of Bibbiena devoted a large section of his modest will to commissioning a painting for the major church of the Aretine monastery of San Bernardo. It was to bear this inscription: "This painting was ordered to be done by Pasquino the son of the former Montagne, its donor." More, next to the figure of Mary the artist was to paint "a figure in the likeness of this person Pasquino" on one side and on the other a figure of his deceased father genuflecting. Above each of them the painting was to say, "Here is Montagne, the Blacksmith; here is Pasquino [the son of] Montagne."[143] In the same year, a condottiere (*Constabularius equitum stipendiariorum*) from a village outside Liège, but a long-time resident of Arezzo, left all of his armor to the confraternity of the Misericordia in Arezzo—all, that is, except his helmet, which together with his other insignia (*cum aliis suis signatibus*) was to be kept everlastingly above his tomb to be constructed in the Aretine church of the Servites. His ardor for earthly memory outstripping the self-indulgence of the blacksmith's son, the soldier did not bother at all with religious figures in an altarpiece he commissioned for the village parish of his birthplace, requesting instead his own figure alone to appear above the altar. Thus, he cast himself as the saintly figure for future parishioners to venerate.[144] The image cut by the laconic terms of his testament portrays a man straight from the pages of Burck-hardt's *Civilization of the Renaissance in Italy*. He left behind five illegitimate children, to whom he bequeathed unequal sums of money.

Similar impressions can be gleaned from a cursory glance through the Florentine testaments, where art commissions and efforts at indi-vidual and familial immortalization appear as early as the first years of the Trecento. Some of these are remarkable for any period and all the more so against the ascetic backdrop of the early Trecento testamentary practices of Siena just 60 kilometers to the south. For instance, in 1312 a Ricchuccus f.q. Puccii from the parish of Santa Maria Novella sought to preserve his memory by attaching it to works of art. At five lire a year he financed oil to be burnt continually in the church of Santa Maria Novella under the crucifix "made by the distinguished painter named Giottus Bondonis." He also provided for oil to fill a lamp under the "large painting of the blessed Virgin in the same church." A third gift of 20 soldi went to illuminate another painting in the Dominican church of Prato previously commissioned by this testator and again painted by the "egregious" Giottus Bondonis.[145] In the year of the Black Death, 1348, a merchant from the parish of San Pancrazio, Turinus f.q. Baldese, left the extraordinary sum of one thousand lire "for the honor of God, the Virgin and the entire celestial court" to be spent on a painting of "the entire history of the Old Testament from beginning to end." For its "execution" the testator left the plans to the discretion of the famous Dominican spiritual writer Jacopo Passavanti.[146]

As the example of the blacksmith's son's commission suggests, an obsession with leaving lasting marks on earthly posterity was not confined to the testaments of the rich and prominent of Arezzo or Florence. In 1343 a Florentine tavernkeeper who doubled as a gravedigger gave a field in the rural suburb of Novoli to the hospital of Santa Maria della Scala but required the brothers of the hospital to construct a "walled" statue of the Madonna and Child on the road in front. The Madonna was to be constructed with bricks, mortar, and stones and to stand at least six *"brachiorum . . . in altitudinis super terram"* (about 15 feet high).[147]

These early testamentary commissions were not always so monu-mental. Several Florentines and Aretines stipulated that the beds they bequeathed to hospitals should be painted with coats of arms and other family regalia. In one case, a stablemaster, Nutius f.q. Dietiguardi, left 14 lire for the difficult task of adorning his bed, to be bequeathed to the poor lying in the hospital of Borgo San Lorenzo, "with an image in the likeness of the majesty of God."[148] Other Trecento testaments from Arezzo and Florence demanded art that has literally gone up in smoke: wax images of the Madonna or family coats of arms to be painted on candles and candlestick holders to be stuck in churches, monasteries, and hospitals.

In the face of sermons delivered by mendicant preachers condemning the earthly hubris grounded in temporal properties and family pride, these devotional acts attest to testators' zeal to extend their earthly traces and to immortalize their names, at least for Arezzo and Florence and later, as we shall discover, for Perugia. In Siena, attempts to preserve the memory of lineages by plastering holy places with family coats of arms date only from the end of the Quattrocento and never penetrated the testaments of artisans. In Florence, the practice appeared early, even among members of the laboring classes. The 1368 testament of a wool carder who did not even possess a family name required the *hospitalarius* of Santa Maria Nuova to paint his "arms" on a torch, which he gave to the hospital and which was to be kept burning on the hospital's altar every Sunday.[149]

The Localization of Culture and Its Convergence

These Aretine and Florentine examples of testamentary art patronage and preoccupations with earthly memory do not prove Siena the exception and Arezzo and Florence the norm. As we shall see, the liquidation of property, the scattering of pious gifts to numerous ecclesiastical entities, and the conscious obliteration of ties to earthly forms of remembrance were even more pronounced in Pisa and Assisi. Nor do Perugia and Assisi form a uniform "Umbrian" model, as I thought they might when I undertook this project. The birthplace of the mid-thirteenth-century flagellants and the crucible of more radical forms of religiosity that followed Saint Francis's example do not form a convenient foil for viewing Tuscan piety and culture (as has been often assumed).[150] The differences between these two capitals of art and religion, though they were separated by a mere twenty kilometers, were as sharp as the differences between Siena and Arezzo.

One theme of this book is to illustrate this extraordinary localization of culture from the late Duecento through the first two-thirds of the Trecento, at least as seen from the testaments of townsmen and villagers, ranging from local notables bearing family names familiar to historians—

the Tarlati of Arezzo, the Upezzingi of Pisa, the Oddi of Perugia, the Guicciardini of Florence—to those whose final decisions over property show worlds barely beyond a state of dire misery. Certainly, other sources of culture, such as notarial script, formula books, storytelling (*il novellistico*), or the sermons of mendicant preachers, would trace different geographies. But, as Francesco Tateo has argued, drawing specific geographical lines to demarcate mentalities and customs in Tuscany from vernacular literary sources "would be misleading for many reasons."[151] Moreover, how would the historian even begin to pinpoint spatially a preacher such as Giordano da Rivolta, who was born between 1260 and 1265 either in Pisa or in the nearby village of Rivolta, joined the Dominican order of Pisa in 1280, studied at Pisa, Bologna, and Paris, joined the Florentine *studium* at Santa Maria Novella in 1303, became embroiled in the political and religious conflicts of Florence, returned to lecture at Pisa in 1311, and died in Piacenza in the same year while en route to Paris;[152] or the even more itinerant San Bernardino, who was born in Massa Marittima, a provincial town in southern Tuscany, came to Siena as a small child in the custody of his paternal aunts and uncles, entered several orders in Siena, became Vicario di Toscana of the Observant Franciscans in 1405, was transferred to Fiesole, began his career as an itinerant preacher in Genoa in 1417, and traveled throughout Italy until his death in 1444 in L'Aquila?[153]

The localization of culture detailed in this book does not, however, pose as an argument for a pointillist empiricism. The broad patterns of similarities and contrasts, instead, divide these cities into two groups that were historically specific, enduring from the late thirteenth century through the plague of 1362-63, which ravaged all six of these city-states alike.[154] While this book unabashedly presents an explanation for the changes of the late Trecento, it does not offer a complete explanation of the earlier groupings of the two sets of cities. From the evidence here assembled, these geographical patterns appear not to have been matters of propinquity, political regime, commercialization, type of economy, education, the prominence of Dominicans versus Franciscans, or the results of distant historical residues such as pre-Roman tribal or early medieval settlement patterns, laws, and customs from a Lombard or a Byzantine past or a more recent cultural past stemming from the international allegiances of the Guelphs and Ghibellines. Instead, Chapter 5 suggests that a better key to the differences in piety and self-consciousness found in these cities lies in the contemporaneous strength of the male lineage and customs of inheritance based on a masculine ideology.

The distances and differences between the cultures of these city-states, however, did not remain constant over time. Instead, my statistics plot a convergence of cultures that cut across political boundaries and even the regions between Tuscany and Umbria over the course of the Trecento and particularly at the pivotal point of the recurrence of pestilence in 1362–63 and immediately thereafter, when the patterns of piety changed in all of these city-states. By the mid-1360s, the long lists of itemized pious gifts conveying paltry sums and distributed to numerous causes (which to greater or lesser degrees had characterized the legacies of all of these towns in the early Trecento) suddenly all but disappeared. Moreover, even in Perugia, Arezzo, and Florence, where some testators early on had been preoccupied with earthly remembrance, had commissioned private family chapels and altarpieces, and had attempted to control the flow of landed properties down the male line, 1363 and the years thereafter registered a profound change in the direction of this-worldly obsessions with salvation and remembrance.

The number of pious bequests in all six towns fell sharply. In fact, those towns that began the century by scattering and fragmenting their pious bequests the most (Pisa, Siena, and Assisi) ended it with fewer charitable gifts per testator. And although testators in Arezzo, Florence, and Perugia commissioned works of art in their wills from the earliest decades of the Trecento, the number of commissions skyrocketed in the 1360s and 1370s with new groups of artisans, workers, and even peasants stockpiling their pious revenues to leave a lasting mark in their parishes or in local monasteries. Testators, moreover, turned increasingly from the laconic lists of itemized bequests to the clauses regulating and conditioning their final bequests to their universal heirs. Similar to those testators in Cinquecento Siena, which is beyond the period I cover, these late Trecento and early Quattrocento testators—whether patricians or peasants—became increasingly obsessed with controlling from the grave the fate of their heirs and property.[155]

Black Death Studies

The centerpiece of this book is the Black Death of 1348 and its recurrence in 1362–63.[156] This may wrongly suggest epidemiological issues, that is, the causes and the spread of the late medieval pestilence.[157] Indeed, this topic took center stage through the 1960s with the interdisciplinary marriage of medical and social history. This subject may also mislead the reader in other directions, which engaged the attention of historians in the 1950s and early 60s: the reactions of municipalities[158] and the social and economic consequences of the Black Death from 1348 to 1500.[159] Instead, the reactions to plague which this book seeks to uncover are psychological and cultural. Such an inquiry is not new:[160] by the late 1970s, the focus of work on the Black Death already pointed in this direction. In a conference on the Black Death held in 1977, 15 of 30 papers considered the cultural and psychological side of the great medieval pestilence.[161]

This book, however, takes a fundamentally different approach to "cultural history" from the published papers of that conference and employs different sources and methods. The evidentiary basis of their cultural history was works of art and literature, from Giovanni Boccaccio's *Decameron* to little-known sermons. From single works, such as a newly discovered chronicle or the fresco series *The Triumph of Death,* which decorated the Pisan Mausoleum, the Camposanto, these historians attempted to extrapolate more general attitudes embedded in the society from which these artifacts issued. These studies, moreover, concentrated on the years of the plagues themselves; they did not examine the *longue* or even the *moyenne durée* or view trends and patterns of change.[162] By scrutinizing nearly thirty-four hundred testaments from the earliest notarized wills through the first twenty-five years of the Quattrocento, this study pushes the cultural and social level of analysis beyond the reaches of that image formed from the scattered remains of literary or artistic evidence. In addition, the plurisecular scope of my investigation, unlike the glimpse afforded by the commissioning of a single altarpiece or narrative cycle (no matter how important), the preaching of a sermon, or the composition of a literary masterpiece, makes it possible to compare trends over time and big patterns across geography. A statistical analysis of the testamentary evidence from towns in Tuscany and Umbria with different political regimes, different population sizes, and different economies runs counter to "the current consensus . . . that the massive plague outbreaks of the 14th century . . . neither created nor radically changed existing social, economic, and cultural trends."[163]

Although not much may have changed in the minds and wills of ordinary merchants, artisans, and villagers in the summer months of horror wrought by the unprecedented mortality of 1348, the trend over the late Trecento, its experience of recurring waves of pestilence, is unmistakable. While patterns of piety were worlds apart between Siena and Arezzo, Florence and Pisa, and Assisi and next-door Perugia, by the last decades of the Trecento these towns uncannily began to resemble one another in their patterns of piety and in their desires for salvation despite radical differences in their economic and political histories.

This book's organization follows in part a statistical rationale: after this introduction to the problems and prospects of the comparative analysis of mentalities, the methods of study, and the socioeconomic contexts of the six cities, Chapter 2 examines testators' choices of beneficiaries and makes use of all the testaments, including a smattering of codicils and fragments. This chapter challenges the now general conclusion that charity shifted with the early Renaissance from the old church beneficiaries and ideals of penitence to organizations aimed at assuaging social problems of the present world, principally hospitals and lay religious confraternities. Chapter 3 lays out the general paradigm from which the remainder of the book follows. Instead of a change in the choice of beneficiaries, testators changed their manner of testamentary giving in the early Renaissance. A cult of remembrance spread through all these towns with or soon after the second strike of pestilence in 1362–63. My analysis of pious bequests finds that underlying this diachronic similarity, the towns can be divided into two camps that cut across lines once thought to be fundamental boundaries in the cultural history of central Italy: Umbria versus Tuscany, Florence versus Siena, or the peculiarity of Florence and its dominance in the formation of Renaissance culture. This investigation of the structure of pious bequests considers only complete testaments, which, however, decreases the sample size only slightly.[164] From these analyses based on over twenty thousand legacies, the data base then shrinks more significantly in my examination of burial patterns, restrictions on property, demand for artwork, and finally painting. After an investigation of concerns over the body and burial, Chapter 5 turns to those gifts left to nonpious ends—kin and friends—and finds patterns of giving that parallel the differences in the six cities uncovered through the analysis of the pious bequests. The second onslaught of pestilence again emerges as a turning point—this time in testators' attachment to their ancestral property and worldly gains and in their desires to rule their progeny and future generations of heirs from the grave. The same sets of differences across geography and changes over time inform Chapter 6—an investigation into testamentary works of art ranging from candlestick holders, engraved chalices, and wax images costing several shillings to commissions for sculpted effigies, chapels, monasteries, and fresco cycles amounting to hundreds of florins. The final chapter concentrates on commissions for paintings, examining changes in demand, prices, and compositions. It sets on end an interpretation of painting and its reflections about spirituality after the Black Death that has largely held firm from Millard Meiss's thesis of 1951 (if not earlier) through his critics of the 1980s.

As the reader will find, some of the cells for comparison in the latter half of this book are small—such as examples of the use of entail, *ius patronatus* of family chapels, the number of chalices with family coats of arms, or paintings bearing price tags in the first decades of the Quattrocento. Taken in isolation, these scattered statistics and illustrative materials can be little more than suggestive. I do not intend, however, that these illustrations should be seen in isolation but rather that they be viewed in the larger contexts of spatial differences and change over time set out in the opening chapters of this book from the full deck of data and supplemented in later chapters by further statistical analyses of trends ranging from testamentary choices of ancestral graves to the prices offered for altarpieces. By combining a serial analysis of testaments with the comparative method, this study draws a direct link between the experience of pestilence and cultural change. It points to the rise of a Renaissance psychology, which Jacob Burckhardt defined 130 years ago as the preoccupation with "fame and glory," and which Renaissance historians of art, philosophy, literature, politics, and even economics have often since made the cornerstone of their analyses.[165] While my point of departure might be defined as Burkhardtian, the reader will find that my conclusions recast that "Renaissance."

I

The Structure of Piety

2

Pious Choices

A certain fellow approaching death wished to draw up his testament. It was summer and mortality so rampant that wives refused to come near their husbands, children fled their fathers and brothers ran from one another, since as those who saw it know, that plague hit hard. And seeing himself abandoned by all his kin, he made the notary write that his sons and heirs every year on the feast day of Saint Jacob in July must give a basket filled with one *staio* of sliced pears to the flies in a certain place designated by him . . . attesting that "in this my present illness I have received assistance from neither friend nor kin; all have abandoned me, except the flies."

— Franco Sacchetti, *Il Trecentonovelle*

 eath and Property in Siena discusses at length the problems and possibilities of quantifying the pious choices made in last wills and testaments as "opinion polls" of piety, to measure wide shifts in charity over long time periods. French historians—Michel Vovelle, Pierre Chaunu, François Lebrun, Jacques Chiffoleau, and others—have pioneered the use and quantification of the will for these purposes.[1] They have thus far confined their analyses, however, to pious preambles and certain key pious bequests for masses, religious confraternities, and burial processions. They have not quantified the itemized pious choices that almost every late medieval or early modern will contained—whether to give money or property to a monastery instead of a hospital; a religious confraternity rather than a parish church; or a dowry fund as opposed to clothing, pennies, and bread to the "poor of Christ."

Historians of late medieval and early Renaissance Tuscany, on the other hand, have attached central importance to changes in the patronage and foundation of different ecclesiastical beneficiaries for evaluating changes in mentality. David Herlihy, Gene Brucker, Marvin Becker, and, most recently, Philip Gavitt have found a general transformation in piety from the stress on penitence and ascetic values, exemplified by the patronage of Benedictine monasteries and nunneries, to a religiosity focused on easing suffering in the present, living world—care for the sick and charity for the poor, expressed largely through the foundation of hospitals and the participation in religious confraternities. The chronology for this transformation remains hazy. In some of Becker's studies, the change seems to occur early on, perhaps as early as the twelfth century;[2] in others, it comes later.[3] For Herlihy, the shift begins as early as the opening decade of the Trecento, but its impact—the emergence of "civic Christianity"—comes only after the plague, indeed because of the ensuing social and demographic dislocations. The turn from the asceticism of the old monastic orders to social responsibility and "cere- monial magnificence" parallels Hans Baron's "civic humanism," reaching full fruition in the early Quattrocento.[4] Similarly, Gavitt sometimes locates the transformation in "charitable giving" for Renaissance Florence during the aftermath of the Black Death of 1348, other times more loosely during the fifteenth century when, according to him, charity became "more laicized or more rationalized."[5]

The conclusions of these historians do not come from weighing the testamentary choices of peasants, artisans, and petty merchants. Rather, they emerge from evidence on (1) the foundations of institutions and the actions of big benefactors, such as the merchant-prince of Prato, Francesco Datini,[6] and (2) shifts in the inventories of property and the financial well-being of large ecclesiastical entities.[7] The trends set by big benefactors and the changes in fortune of large church foundations may indeed reflect fundamental societal changes in attitudes toward charity. At the same time, however, one gift or foundation by a Francesco Datini or a Cosimo de' Medici could dwarf the pious impulses of hundreds of peasants and artisans.

My quantification of pious choices from the Sienese testaments led to conclusions at variance with others using different sources which focused largely on the north of Tuscany—the cities and territories of Florence and Pistoia. For the south, I did not find striking shifts in the pious choices of ordinary citizens and villagers. Fluctuations were mostly short- term. By the end of the Quattrocento the large blocks of patronage reflected in these documents had not changed. Parishes, monasteries, hospitals, and confraternities continued to draw pious gifts well into the fifteenth century with patterns similar to those of the seventy-five-year period preceding the Black Death. The composition of pious choices demarcated only two significant trends, which became distinctive in the Quattrocento—the decline in bequests to nuns and a change in social charity, away from indiscriminate handouts of clothing, coins, and bread for the "poor of Christ" to the foundation of dowry funds for a few carefully selected young virgins of "good habits."

My analysis of the choices made in late medieval and early Renaissance Sienese wills ended, however, in a quandary. Did the differences between my conclusions and those of other Renaissance scholars result from differences in evidence and the methods employed, or did they reflect differences in pious practices and mentality between the Florentine-dominated north and the Sienese south? Were the sentiments voiced by ordinary townsmen and villagers through their pious choices simply the cultural underside of what the art historians and generalists had been preaching for years: had Siena reacted against the Renaissance as it developed in Florence, turning her back on the fifteenth century?[8]

Parishes and Monasteries

Now that I have assembled comparable testamentary data for Florence and four other towns of central Italy, it is possible to examine these differences. From the perspective, not of Leonardo Bruni or Cosimo de' Medici, but of a broader population of property holders including peasants and poor widows, was Florence the forerunner of the Renaissance? The tally of pious choices from Florence does not show striking differences from the patterns in Siena. (See tables 1 and 2.) The share of pious gifts culled by the neighborhood parish or its priest fluctuated between one-sixth and one-quarter from the thirteenth through the early fifteenth century. But no clear trend emerges toward or away from these neighborhood-based sources of charity and salvation. The mendicant houses—the Franciscans of Santa Croce, the Dominicans of Santa Maria Novella and several smaller churches (such as San Pietro Murrone), the Servites at Santissima Annunziata, the Carmelites across the Arno, and the Augustinians at Santo Spirito—were slightly more successful than the parishes in gathering gifts from the pious over the long haul. In fact, of the pious institutions found in the ledgers of Florentine testaments, they were usually the most important charitable institutions, gathering one-quarter of the Florentine pious bequests. Yet, again, no

Table 1.
Pious Choices

Period	Misc.	Parishes	Mendicant Orders	Monasteries	Nunneries	Hospitals	Confraternities	"Poor of Christ"	Dowry Funds	Servants	Total
AREZZO											
< 1275											
1276–1300											
1301–25	97	102	102	3	155	62	69	19	0	5	614
1326–47	105	128	183	22	132	131	134	31	3	10	879
1348	83	126	109	30	47	60	85	42	1	25	608
1349–62	63	101	103	29	82	37	66	11	0	8	500
1363	45	91	63	23	57	42	61	15	2	4	403
1364–75	73	83	120	31	64	49	61	2	8	11	502
1376–1400	56	70	92	12	32	24	46	30	8	1	371
1401–25	48	107	89	14	18	42	56	10	10	4	398
Total	570	808	861	164	587	447	578	160	32	68	4,275
ASSISI											
< 1275	9	7	28	9	36	15	2	6	0	1	113
1276–1300	12	21	76	26	118	37	8	13	0	4	315
1301–25	16	13	56	8	61	10	5	6	1	7	183
1326–47	11	8	100	9	59	8	12	6	0	6	219
1348	12	25	67	11	30	9	12	5	2	1	174
1349–62	1	9	23	6	10	9	10	4	3	4	79
1363											
1364–75	5	6	32	1	8	1	3	0	1	0	57
1376–1400	13	20	65	1	20	2	22	5	6	2	156
1401–25	49	31	195	8	40	3	20	2	1	5	354
Total	128	140	642	79	382	94	94	47	14	30	1,650
FLORENCE											
< 1275	7	21	22	11	30	10	2	1	0	2	106
1276–1300	47	70	106	10	88	25	14	18	1	8	387
1301–25	47	82	120	28	93	56	26	24	2	9	487
1326–47	30	54	101	26	28	52	35	23	2	4	355
1348	51	86	116	30	38	66	62	28	1	12	490
1349–62	10	45	39	11	17	29	19	15	0	3	188
1363	44	62	92	34	41	72	36	24	5	11	421
1364–75	35	71	100	19	26	50	34	19	9	7	370
1376–1400	22	78	96	39	26	55	37	15	17	11	396
1401–25	9	70	47	19	15	59	27	11	22	9	288
Total	302	639	839	227	402	474	292	178	59	76	3,488
PERUGIA											
< 1275	0	0	3	0	0	0	0	0	0	0	3
1276–1300	1	2	0	0	1	0	0	2	1	0	7
1301–25	5	26	27	5	24	14	6	2	0	1	110
1326–47	31	77	31	18	16	35	14	29	2	5	258
1348	15	74	70	19	71	43	40	30	6	4	372
1349–62	4	10	31	13	2	2	1	11	3	2	79
1363	3	47	38	13	8	4	11	14	3	3	144
1364–75	5	55	51	15	3	8	11	19	6	10	183
1376–99	43	148	251	39	33	44	26	62	48	44	738
1400–1425	27	49	170	23	20	21	13	12	12	14	361
Total	134	488	672	145	178	171	122	181	81	83	2,255

Table 1.
Continued

Period	Misc.	Parishes	Mendicant Orders	Monasteries	Nunneries	Hospitals	Confraternities	"Poor of Christ"	Dowry Funds	Servants	Total
PISA											
< 1275	21	19	13	16	18	22	0	12	0	2	123
1276–1300	93	67	101	54	90	101	6	47	1	14	574
1301–25	434	359	519	234	403	709	45	230	12	54	2,999
1326–47	114	112	254	56	95	155	6	86	10	18	906
1348	20	20	27	11	12	11	0	11	2	3	117
1349–62	80	96	108	41	38	100	4	40	6	6	519
1363	40	39	155	44	36	53	5	38	7	4	421
1364–75	34	57	70	13	4	26	4	13	6	12	239
1376–1400	104	114	115	39	15	65	8	27	25	10	522
> 1400	58	35	26	13	12	18	6	6	4	3	181
Total	998	918	1,388	521	723	1,260	84	510	73	126	6,601
SIENA											
< 1275	49	62	27	28	35	41	0	25	0	3	270
1276–1300	77	58	58	34	69	47	2	50	0	3	398
1301–25	81	92	77	96	97	85	13	67	1	5	614
1326–47	82	91	110	103	62	95	20	55	1	9	628
1348	38	105	52	56	13	34	12	49	2	5	366
1349–62	18	26	72	56	12	22	11	25	1	8	251
1363	6	13	16	11	3	13	5	6	0	4	77
1364–75	12	21	16	21	8	9	2	9	2	4	104
1376–99	25	27	21	32	3	22	19	23	11	1	184
1400–1425	39	51	27	14	8	15	5	14	18	5	196
Total	427	546	476	451	310	383	89	323	36	47	3,088
TOTAL											
< 1275	86	109	93	64	119	88	4	44	0	8	615
1276–1300	230	218	341	124	366	210	30	130	3	29	1,681
1301–25	680	674	901	374	833	936	164	348	16	81	5,007
1326–47	373	470	779	234	392	476	221	230	18	52	3,245
1348	219	436	441	157	211	223	211	165	14	50	2,127
1349–62	176	287	376	156	161	199	111	106	13	31	1,616
1363	138	252	364	125	145	184	118	97	17	26	1,466
1364–75	164	293	389	100	113	143	115	62	32	44	1,455
1376–99	263	457	640	162	129	212	158	162	115	69	2,367
1400–1425	230	343	554	91	113	158	127	55	67	40	1,778
Total	2,559	3,539	4,878	1,587	2,582	2,829	1,259	1,399	295	430	21,357

Table 2.

Pious Choices
(Percentages)

Period	Misc.	Parishes	Mendicant Orders	Monasteries	Nunneries	Hospitals	Confraternities	"Poor of Christ"	Dowry Funds	Servants
AREZZO										
< 1275										
1276–1300										
1301–25	15.80	16.61	16.61	0.49	25.24	10.10	11.24	3.09	0.00	0.81
1326–47	11.95	14.56	20.82	2.50	15.02	14.90	15.24	3.53	0.34	1.14
1348	13.65	20.72	17.93	4.93	7.73	9.87	13.98	6.91	0.16	4.11
1349–62	12.60	20.20	20.60	5.80	16.40	7.40	13.20	2.20	0.00	1.60
1363	11.17	22.58	15.63	5.71	14.14	10.42	15.14	3.72	0.50	0.99
1364–75	14.54	16.53	23.90	6.18	12.75	9.76	12.15	0.40	1.59	2.19
1376–1400	15.09	18.87	24.80	3.23	8.63	6.47	12.40	8.09	2.16	0.27
1401–25	12.06	26.88	22.36	3.52	4.52	10.55	14.07	2.51	2.51	1.01
Total	13.33	18.90	20.14	3.84	13.73	10.46	13.52	3.74	0.75	1.59
ASSISI										
< 1275	7.96	6.19	24.78	7.96	31.86	13.27	1.77	5.31	0.00	0.88
1276–1300	3.81	6.67	24.13	8.25	37.46	11.75	2.54	4.13	0.00	1.27
1301–25	8.74	7.10	30.60	4.37	33.33	5.46	2.73	3.28	0.55	3.83
1326–47	5.02	3.65	45.66	4.11	26.94	3.65	5.48	2.74	0.00	2.74
1348	6.90	14.37	38.51	6.32	17.24	5.17	6.90	2.87	1.15	0.57
1349–62	1.27	11.39	29.11	7.59	12.66	11.39	12.66	5.06	3.80	5.06
1363										
1364–75	8.77	10.53	56.14	1.75	14.04	1.75	5.26	0.00	1.75	0.00
1376–1400	8.33	12.82	41.67	0.64	12.82	1.28	14.10	3.21	3.85	1.28
1401–25	13.84	8.76	55.08	2.26	11.30	0.85	5.65	0.56	0.28	1.41
Total	7.76	8.48	38.91	4.79	23.15	5.70	5.70	2.85	0.85	1.82
FLORENCE										
< 1275	6.60	19.81	20.75	10.38	28.30	9.43	1.89	0.94	0.00	1.89
1276–1300	12.14	18.09	27.39	2.58	22.74	6.46	3.62	4.65	0.26	2.07
1301–25	9.65	16.84	24.64	5.75	19.10	11.50	5.34	4.93	0.41	1.85
1326–47	8.45	15.21	28.45	7.32	7.89	14.65	9.86	6.48	0.56	1.13
1348	10.41	17.55	23.67	6.12	7.76	13.47	12.65	5.71	0.20	2.45
1349–62	5.32	23.94	20.74	5.85	9.04	15.43	10.11	7.98	0.00	1.60
1363	10.45	14.73	21.85	8.08	9.74	17.10	8.55	5.70	1.19	2.61
1364–75	9.46	19.19	27.03	5.14	7.03	13.51	9.19	5.14	2.43	1.89
1376–1400	5.56	19.70	24.24	9.85	6.57	13.89	9.34	3.79	4.29	2.78
1401–25	3.13	24.31	16.32	6.60	5.21	20.49	9.38	3.82	7.64	3.13
Total	8.66	18.32	24.05	6.51	11.53	13.59	8.37	5.10	1.69	2.18
PERUGIA										
< 1275	0.00	0.00	100.00	0.00	0.00	0.00	0.00	0.00	0.00	0.00
1276–1300	14.29	28.57	0.00	0.00	14.29	0.00	0.00	28.57	14.29	0.00
1301–25	4.55	23.64	24.55	4.55	21.82	12.73	5.45	1.82	0.00	0.91
1326–47	12.02	29.84	12.02	6.98	6.20	13.57	5.43	11.24	0.78	1.94
1348	4.03	19.89	18.82	5.11	19.09	11.56	10.75	8.06	1.61	1.08
1349–62	5.06	12.66	39.24	16.46	2.53	2.53	1.27	13.92	3.80	2.53
1363	2.08	32.64	26.39	9.03	5.56	2.78	7.64	9.72	2.08	2.08
1364–75	2.73	30.05	27.87	8.20	1.64	4.37	6.01	10.38	3.28	5.46
1376–99	5.83	20.05	34.01	5.28	4.47	5.96	3.52	8.40	6.50	5.96
1400–1425	7.48	13.57	47.09	6.37	5.54	5.82	3.60	3.32	3.32	3.88
Total	5.94	21.64	29.80	6.43	7.89	7.58	5.41	8.03	3.59	3.68

Table 2.
Continued

Period	Misc.	Parishes	Mendicant Orders	Monasteries	Nunneries	Hospitals	Confraternities	"Poor of Christ"	Dowry Funds	Servants
PISA										
< 1275	17.07	15.45	10.57	13.01	14.63	17.89	0.00	9.76	0.00	1.63
1276–1300	16.20	11.67	17.60	9.41	15.68	17.60	1.05	8.19	0.17	2.44
1301–25	14.47	11.97	17.31	7.80	13.44	23.64	1.50	7.67	0.40	1.80
1326–47	12.58	12.36	28.04	6.18	10.49	17.11	0.66	9.49	1.10	1.99
1348	17.09	17.09	23.08	9.40	10.26	9.40	0.00	9.40	1.71	2.56
1349–61	15.41	18.50	20.81	7.90	7.32	19.27	0.77	7.71	1.16	1.16
1362	9.50	9.26	36.82	10.45	8.55	12.59	1.19	1.66	1.66	5.02
1363–75	14.23	23.85	29.29	5.44	1.67	10.88	1.67	5.44	2.51	5.02
1376–1400	19.92	21.84	22.03	7.47	2.87	12.45	1.53	5.17	4.79	1.92
1401–25	32.04	19.34	14.36	7.18	6.63	9.94	3.31	3.31	2.21	1.66
Total	15.12	13.91	21.03	7.89	10.95	19.09	1.27	7.73	1.11	1.91
SIENA										
< 1275	18.15	22.96	10.00	10.37	12.96	15.19	0.00	9.26	0.00	1.11
1276–1300	19.35	14.57	14.57	8.54	17.34	11.81	0.50	12.56	0.00	0.75
1301–25	13.19	14.98	12.54	15.64	15.80	13.84	2.12	10.91	0.16	0.81
1326–47	13.06	14.49	17.52	16.40	9.87	15.13	3.18	8.76	0.16	1.43
1348	10.38	28.69	14.21	15.30	3.55	9.29	3.28	13.39	0.55	1.37
1349–62	7.17	10.36	28.69	22.31	4.78	8.76	4.38	9.96	0.40	3.19
1363	7.79	16.88	20.78	14.29	3.90	16.88	6.49	7.79	0.00	5.19
1364–75	11.54	20.19	15.38	20.19	7.69	8.65	1.92	8.65	1.92	3.85
1376–1400	13.59	14.67	11.41	17.39	1.63	11.96	10.33	12.50	5.98	0.54
1401–25	19.90	26.02	13.78	7.14	4.08	7.65	2.55	7.14	9.18	2.55
Total	13.83	17.68	15.41	14.60	10.04	12.40	2.88	10.46	1.17	1.52
TOTAL										
< 1275	0.14	0.18	0.15	0.10	0.19	0.14	0.01	0.07	0.00	0.01
1276–1300	0.14	0.13	0.20	0.07	0.22	0.12	0.02	0.08	0.00	0.02
1301–25	0.14	0.13	0.18	0.07	0.17	0.19	0.03	0.07	0.00	0.02
1326–47	0.11	0.14	0.24	0.07	0.12	0.15	0.07	0.07	0.01	0.02
1348	0.10	0.20	0.21	0.07	0.10	0.10	0.10	0.08	0.01	0.02
1349–62	0.11	0.18	0.23	0.10	0.10	0.12	0.07	0.07	0.01	0.02
1363	0.09	0.17	0.25	0.09	0.10	0.13	0.08	0.07	0.01	0.02
1364–75	0.11	0.20	0.27	0.07	0.08	0.10	0.08	0.04	0.02	0.03
1376–1400	0.11	0.19	0.27	0.07	0.05	0.09	0.07	0.07	0.05	0.03
1401–25	0.13	0.19	0.31	0.05	0.06	0.09	0.07	0.03	0.04	0.02
Total	0.12	0.17	0.23	0.07	0.12	0.13	0.06	0.07	0.01	0.02

clear trend appears; their popularity, despite changes in the spiritual directions of these houses, reforms, and counter reforms, remained roughly stationary from the thirteenth through the early fifteenth century. Nor do gifts to other monasteries, mostly Benedictine tied to the city's most ancient parish churches as well as Carthusian and Cistercian monasteries in the surrounding countryside, show a Florentine population closing its pocketbook to these ancient and venerable institutions.

Given the recent literature on the directions of change in Renaissance piety, we might well have expected a shift in monastic support away from the old houses toward the friars, who were intimately involved with the social problems of the expanding commercial centers in northern and central Italy. These new friaries were more than monasteries; they incorporated within their walls hospitals, to which testators often earmarked their gifts, as well as building funds (the *opera*) which, through the early Quattrocento, sustained lavish building programs and patronized frescoes, panel paintings, and their restoration.[9] Yet the proportion of legacies to these institutions of a more "civic Christian" bent do not uncover a major shift in mentality after the Black Death or even into the early Quattrocento.

Nor do these big blocks of pious patronage—the parish church and the monasteries—show decisive trends for the other cities in my analysis. In support of the neighborhood church, the mendicant orders, and monasteries, the charitable profile of the Aretines and Pisans closely resembled that of the Sienese and the Florentines. The mendicant orders received slightly more in Florence (nearly one-quarter of all pious gifts as opposed to one in five gifts in Arezzo and Pisa).

Within the ranks of the mendicants, differences do arise. The Dominicans, principally from the monastery of Santa Maria Novella, dominated the souls of Florentines;[10] 43 percent of the bequests to mendicants ended in the hands of this order, while the Franciscans claimed a quarter,[11] followed by the Servites (12 percent), the Augustinians (10 percent), and the Carmelites (7 percent).[12] Nor did these percentages change appreciably over the course of the fourteenth and early fifteenth centuries.[13] Pisa, on the other hand, appears from these data more as a Franciscan than a Dominican city, despite "the succession of eminent Dominicans" at Santa Caterina, such as Giordano da Rivolta, Domenico Cavalca, and Bartolomeo da San Concordio.[14] The minor friars drew one-third of all pious gifts, as opposed to 29 percent given to the Dominican preachers, followed by the Augustinians (20 percent) and the Carmelites (17 percent).[15] In contrast, the Servite order hardly made a showing, receiving only ten gifts over the four centuries of documents (less than one percent). The composition of mendicant bequests in Arezzo forms yet another pattern. Like Siena and Pisa, Arezzo was a Franciscan town. More than one-third of the mendicant charities ended in the hands of these minor friars.[16] But here, the Dominicans were not even decisively the second order in town; instead, they shared that position with the Augustinians, each attracting 29 percent of the mendicant bequests, followed by the Servites (14 percent) and finally the Carmelites (8 percent).[17] The relative weakness of the Dominicans in Arezzo is reflected architecturally. In contrast to San Francesco's imposing "monumentality and spaciousness" (especially before the disastrous renovations of the 1870s), the Dominican church was considerably smaller and, according to Mario Salmi, "more withdrawn."[18]

The old orders of monks (mostly Benedictines and mostly tied to ancient parish churches), like their more successful and more worldly mendicant brethren, do not show significant or striking transformations over time. Nor do any of the differences among the cities suggest possible broad contrasts in the patterns of piety across the urban geography of Tuscany. These older houses (with the exception of the Benedictine Olivetani, founded by Sienese noblemen in the fourteenth century) received slightly fewer gifts in Arezzo than in Pisa (4 percent versus 8 percent) or in Florence (7 percent). Pisans gave slightly less to their parishes than did Aretines (14 percent versus 19 percent) or Florentines (18 percent). No events such as the famines of the second decade of the fourteenth century, the Black Death of 1348 and 1363, or the formation of an early Renaissance culture in the early Quattrocento marked a watershed in the allocation of gifts to these largest blocks of charitable beneficiaries. Consistently through time and from city to city in Tuscany the mendicants, monasteries, and parishes, considered together, drew one-half of all charitable contributions.

Umbria, on the other hand, varied slightly from the picture portrayed by the Tuscan towns. First, in Franciscan-dominated Assisi, the parish amassed significantly fewer pious bequests than in Tuscany and less than half of what the parish could attract in Florence, Arezzo, or Pisa. But gifts to the parish did not constitute a Tuscan versus an Umbrian pattern of charity or suggest possible differences in neighborhood alliances. The town that was literally the most parochial in its choice of endowments was neighboring Perugia, where local churches garnered the highest percentage of total pious bequests over time for all six cities (22 percent). With the recurrence of plague in 1363, this percentage reached its acme for any of the towns—33 percent. The second coming of pestilence, however, did not demarcate a decisive change in pious choices. As in Tuscany, the changes fluctuated but without a clear direction.

When we consider monasteries and friaries, however, an Umbrian pattern does emerge. First, for the oversized village that Saint Francis catapulted into the world history of religions, the mendicants dominated pious last giving to a greater degree than can be found in any of the

Tuscan towns. Perhaps not surprisingly, the mendicants here were almost exclusively Franciscans. Yet the extent of their monopoly is remarkable: 99.97 percent of all pious bequests to the mendicant orders went to Franciscans. Of 642 pious legacies for orders both in the city and the countryside only five went to non-Franciscans (all to houses beyond the territory of Assisi).

The selective survival of sources might explain in part this exceptional domination of the Franciscans in Assisi. The earliest notarized protocols date only from the plague year 1374. Before that year, only a handful of testaments came from the cathedral archive of San Ruffino. Instead, the Mother Basilica was the supplier of this remarkable set of early *pergamene,* and thus we might question whether this sample seriously overstates the importance of the Franciscans and particularly of gifts to their "Sacro Convento." The Mother Church, however, was not the only Franciscan house vying for pious presents from the Assisani. The church in the lowlands just below Assisi, Santa Maria degli Angeli, also called the Porziuncola, which still today encloses the straw-hut cell where Saint Francis died, drew fully one-quarter of all bequests to Franciscans;[19] next, the church of San Damiano, where Saint Francis first heard his calling in the summer of 1205 and where Saint Clare established the first church of the Poor Clares, culled ten percent of these legacies;[20] then, with 6 percent, came the Franciscan hermits (*carcerati*), called *fraticelli* in the earliest documents, who stayed on the mountaintop of Monte Subàsio to the east of the city.[21] Finally, these testators regularly gave to a number of Franciscan houses in the district, such as San Corrado de Insula and Santa Maria de Rochezola, or Rocheciola (8 percent).[22]

Assisi also differs from the Tuscan model in a way that runs completely against the evidentiary bias. Quite unexpectedly, the mendicants (here really the Franciscans) more than doubled their claims on the pious, progressing from 24 percent in the last years of the thirteenth century to 55 percent in the early Quattrocento. The largest increase came sometime after the plague of 1363. Unfortunately, only three testaments could be found in all the archives in Assisi for this plague year. But soon afterward, 1364–1375, gifts to the Franciscans (including the churches and friaries of San Francesco, Santa Maria degli Angeli, San Damiano, and the *carcerati* at Monte Subàsio) jumped from 29 to 56 percent. Thus the highest percentages of gifts to Franciscans came after the *pergamene* collections of testaments from the Sacro Convento had dried to a trickle, and when wills from the public notary books, unconnected with any religious organization, supplied this sample almost exclusively.

These changes cannot be explained simply by the change in Franciscan rule, when Pope John XXII and the secretary general of the order "moved in unison to destroy the Spiritualists."[23] The increase of gifts found in these testaments began after the heroic period of Saint Francis and his immediate followers and continued until well after John's Bull, *Gloriosam ecclesiam* of 23 January 1317, legalized the order's retention of pious legacies.

While the lopsided domination of the Franciscans in the historically anomalous Assisi may not be surprising, the importance of the mendicants in Perugia suggests that the friaries may have established a stronger foothold in Umbria than in Tuscany, perhaps stronger than anywhere else in late medieval Italy. In Perugia, in contrast to Assisi, legacies went to all the mendicants—the Dominicans, Augustinians, Servites, and Carmelites, as well as the Franciscans. In fact, the Dominicans predominated, culling 44 percent of the bequests to mendicants, as against their Franciscan confrères' 36 percent.[24] The Augustinians (11 percent), the Servites (9 percent), and finally the much weaker Carmelites (one percent) trailed these powerful organizations.[25]

Unlike Assisi, where the parish was weak and hospitals not as central to the religious life as elsewhere, a plethora of religious institutions crowded the religious landscape in Perugia as in the large Tuscan towns in my sample. Not only did the numerous parishes in Perugia attract more bequests over the long haul than did those in any of the other five towns, the pious legacies of Perugia reveal numerous hospitals organized around the guilds, the popularity of other monasteries, especially the new Benedictine order of the Olivetani, as well as over fifteen nunneries, and the existence of a rich life of religious confraternities. Nonetheless, as in Assisi, mendicants dominated as beneficiaries to an extent not found in any of the Tuscan towns; one out of every three gifts ended up in their hands. Their popularity, moreover, was not static; instead, as in Assisi, it grew after the Black Death until nearly one out of every two pious bequests (47 percent) fell into these coffers by the end of the period I studied.

Nunneries

Of those religious institutions founded largely in the central Middle Ages and which reflect the older views of penitence and asceticism, only the women's houses show a clear trend in Tuscany over this two hundred-year period. From attracting over one-quarter of all pious bequests, more than any other institution, in the earliest documents (until 1275), their share shrank steadily over time until, by the early Quattrocento, Florentines gave only one-twentieth of their pious legacies to them. The sharpest fall in the Florentine convents' ability to attract monies and properties from those seeking salvation came well before the demographic collapse wrought by the Black Death. Between 1301– 25 and 1326–47, their share declined by half from nearly 20 to less than 10 percent of all final gifts. As against Siena, however, where nunneries disappeared almost completely from the itemized lists of pious bequests, in Florence a plethora of houses persisted into the Quattrocento.[26] The decline in number in Florence did not result from a single house or a small group of convents consolidating property, absorbing smaller houses and thereby attracting large pious properties that earlier might have been fragmented into more numerous but smaller gifts to a large array of nunneries. Did the decline in sponsoring nunneries depend on under-lying demographic causes—a change in society's conception of the role of women in a period of population stagnation? David Herlihy and others have shown convincingly that the Tuscan population was on the wane well before the catastrophe of 1348; the apex of population may have even preceded the turn of the fourteenth century.[27] But these demo-graphic historians have argued that the decades leading to 1348 may have been the most depressed of the central and late Middle Ages. Because of the severe problems of relative overpopulation and under- and unemployment, no demographic or economic rationale should have convinced pious artisans, peasants, or merchants circa 1325 to have become suddenly pro-populationist, reversing their image of women from ascetics to be shielded from the worldly dangers of sex to mothers of "good custom" capable of raising large families. Moreover, no cross-over to dowry funds becomes evident in these early documents for any of the six cities. In Florence, where testamentary dowry funds would later become the most pronounced, they began to mount in importance only toward the end of my period, in the last years of the Trecento.

Nor was this secular decline of nunneries peculiar to Siena and Florence. Its timing, however, varied from place to place. The importance of nunneries was most evident in the testaments from Assisi. In the earliest documents until 1275, they received one-third of all pious be-quests, and in the last years of the thirteenth century, their strength reached an all-time high for all six of these cities (37 percent). It then tapered off following the Black Death, but the decline was not as dramatic as elsewhere. In the early Quattrocento, Assisani still gave over one-tenth of their pious bequests to women's convents.

By contrast, those in neighboring Perugia gave the least to nuns. But, as in the other towns, convents declined in Perugia over the course of the Trecento and particularly after the Black Death. They peaked in the last years of the Duecento, attracting slightly more than one of every five pious bequests. This level was momentarily approached again in the year of the Black Death (19 percent), but immediately afterward it plummeted to 3 percent. Although the nuns attracted 6 percent of all legacies after 1400, certainly this figure marked no return to their pre-Black Death charitable importance.

In Pisa, their decline was more gradual than in Florence until the plague of 1362. Thereafter, the draw of the convents dropped to a negligible 2 percent of their pious legacies. In Arezzo, a sharp decline set in still later—in the last quarter of the Trecento and the early years of the Quattrocento.

Hospitals

To examine the other supposed side of piety—the this-worldly sustenance of the sick and poor—we should look at legacies to hospitals and religious confraternities. Yet, it is never easy to divide these institutions into tidy categories—those aimed at alleviating earthly suffering and those devoted to asceticism and penitence. While the mendicant houses staffed infirmaries, the objectives of the medieval hospital were not identical to those of its modern progeny. Medieval and early modern hospitals could function as wayside hostels for pilgrims as well as caring for the poor; they also performed sacramental duties.[28] Similarly, that other group of pious entities which has been associated with a more this-worldly religiosity—lay confraternities—and which increased in number and possibly in membership from the early thirteenth century through the Renaissance, attracted members not only for charitable purposes but for the devotional singing of praises of Mary or Christ (laude) and for rites of flagellation. In fact, in all six cities, confraternities devoted to this form of "discipline"—the disciplinati—dominated in number those engaged in praising the Lord through their songs and psalms—the laudesi.[29]

Across these rough lines of demarcation, does Florence show a more distinctive Renaissance pattern in its bequests to these this-worldly religious institutions than the possibly more provincial and backward

looking Siena? The numerous hospitals of Florence accumulated proportionately more pious bequests over time. From 6 percent of all pious
legacies during the last years of the thirteenth century, that proportion
trebled during the plague year of 1363, then by the opening years of
the fifteenth century increased to 20 percent.

For Siena, gifts to hospitals followed a similar trajectory, at least until
1363, when the proportion of hospital gifts was almost exactly the same
as that found in Florence. But then the numbers of bequests to Sienese
hospitals tumbled to less than half the earlier proportion by the first years
of the fifteenth century. This fall does not, however, accurately reflect a
turning of Sienese pious impulses away from the hospital. Instead, another process, if not originally spawned then certainly accelerated by
the financial dislocations following the plagues and demographic decline,
was well under way during the last decades of the fourteenth century.
The powerful, quasi-state-run hospital of Santa Maria della Scala began
to gobble up a myriad of smaller hospitals;[30] others such as the Misericordia came on hard times and ultimately filed for bankruptcy, becoming the *Sapienza* of the University of Siena at the beginning of the
fifteenth century.[31]

As a result, fewer hospitals remained on the ecclesiastical horizon in
post-1363 Siena, ready with their hands extended to the pious of Siena
and its territory. At the same time, the prestige and wealth of its principal
hospital mounted, and the size and values of its testamentary gifts reflected
this change. This single institution more than compensated for the loss
in pious gifts due to the disappearance of the jumble of small hospices
and wayside stations for the sick which, before the Black Death, had
crowded the ecclesiastical map of Siena. In terms of the value of gifts,
the proportion of gifts to hospitals in Siena actually increased from the
plague year of 1363 to the first quarter of the fifteenth century (from under
13 percent of all monetized gifts to over 18 percent).[32]

Did Florence's principal hospital, Santa Maria Nuova (founded by
Falco Portinari in 1288),[33] follow a similar pattern of concentration and
monopolization? A superficial reading of the testaments does not suggest
this, and Giuliano Pinto has recently remarked that "the case of Florence"
was different from that of Siena. "No single grand hospital" dominated
in the Arno city; rather, these services were divided among three or
four institutions with different fields of specialization.[34] In support of this
view, important hospitals, such as San Gallo (founded in 1218)[35] in the
north of the city and its neighbor, Santa Maria della Scala in the via
San Gallo, did not decline noticeably after the plague of 1363 as far as

the testamentary choices disclose. And numerous smaller institutions that catered to the ill and the poor—Santa Maria Maddalena, the hospital del Serre, San Biagio (located in one of the most impoverished districts of the city, Verzaia),[36] the Misericordia across from the Baptistry, the hospital of the Pinzocheri (most likely, San Paolo),[37] San Matteo in via del Cocomero,[38] San Lotto, San Salvi, San Miniato—persisted as the beneficiaries of Florentine legacies. The early Quattrocento in Florence, unlike Siena, even saw the first appearance in last wills of new city hospitals, which would become increasingly important through the Renaissance. In 1417 a widow from the magnate lineage of the Tornaquinci gave 20 florins to the hospital of Ser Bonifazio.[39] The hospital for the poor, San Paolo (although a much older institution), first appears in these documents under this name with a pious bequest only in 1417.[40] And the hospital of the Innocenti, called in the document the *"hospitale puerorum de gittategli"* and whose Brunelleschi arches in the piazza of Santissima Annunziata gave rise to a model of Renaissance public architecture, first appeared in the testament of a wine seller in 1423.[41]

Counting the appearances of hospitals in these documents before and after 1363 does not seem to change the picture. From the earliest Florentine documents to the second occurrence of pestilence, 26 different hospitals appear as the objects of charity. Afterward, at least 20 remained. The frequency of gifts to Florence's main hospital in relation to all the others, however, tells another story. Before the second plague, Santa Maria Nuova accounted for little more than one-third of hospital bequests; afterward, its share grew to 78 percent.[42] This change, moreover, cannot be attributed to biases in the selection of documents. As most social and political historians of late medieval Florence know, the *Diplomatico,* or set of loose parchment rolls, once preserved by the hospital of Santa Maria Nuova forms the largest and richest of these parchment archives, assembled by archivists during the rule of the Lorrainians and placed in the hands of the state archives at the end of the eighteenth century. To avoid a bias in the direction of gifts to hospitals, I sampled this collection of *pergamene* sparingly. Of 653 testaments selected for the Florentine sample, 174 come from this vast archive containing possibly over a thousand last wills for the periods under scrutiny.[43] But if those documents originating from Santa Maria's archive are removed from the sample, the differences over time become even more striking: from the remaining documents Santa Maria Nuova drew slightly less than one-quarter of all hospital gifts before the second plague and over two-thirds afterward.[44]

When these statistics are broken down still farther, a history of concentration comes into bold relief paralleling and even exceeding the history of Siena's central hospital, Santa Maria della Scala. Before 1326, Santa Maria Nuova collected only 15 percent of all pious gifts. It was then not even the most popular of Florence's hospitals. San Gallo, tucked away in the northernmost point of the fourteenth-century city, received more than double the number and accounted for nearly one-third of the legacies given to hospitals. Moreover, in the earliest documents, various small hospitals and hospices in the countryside together attracted more bequests from city testators than Santa Maria Nuova.[45] Even a small hospital such as San Bartolommeo de Mugnone, not particularly well remembered in the annals of Florentine charities, received half as many gifts as Santa Maria Nuova. But in the quarter-century preceding the Black Death, San Gallo quickly lost its early hegemony, its share declining sharply to only 6 percent of these pious legacies, and it disappeared altogether from the lists of charitable legacies by the last 25 years of my analysis. In its place, Santa Maria Nuova emerged as Florence's principal hospital, reaping 42 percent of all hospital legacies between 1326 and 1348. In the year of the plague's first strike, its share increased, but not significantly, to 44 percent. Then, in the interval between the plagues of 1348 and 1363, its popularity jumped significantly to 69 percent.[46] After maintaining this high level in the plague year of 1363 (71 percent), its proportion again soared in the 1364-1400 period, when it attained 85 percent of all hospital legacies. In the final years of this survey, 1401-25, its share dropped slightly to 75 percent.[47] This last figure still represents a higher concentration of gifts than Siena's commune-backed hospital ever managed to attract during the six hundred years traced in my *Death and Property in Siena*. At its apex in the fifteenth century,[48] Siena's Santa Maria della Scala amassed two-thirds of all hospital legacies.

As in Siena, so in Florence the concentration of hospital bequests to a single institution masked testators' desires in the latter part of the Trecento to contribute substantially greater shares of their pious endowments to hospitals. Where in the earliest documents Florentines gave only one percent of their pious properties to hospitals (see table 3), this figure increased to 9 percent in 1348 and remained roughly the same for the next 15 years. Then, when the plague returned in the summer months of 1363, the proportion of wealth directed toward them soared to 40 percent. In the ensuing 12 years, it increased still farther to 42 percent. By the early Quattrocento, these proportions had tapered off; still, Florentines of the early Renaissance were giving one-third of the values of their last charities to hospitals and two-thirds of that to a single institution, Santa Maria Nuova.

Was the progressive concentration and monopolization of hospital services at Florence and Siena exceptional? For Pisa, the frequency of hospital legacies did not follow the path of civic Christianity plotted roughly by the Florentine ones. From the earliest documents until 1275, hospitals already drew 18 percent of all Pisan pious bequests, a share higher than that obtained by the combined hospitals of Siena for any period through the six centuries charted by my earlier study. In the 1326–47 period, the Pisan hospitals, just as the Florentine ones were beginning their ascent, peaked with nearly a quarter of all pious bequests, the highest proportion found for hospital gifts in any period and any city studied here. Afterward the figure fluctuated, but the direction of change was unmistakably downward, especially with the recurrence of pestilence in 1362, when it dropped to 13 percent before sliding to a low of 10 percent in the opening years of the Quattrocento—one-half the share of Florentine hospitals for these years.

Before concluding that the pious choices of Pisan testators ran against a supposed Renaissance trend, I need to raise two questions. As in Siena, did the centralization of a single hospital mask a trend toward increasing contributions in larger parcels to the hospitals of Pisa? And have biases in the selection of documents skewed my perceptions? In Pisa, because of the paucity of early notarial books and testaments,[49] I could not avoid relying on the rich notarial collections preserved in the archives of this city's principal hospital, founded in 1257 by Pope Alexander IV to end a 16-year excommunication of the maritime commune and called over time by various names—the Misericordia, Santa Chiara, L'Ospedale Nuovo, L'Ospedale del Papa Alessandro VI.[50] (I shall refer to it as the hospital of Santa Chiara). Eighty-eight percent of the testaments before 1326 derive from notarial books kept originally by this principal hospital. Afterward, their proportion falls off just when other collections begin to increase (particularly the notarial protocols now housed in the state archives of Florence). In the 1326–47 period, 42 percent of the testaments derived from the *notarile* of Santa Chiara; for the Black Death and afterward, its share dropped to 18 percent of the Pisan sample.[51] Unlike the *pergamene* collections, which occasionally would excerpt those portions of a testament pertaining directly to the monastery, hospital, or confraternity conserving it, these notarial books contain complete testaments, from the preamble through the numerous itemized bequests

Table 3.
The Values of Bequests to Hospitals

	No. Pious Bequests to Hospitals	No. Hospital Bequests Monetized	Proportion of Hospital Bequests Monetized	Average Price of Hospital Bequests (Florins)	Hypothesized Amount of Hospital Bequests (Florins)	No. of All Pious Bequests	No. of All Pious Bequests Monetized	Proportion of All Pious Bequests Monetized	Average Price of All Bequests (Florins)	Hypothesized Amount of All Pious Bequests (Florins)	Ratio of Values of Hospital Bequests to All Pious Bequests
AREZZO											
< 1326	62	51	0.82	0.34	21.08	614	516	0.84	1.84	1,129.76	0.02
1326–47	131	110	0.84	2.53	331.43	879	714	0.81	4.20	3,691.80	0.09
1348	60	37	0.62	1.27	76.20	608	374	0.62	19.84	12,062.72	0.01
1349–61	37	30	0.81	1.53	56.61	500	397	0.79	5.36	2,680.00	0.02
1362	42	29	0.69	14.65	615.30	403	291	0.72	10.54	4,247.62	0.14
1363–75	49	37	0.76	5.10	249.90	502	357	0.71	8.89	4,462.78	0.06
1376–1400	24	14	0.58	3.42	82.08	371	251	0.68	11.45	4,247.95	0.02
1401–25	42	29	0.69	2.88	120.96	398	240	0.60	14.02	5,579.96	0.02
ASSISI											
< 1326	52	52	1.00	1.01	52.52	611	579	0.95	3.04	1,857.44	0.03
1326–47	8	8	1.00	0.27	2.16	219	191	0.87	4.42	967.98	0.00
1348	9	4	0.44	0.26	2.34	174	124	0.71	6.41	1,115.34	0.00
1349–62	9	5	0.56	34.79	313.11	79	53	0.67	10.44	824.76	0.38
1363											
1364–75	1	1	1.00	4.00	4.00	57	50	0.88	3.11	177.27	0.02
1376–1400	2	1	0.50	0.26	0.52	156	107	0.69	4.88	761.28	0.00
1401–25	3	1	0.33	5.00	15.00	354	205	0.58	3.95	1,398.30	0.01
FLORENCE											
< 1326	91	80	0.88	6.53	594.23	980	891	0.91	16.59	16,258.20	0.04
1326–47	52	29	0.56	1.29	67.08	355	284	0.80	13.46	4,778.30	0.01
1348	66	46	0.70	22.56	1,488.96	490	414	0.84	34.51	16,909.90	0.09
1349–61	29	14	0.48	22.44	650.76	188	119	0.63	45.06	8,471.28	0.08
1362	72	30	0.42	61.09	4,398.48	421	315	0.75	26.15	11,009.15	0.40
1363–75	50	13	0.26	92.53	4,626.50	370	255	0.69	29.55	10,933.50	0.42
1376–1400	55	20	0.36	46.31	2,547.05	396	257	0.65	25.32	10,026.72	0.25
1401–25	59	23	0.39	129.09	7,616.31	307	184	0.60	80.62	24,750.34	0.31
PERUGIA											
< 1326	14	8	0.57	2.75	38.50	120	102	0.85	5.55	666.00	0.06
1326–47	35	29	0.83	19.14	669.90	312	264	0.85	5.93	1,850.16	0.36
1348	44	28	0.64	4.56	200.64	372	310	0.83	6.65	2,473.80	0.08
1349–61	2	1	0.50	1.60	3.20	79	62	0.78	26.92	2,126.68	0.00
1362	4	0	0.00	0.00	0.00	144	99	0.69	11.62	1,673.28	0.00
1363–75	8	5	0.63	4.60	36.80	183	151	0.83	9.52	1,742.16	0.02
1376–1394	43	20	0.47	46.70	2,008.10	738	437	0.59	22.14	16,339.32	0.12
1400–1425	21	8	0.38	23.84	500.64	361	156	0.43	33.39	12,053.79	0.04

Table 3.
(Continued)

	No. Pious Bequests to Hospitals	No. Hospital Bequests Monetized	Proportion of Hospital Bequests Monetized	Average Price of Hospital Bequests (Florins)	Hypothesized Amount of Hospital Bequests (Florins)	No. of All Pious Bequests	No. of All Pious Bequests Monetized	Proportion of All Pious Bequests Monetized	Average Price of All Bequests (Florins)	Hypothesized Amount of All Pious Bequests (Florins)	Ratio of Values of Hospital Bequests to All Pious Bequests
PISA											
< 1326	832	722	0.87	3.40	2,828.80	3,696	3,271	0.89	3.23	10,565.33	0.27
1326–47	155	102	0.66	4.14	641.70	906	730	0.81	13.57	9,906.10	0.06
1348	11	5	0.45	1.57	17.27	117	83	0.71	4.99	414.17	0.04
1349–61	100	54	0.54	2.90	290.00	519	352	0.68	22.97	8,085.44	0.04
1362	53	44	0.83	2.72	144.16	421	328	0.78	7.21	2,364.88	0.06
1363–75	26	7	0.27	6.57	170.82	239	136	0.57	11.22	1,525.92	0.11
1376–1400	65	18	0.28	16.12	1,047.80	522	264	0.51	19.00	5,016.00	0.21
1401–25	18	7	0.39	10.00	180.00	181	80	0.44	9.69	775.20	0.23
Adj < 1326	42	35	0.83	0.75	31.50	340	280	0.82	4.72	1,321.60	0.02
Adj 1326–	89	80	0.90	3.17	282.13	708	592	0.84	15.63	9,253.00	0.03
SIENA											
< 1326	173	145	0.84	3.50	605.50	1,282	1,107	0.86	9.75	12,499.50	0.05
1326–47	95	72	0.76	67.91	6,451.45	628	516	0.82	14.22	8,930.16	0.72
1348	34	24	0.71	23.02	782.68	366	280	0.77	8.26	3,023.16	0.26
1349–62	22	18	0.82	6.35	139.70	251	217	0.86	7.23	1,814.73	0.08
1363	13	11	0.85	10.26	133.38	77	64	0.83	13.60	1,047.20	0.13
1364–75	9	3	0.33	34.67	312.03	104	79	0.76	9.83	1,022.32	0.31
1376–1400	22	7	0.32	324.91	7,148.02	184	103	0.56	42.48	7,816.32	0.91
1401–25	15	11	0.73	71.09	1,066.35	196	138	0.70	24.44	4,790.24	0.22

to the concluding sections channeling the residual properties and responsibilities to the universal heirs, whether or not they conveyed properties to the hospital.[52] In fact, these notarial books do possess testaments (although few in number) that conveyed nothing to the hospital. According to Michele Luzzati, these protocols contain not only the "private" transactions of the hospital but present a "mixture" of public and private business as was common practice among early notaries attached to large religious corporations.[53]

Nonetheless, these sources, kept most likely by the hospital's own scribes, do reflect a bias toward hospital business.[54] Hospitals in general (not only Santa Chiara) received 23.5 percent of all pious bequests from the earliest records until 1325. Of the smattering of documents from other sources before this date (a mere 34 testaments), the hospitals' share was nearly half this (12 percent).[55] Moreover, if only the records from other archives are considered, Pisans' contributions to hospitals show neither a secular decline nor the ascent of civic Christianity; instead, they trace a flat course similar to Siena's. In the period after 1325, the share to Pisa's hospitals declined insignificantly, from 12 to 11 percent of all pious gifts.[56] Thus, even if hospitals did not wane in popularity before the Black Death, the choices of Pisan testators do not reflect (at least at this point in the analysis) an upward turn from the period of the Black Death through the early Quattrocento.

But beneath the surface of these stable proportions over time, could there have been occurring a concentration and centralization of hospital services in the so-called new hospital, Santa Chiara? Even though 88 percent of the testaments until 1325 come from notarial books once a part of this hospital's archives and afterward fell off sharply, the trend line of bequests, nonetheless, charts a process of concentration over time parallel to that in Siena and Florence. When all the documents are considered, Santa Chiara absorbed 43 percent of all hospital legacies before 1325.[57] In these documents a number of hospitals appeared consistently as the objects of testamentary devotion, even though the bias was certainly in the direction of Pisa's principal hospital. The orphans' hospitals (trovatelli) of Santo Spirito and San Domenico received 154 gifts (19 percent of all gifts to hospitals);[58] the women's hospital of San Giovanni in the parish of San Marco, 101 gifts (12 percent); the hospital of Sant'Asnello, 88 (11 percent); the lepers' hospital, Saint Lazarus, 40 (5 percent); and 36 other hospitals in the city and countryside of Pisa divided the remainder. In the quarter-century preceding the Black Death, Santa Chiara's share rose to 52 percent; it then climbed to 60 percent in the period of the Black Death until the pestilence recurred in 1362, when it dropped momentarily to 38 percent,[59] only to jump to 65 percent in the 1363–75 period, then to a high of 77 percent by the end of the century, though few documents at this point still derived from Santa Chiara's archival chambers.[60] By the beginning of the Quattrocento, the number of hospitals drawing pious bequests had diminished from 36 to only 3: one in the countryside, the lepers' hospital, and Santa Chiara.[61]

If the mass of testaments from this hospital's archives is excluded, the trend of concentration becomes, as one might expect, more accentuated. Instead of 43 percent of all hospital gifts, Santa Chiara drew 30 percent in the earliest documents until 1325; from then to the Black

Death, the proportion actually fell to 28 percent, but afterward, it jumped to the same level plotted by the entire sample of Pisan testaments (comprising now almost exclusively wills from various ecclesiastical collections and most importantly from public notarial chartularies housed in Florence).[62]

As in Siena and Florence, so in Pisa the force of a single hospital succeeded in weeding out the plethora of lesser hospitals and hospices in the city and countryside during the late thirteenth and early fourteenth centuries. Santa Chiara's gradual monopolization, which began well before the Black Death, and perhaps as early as the turn of the fourteenth century, masked an upward trend in the value of Pisan bequests to hospitals. Even as the number of legacies to hospitals declined, their share in the total value of pious bequests increased steadily from at least as early as the recurrence of the plague in 1362 through the opening decades of the Quattrocento. That share rose from 4 percent in the year of the Black Death to 6 percent on the plague's return. Then it nearly doubled (11 percent) in the years immediately following the plague, and nearly doubled again (21 percent) in the last decades of the Trecento. By the Quattrocento, the hospitals of Pisa, now almost exclusively accounted for by Santa Chiara, captured almost a quarter of all pious legacies (23 percent).

The only period when this portion was exceeded was the initial years of the Pisan documentation, from the twelfth century until 1325. Let us remember, however, that 88 percent of these testaments for that time bracket came from the notarial books of Santa Chiara. Even in the preceding period, when the value of gifts to hospitals had fallen to 6 percent of all pious values, more than half of the documents used in this study derived from Santa Chiara. If only those documents originating from sources other than Pisa's hospital are used, a different picture emerges. The period before 1326 appears not as the peak of hospital piety but as the period when testators gave their lowest share of their last gifts in terms of value to hospitals (2 percent). Nor did the picture then change significantly in the years leading to the Black Death; between 1326 and 1348, Pisans gave only 3 percent of their pious legacies to hospitals, even though they continued to give at least token amounts to numerous different hospitals in the city and territory of Pisa. Thus, the values of pious charities in Pisa plot a trend in marked contrast to the one described by the frequency of bequests. Instead of a flat line or even a decline in their sponsoring, the value of their pious legacies progresses from as low as 2 percent of the Pisans' portfolios of piety in the earliest surviving testaments to 25 percent by the last years of analysis. Here, the crucial turning point was not the Black Death of 1348 but instead the years immediately following the second outbreak of pestilence (for Pisa) in 1362.

The trend in endowing hospitals in Pisa as well as Florence and, to a slightly lesser extent, Siena may indeed underlie a general Tuscan advance toward a civic Christianity on the eve of the Quattrocento. It did not, however, result from a new flurry of hospital foundations after the Black Death, as Herlihy, Goldthwaite and Rearick, and Becker have assumed.[63] A different process was at work, one of centralization and monopolization of hospital services by institutions that had been founded earlier, in the thirteenth century, when the practice of drafting last wills and testaments begins to filter through the social ranks of these central Italian communes. The new monopolistic hospitals—Santa Maria della Scala in Siena, Santa Maria Nuova in Florence, and Santa Chiara in Pisa—gathered momentum in the mid-Trecento, gaining the appeal of those contemplating the afterlife while weeding out what had once been a wide array of small hospitals and hospices scattered throughout these late medieval city-states.

Does Arezzo fit this general pattern of hospital expansion? Again, the mere numbers of hospital legacies hardly show a shift in piety in the direction of funding hospitals. Beginning with the earliest years until 1325 (for Arezzo, the earliest testaments found for this study come only in 1305), the Aretines were already endowing their hospitals with 10 percent of their pious legacies, and the proportion reached its apex (15 percent) preceding the Black Death. Then, after dipping to 7 percent in the summer months of 1348, it rebounded to 10 percent and in the early years of the Quattrocento finished at 11 percent of all pious gifts.

Does the flatness of this line result from evidentiary problems similar to Pisa's? Did a single entity monopolizing hospital services mask a steady Aretine trend toward the increased patronage of hospitals in the testaments of ordinary townsmen and villagers? In Arezzo, as in Florence and Siena, my sample of last wills derives from a number of archive and various *diplomatico* collections assembled in the state archives by the late eighteenth-century Hapsburgs. But the problem of assessing changes in the complex of hospitals drawing legacies from the pious in Arezzo is of a different character: how to categorize one of the richest and most prominent of Aretine charities, the lay fraternity called the Misericordia?[64]

As already mentioned, the institutional line dividing ecclesiastical entities was not always a sharp one. Just as hospitals served at once to shelter pilgrims, distribute alms to the poor, and perform sacramental functions, as well as to care for the sick, religious lay confraternities often built and governed hospitals. Arezzo's Misericordia presents such a problem: do we categorize it as a lay confraternity or a hospital?

My answer was to take the documents at their word. If the testator gave property or money to the "Confraternity of the Misericordia," I tallied the bequest as a gift to a confraternity. If instead the bequest was directed to the "Hospital of the Misericordia," I considered it as a hospital legacy. In administering the pious property, little difference may have resulted from the notary's or testator's description. Nonetheless, most contributions to the Misericordia (84 percent) signaled it not as a hospital but as a lay confraternity.[65] This accounting, moreover, corresponds with its institutional history. From its origins, the Misericordia's principal objective was "attendance at the prayers [of the Dominicans], participation in processions and singing songs in honor of the Virgin . . . Charitable practices were entirely secondary at least until the second half of the [thirteenth] century," when the threat of heretical movements—the Cathars, Waldensians, and others—were in serious decline.[66]

Pious gifts to hospitals in Arezzo do not evince a rationalization and concentration of hospital services as found in the other three Tuscan cities. In no period did Aretine legacies to hospitals spread across so wide an array of independent entities as they did in Pisa, Siena, and Florence. Only 8 hospitals appear in the earliest testaments as compared with 28 different Pisan institutions during the same years. Nor did the number sharply diminish over time even after the recurrence of plague in 1363. For Arezzo, the number of these establishments instead rose to 14 in the last quarter of the Trecento and afterward held at 10 in the early Quattrocento.

In the years leading to the Black Death, no dominant or principal hospital emerged in Arezzo. Three hospitals shared in importance—the hospital of the Bishop (the Episcopatus), the "new" hospital of San Giovanni called the Oriente, and the hospital of Santa Maria called the Ponte, with the Misericordia a close fourth.[67] With the Black Death in 1348, the hospital of the Oriente emerged as the principal beneficiary of hospital legacies, absorbing nearly half of the total. Its dominance persisted through the summer months of the next strike of pestilence in 1363, when it garnered 55 percent of these gifts.[68] It maintained its lead through the third strike of pestilence in 1374. But then at the century's end, unlike Santa Maria della Scala, Santa Nuova, and Santa Chiara, which in these years made their most significant strides in dominating the last desires of the pious, the Oriente began losing ground, capturing less than a third of these bequests.[69] In the subsequent years, 1364–75, its share was indistinguishable from that of a number of other institutions of middling size—the hospital of the Annunciation, the Bishop's hospital, the Ponte, the hospital of Saint John the Baptist, the hospital of San Marco, and the Misericordia. In the first years of the Quattrocento, the new hospital of the Annunciation, with one-third of hospital bequests, was Arezzo's most successful hospital in terms of attracting last gifts,[70] followed by the Ponte; only two legacies went to the Oriente.

Even if all legacies to the renowned confraternity of the Misericordia are classified as gifts to a hospital, still no single hospital emerges as hegemonic. Nor do the percentages of legacies show a progressive concentration of bequests around a single hospital at the expense of an array of others. Combining all legacies to the Misericordia, regardless of how they were labeled, still presents a picture more of decline than of concentration and monopolization. The Misericordia so considered reached its highest concentration in the opening years of the Trecento, when it drew 56 percent of all pious bequests.[71] Then its portion shrank steadily to its low-water mark of one out every five bequests to hospitals at the end of the Trecento.[72] This secular trend was then reversed; the combined confraternity-hospital climbed back to 34 percent in the opening years of the Quattrocento[73]—a figure, however, in no way comparable to the concentration achieved by its neighbors Santa Maria della Scala, Santa Maria Nuova, and Santa Chiara. At the end of the Trecento and in the initial years of the Quattrocento, these Tuscan hospitals (as we have seen) were capturing between two-thirds and three-fourths of hospital legacies.

If no single principal hospital here emerges, do the values of pious legacies show, nonetheless, an increase in the wishes to sponsor hospitals? In the year of the Black Death, Aretines gave proportionally less to hospitals than at any other time (one percent of the values of all their pious bequests). In contrast, the return of pestilence in 1363 marked its high point (14 percent of all bequests). However, as it did in the other three Tuscan towns, 1363 did not mark a turning point in Arezzo. By the end of the century and into the fifteenth, the values of Aretine hospital bequests once again sank to their early Trecento levels of only 2 percent of their last charities.

Was Arezzo the exception in its endowment of hospitals, or does it suggest an eastern trend that might relate to developments in Umbria? At first glance, the frequencies of pious choices in the Umbrian towns trace a pattern not unlike that found in Siena, Pisa, and Florence. In the capital of Umbria, the endowment of hospitals reached its apex in the years preceding the Black Death, when one in every four pious legacies went to these institutions and remained roughly the same during the catastrophic summer months of 1348.[74] Once the horrific levels of mortality had subsided, piety expressed through hospital bequests plummeted; hospitals received their smallest share over the long period of this study, capturing only 3 percent of all pious gifts. In the last years of the Trecento, the proportion rose slightly, to 6 percent of pious bequests, where it remained fixed to the end of my analysis, with Perugia's hospitals at the beginning of the Quattrocento receiving under half the number of legacies they had captured at the beginning of the Trecento.

Although over time these hospitals received a smaller share of pious bequests (8 percent) than those in Siena and Pisa, the decline in the number of bequests to Perugian hospitals was not markedly different from that for Pisa and Siena. But in the Tuscan towns, while the number of bequests slid, their values rose. Did the same happen in Perugia? Or does Perugia appears similar to its western neighbor, Arezzo? A glance at historic maps of Perugia[75] or through the archival collections originally preserved by Perugian ecclesiastical institutions immediately suggests that the principal hospital of the city was its Misericordia, which first appears in a document of 1296.[76] In the earliest documents until 1325, this institution did dominate the hospital charities of testating Perugini: it drew 57 percent of their hospital legacies.[77] In the period preceding the Black Death, however, it fell as the most important of hospital beneficiaries.[78] The lepers' hospital on the edge of town received nearly twice as many last gifts, and various hospitals in the countryside together received almost four times as many. In the year of the Black Death, the Misericordia garnered a quarter of all such bequests; yet hospitals outside the city proper captured a greater share. Only in the last years of the Trecento did it again predominate, capturing nearly one in every three last gifts to hospitals.[79] It had not succeeded, however, as had the principal hospitals of Siena, Florence, and Pisa, in swallowing up its smaller rivals. In the last quarter of the Trecento, 18 different hospitals appeared in the ledgers of itemized gifts, 10 of them city institutions. The guild hospitals of the notaries, the druggists, and the wool merchants, as well as the merchants' hospital, all appeared in these years more than once. Only in the opening years of the Quattrocento (when hospitals

collectively received a meager 6 percent of all pious bequests) did the
Misericordia emerge hegemonic, cornering half of all hospital gifts.[80]
This time, however, only two other city hospitals received more than
two gifts—the hospital of Saint Jacob and the notaries' hospital.

Were these years a harbinger of later developments of the fifteenth
century? Was the concentration and monopolization of hospital space
in the city simply a half- or quarter-century behind the pace set by the
Tuscan cities of the west? Only another longitudinal study of piety,
running the course of the Quattrocento, could resolve these questions.
The administrative history of this institution,[81] along with data from the
available prices of pious bequests, however, does not suggest such a
recovery and subsequent monopolization of services in Perugia. Instead,
the values of these legacies roughly followed the lines sketched by hospital
bequests in Arezzo. The portion to hospitals measured by the available
prices peaked for Perugia in the years preceding the Black Death, when
testators endowed these institutions with over one-third of their last
monies. The portion tumbled to 8 percent in 1348 and then failed to
recover. By the end of this century of repeated pestilence, hospitals
attracted the same meager proportions in Perugia as in Arezzo: 2 percent
of all testamentary pious values. This figure, moreover, did not rise above
4 percent with the Quattrocento.

When we move east to Assisi, the importance of hospitals falls still
farther. Only in the days from the earliest documentation to the beginning of the Trecento did the proportions of bequests to hospitals
resemble the patterns found for the other cities. For these periods, the
Assisan hospitals attracted more than 10 percent of testators' pious
investments. In the Trecento these proportions sank, recovering only
momentarily following the Black Death. After the second onslaught of
pestilence, hospitals here managed to attract only negligible numbers of
pious bequests. By the beginning of the Quattrocento, a pious donation
to a hospital proved a rare act of ultimate charity; less than one percent
of pious legacies in the heartland of Saint Francis sponsored the poor
and the sick in hospitals. Only the periods before 1326 present an array
of hospitals from which it is meaningful to assess the importance of a
single institution. In these years, 12 different entities appear; the Communal Hospital of Assisi, founded in 1267,[82] was the most popular, with
37 percent of the donations, followed closely by the lepers' hospital of
Saint Lazarus. In the years preceding the Black Death, only two hospitals
appear in these documents: the Communal Hospital received seven of
eight pious last gifts, the other going to the Hospital of the Germans

(*hospitale Teutonicorum*), located in the Porta Sancti Francisci.[83] But after 1363, the Communal Hospital disappeared from the voluntary itemized lists of bequests, surviving only in the initial formula that mandated all those from the city and *contado* to grant them a canonical 5 or 10 soldi. In value, the contributions to hospitals in Assisi were even more paltry. From the earliest documents to 1325, its hospitals probably reached their high point of pious bequests, which amounted to a meager 3 percent.[84] After the second onslaught of plague, they received less than a percentile of the pious wealth, reaching a negligible one percent only in the Quattrocento.

Assisani gave far less (relative to their other pious legacies) to hospitals than did the residents of any other place studied in this survey. Over time, only 6 percent of their bequests went to hospitals as against 16 percent in Pisa. Measured in values, barely one percent of pious monies in Assisi sponsored institutions for alleviating earthly suffering, while Florentines, after the recurrence of plague in 1363, handed over 40 percent of their itemized last pious monies to them, three-fourths of which went to a single institution. Part of the explanation for hospitals' much lower attraction in Assisi may have been the remarkable Sacro Convento's pull on the souls of this Franciscan city. Indeed, the Mother Church possessed its own infirmary, and on occasion testators earmarked their last pious properties for the friary hospital. To what extent this hospital cared for the lay public of Assisi must await another study. Part of the reason for the decline in the support of hospitals may have lain with communal law, which in the early Trecento appears to have required testators to contribute their canonical portion to the Communal Hospital.[85] A similar legal imposition placed on the Sienese did not, though, inhibit their zeal to sponsor their city's principal hospital.

Hospital Foundations

The growth in importance of hospitals in the three principal cities of Tuscany did not arise from a proliferation of hospitals or from new foundations after the Black Death, as the historiography now suggests.[86] In fact, a search through the documents specifically for hospital foundations may well lead to incorrect perceptions of changes in the importance of hospital sponsorship. Except in Pisa, where only one hospital in this sample was founded after 1348,[87] few foundation charters antedated the Black Death; most came after the plague returned in 1363. Moreover, vast donations to support grandiose construction projects were not the norm in these documents, especially before the recurrence of plague. Clearly exceptional was the Tolomei bequest of numerous landed estates in the Sienese district of Rapolano to the hospital of Santa Maria della Scala, the 1299 bequest of another member of the Tolomei nobility to finance the building and maintenance of four separate hospitals,[88] and even the more obscure and certainly more modest bequest by the rich villager Barone from Buti of his residual estate to found four hospitals, one in the city of Pisa, the others in country villages.[89] Other foundations give the impression that the new institutions dotting the ecclesiastical landscape of late Trecento Tuscany and Umbria were of meager proportions, sponsored by donors of middling levels of wealth. Thus, in the year following the plague of 1374, a Florentine widow, domina Filippa, the daughter of Iacobus di Ser Cambio, directed her heir to sell just two strips of land to finance the "building and construction" of a hospital in the piazza Santa Croce or next to that piazza or in the street called "la via della Vuiola" within two months or else her estate would devolve to the hospital of Santa Maria Nuova.[90] Even more modestly, in 1383 Michelis f.q. Nuti, from the village of Castelnuovo in the Valdarno, left his house to be built into a hospital for "osspitando pauperes Christi" together with "his entire bed and its furnishings."[91] When those from the old Florentine lineages founded hospitals, their constructions were still on a modest scale. In her Black Death testament of 1348, the widow Caterina, a daughter of the ancient Cavalcanti lineage, ordered her executor, who was her parish priest in Sant'Ambrogio, to sell off her "big household goods" (*masseritias grossas*) to pay for the conversion of her house into a hospital for the poor; at the same time the bulk of her estate was to be sold off and "converted into underwear, sheets, blankets and other necessities for the poor" housed in the principal hospital of Florence, Santa Maria Nuova, and to the society of the Misericordia in the *contado* of Florence.[92]

In Arezzo, only one hospital foundation antedated the plague of 1363.[93] The later foundations came from small endowments like those for late Trecento Florence. Typically, one Johannellus Landi, from the village of Chiani, in 1424 gave two "newly constructed" huts (*domunculas*) next to the public road "for the use of a hospital . . . in which the poor of Christ were continually to be cared for."[94] In the testaments from Perugia, the earliest hospital foundation was a contingent one redacted in 1361, when Conte Cecchioli Conti left his estate, if both his sons died, to build a hospital "for feeding, clothing and governing the poor who will live and be cared for in this hospital."[95] The dimensions of such new foundations were specified more precisely in the 1389 testament of another widow, Andrea Gioli Gectarelli, who gave one of her houses in the village of Pilonico for the construction of a hospital. "On the ground floor" were to be placed two beds "well furnished with mattresses, pillows, settees, all of large size . . . for the use of the poor and for their comfort." Naming the hospital *lospedale de Sancte Maria de Monte Morcini,* she placed it in the care (*bona custodia*) of the prior and friars of the Olivetani monastery of Monte Morcino, who were to elect a *hospitalerius* of "honest and good ways, faithful before God to care for the poor . . . suitable for governing this hospital faithfully day and night."[96] Similarly, a Pisan donor, Augustinus f.q. Vanni Fecivi, in 1374 provided that, if his son died before reaching the age of 20, his residual estate was to support the building of a "good and sufficient hospital with four furnished beds for the care of the poor of Jesus Christ."[97]   Hospitals in the modern sense, places to tend to the infirm or house the poor, were not the only foundations that went under the rubric of hospital. In 1327 the Pisan widow Cingha left a third part of her home and two strips of land with a house to build a "house or place" for giving hospitality to a special rank of priests (*sacerdotes forenses*)[98] and for their services (*opus*).[99] Fifteen years later, a canon of the Pisan church, San Lorenzo in Chinzica, specified at the outset of his will that "in the hospital built and constructed by me a *hospitalitus* and a rector of the rank of 'Sacerdos' must always celebrate mass and rule and govern this hospital for wandering priests [*sacerdotes peregrinantes*]."[100]

Only rarely did these laconic testamentary foundations stipulate what bodies would govern and oversee these hospitals, if and when they materialized. We have already seen that at least one testator settled the future status and rule of a foundation—the Perugian widow Andrea, who placed her two-bed hospital under the governance of the Olivetan monastery at Monte Morcino. In the other cases in point, founders of hospitals looked to "the rule and protection" of larger and older hospitals. In 1390 another Perugian, Ranaldutius f.q. Domenici Rinaldi, ordered his executors, after the death of his sister, to build a hospital on his property in the district of nearby Corciano and specified that its "care, protection, and management" be given to the bankers' guild (which ran one of the principal hospitals in the city of Perugia).[101] The choice of governor for a contingent hospital foundation by Pierozius f.q. Ser Federigi of Arezzo was more extraordinary. In his Black Death will of June 1374, he left his rich estate to the Misericordia with numerous conditions; if not met, it would go to Siena's Santa Maria della Scala, provided that the latter build within one year and then govern a hospital in the city of Arezzo to be named Santa Maria della Scala.[102]

In Assisi, where hospitals were weakest as pious beneficiaries, the documents contain two foundations that specified the religious organization that was to govern the new institution, once constructed. Both come from the year 1362 and from the archives of the flagellant confraternity of Santo Stefano. Iacobus f.q. Vanni, called Zuccha, from the porta San Francesco, left a portion of his estate to construct "a certain hospital for sustaining the poor of Christ, pilgrims and the infirm" to be called *"lospedale della pietate"* and to be placed under the "university or college" of the confraternity of *disciplinati*, Santo Stefano.[103] Maragoncellus f.q. Andrutii Ciccarelli Maragonis left his residuary estate to this same society on the condition that the fraternity convert his residence in the porta Perlaxi into a hospital to be named "Maragonis" after him; it was to care for the poor of Christ and "miserabilis persone." Its "protection, governance and control" were given "to the men of this fraternity."[104] To repeat, the smattering of hospital foundations that can be dredged from a survey of thousands of testaments gives an impression that runs counter to the much more massive evidence provided by thousands of individual legacies. The number of hospitals in central Italy was rapidly declining at the moment (ca. 1362-63) that we witness the appearance of these few new foundations of modest dimensions and which, unlike the great foundations of the thirteenth century, most likely experienced low rates of survival.

In conclusion, last gifts to hospitals in these six cities do not plot a general evolution toward civic Christianity. The farther east we look, the less important the hospital appears, especially after the Black Death and into the Quattrocento. Was Umbria simply locked into another system of piety after the Black Death, one that deviated from a Tuscan civic Christianity? Let us now turn to that other pillar of lay involvement with the social as well as spiritual well-being of the present world— the religious confraternity—to see if it supports the geographical pattern traced by the donations to hospitals.

Religious Confraternities

These organizations assembled lay brethren as diverse in composition as magnates and artisan-workers of the wool industry in what Ronald Weissman has described as modules for governmental education.[105] Be-

yond the lessons of scrutinies and other electoral procedures and experience in governing small organizations, members of these lay groups
practiced new forms of devotion, whose roots can be traced to the low
Middle Ages but which began to sweep through central and northern
Italy as early as the 1260 flagellant movements. While citywide confraternities may have characterized the earliest of these groups in places
such as Borgo San Sepolcro and Arezzo, by the Trecento they can be
divided into two basic categories—the *laudesi,* who sang the praises of
the Lord, and, perhaps slightly later, the *disciplinati,* [106] who re-created
the suffering of Christ by communal and processional whipping. [107] Both
types (although they might include priests who could perform the mass)
extended the lay religious experience beyond a passive reception of
liturgy and devotion coming through the church hierarchy from the
pope and bishops down to the flocks in village and neighborhood parishes.
Both, moreover, brought their memberships into direct action in assuaging immediate problems of the social world created by the late
medieval expansion in population and growth of commerce—poverty,
criminality, the homeless, and unwed, unattached impoverished girls. [108]

Lay societies, whether flagellant or *laudesi,* did not appear in Sienese
bequests until the beginning of the Trecento. In Pisa, Assisi, and Florence,
earlier donations to these societies seep into the surviving testaments.
In fact, Assisani, who sponsored hospitals the least, provided many of
the earliest legacies to religious confraternities. In 1267, a domina Becta
gave one of the first found for all six towns: 10 soldi to the *fraternitas
clericorum.* [109] This society of clergymen appeared as a beneficiary of small
monetary sums ranging from 5 to 40 soldi in another nine testaments
between 1267 and 1286. [110]

The very earliest gifts to a lay religious society came, however, from
a Florentine testator in the year following the flagellant movement of
1260: one *Magister* Salvio, from Laburella but residing in the parish of
Santa Maria Novella, gave 20 soldi to the Company of the Bigallo, [111]
located across from the baptistry. [112] Before 1301, Florentines left another
15 bequests to such groups: three to the Company of Orsanmichele; [113]
two to the company called the *mediocri* of Santa Maria della Croce, who
congregated in the church of San Simone near the piazza of Santa Croce;
one to the Bigallo; one to the Company of Santa Maria Novella; one to
a society called the Maioris; one to the *disciplinati* who congregated in
the Augustinian friary; one to the Company of Santa Maria dei Servi;
one to the Company of San Niccolò; and two to companies in the

countryside—the Society of the Blessed Mary in Mezzano (near Impruneta) and the Society of the Blessed Mary in the *plebis* of Santa Maria
Impruneta.[114]

In Pisa, six legacies went to four societies before 1301—the fraternity
of priests, the fraternity of Saint Francis, the parish fraternity of Santa
Lucia de Ricucchio, and a society of priests in the Val di Serchio. In
Arezzo, where none of the testaments for this sample antedate 1305,
the religious confraternity was already at the outset of this documentation
a significant beneficiary, suggesting that it perhaps had played a rich part
in the spiritual lives of the Aretines back into the Duecento.[115] In fact,
the earliest testament found in this sample conveyed a gift to a lay
society—two giant candles (*torchios*) weighing 24 pounds to the fraternity
of the Misericordia.[116] In the first 20 years of Aretine testaments, 11
percent of all pious bequests sponsored religious confraternities, 69
bequests to 10 different societies. Although most went to the famous
Misericordia (38),[117] other societies, such as the confraternity of priests,
the *laudesi* of Saint Augustine, the *laudesi* of San Domenico, and the
laudesi of Saint Francis received multiple gifts. In addition, five Aretine
testators gave vague blanket bequests of as little as 12 pennies to each
of the *laudesi* societies in the city and territory, suggesting that too many
of them may have been scattered through the district for the notary to
bother enumerating.[118]

Ordinary testators' bequests to religious confraternities do not rein-
force the picture of social responsibility and piety formed by the legacies
to hospitals. An east/west Tuscan versus Umbrian development of piety
no longer holds. Confraternities in Assisi, where hospitals were weakest,
attracted 6 percent of all pious gifts over time, which ranked Assisi third
of these six towns. Curiously, these societies fared about the same in
Perugia, which spurred the flagellant movement in the 1260s[119]—5 percent of all pious gifts. Most popular of the Assisan societies were the
fraternity of clerics (19 legacies), followed by the Society of the Rosary
(9), the fraternity of Saint Anthony (8), and the fraternity of Saint Francis
(8). In Perugia the Dominican flagellants led the list (20), followed by the
disciplinati of St. Peter, the Abbot (16), and the *disciplinati* of Saint Anthony,
who maintained a confraternal hospital (15). Over the course of these
records, 22 separate urban societies appear, and 20 legacies endowed
confraternities in the countryside.

In contrast, bequests to confraternities generally remained low in
those towns where bequests to hospitals were numerous. Sienese lay
societies received less than 3 percent of all pious gifts. In Pisa, where

more bequests went to hospitals than in any other city, the confraternity fared the worst, gathering a negligible one percent of all last gifts. In the easternmost region of Tuscany, Arezzo and its *contado,* where the limited support for hospitals suggested an Umbrian mode of pious behavior, confraternities were more important than in any other city, attracting almost double the legacies found elsewhere: 14 percent of all Aretine charitable bequests endowed these new devotional societies. To be sure, the renowned Misericordia (called the *Laici*) accounted early on for a large portion of these bequests: nearly half of them (270 legacies) supported this citywide super-confraternity.[120] But even if these gifts are wholly discounted, Arezzo still emerges as the mecca of confraternities among the six cities. Thirty different devotional societies for the city alone sprinkle these lists of pious legacies. After the Misericordia, the most popular was the society of clerics (30 bequests), followed by the *disciplinati* of Santa Trinità (24), the *laudesi* of San Domenico (27), the *laudesi* of Sant'Agostino (22), the Franciscan *laudesi* (21), and the *disciplinati* of Santa Maria Annunciata (21). In addition, the Aretines bequeathed 46 gifts to numerous societies in the countryside. In contrast, only one confraternity in Pisa drew more than 20 legacies over the time span of this study—the confraternity of clergymen (21 gifts)—and only nine urban brotherhoods appear in Pisan documents, even though Pisan pious legacies outnumbered Aretine by one-and-one-half times.

These trends for the six cities do not, however, consistently chart a negative correlation between devotion to the hospital and to the confraternity. Florence, which gave most lavishly to hospitals in terms of the values of legacies, at the same time sponsored a rich confraternal life, surpassed only by Arezzo's. Eight percent of all pious gifts in Florence ended in the coffers of these societies. The most popular by far was the Company of Orsanmichele (84 legacies), which often served in Florentine testaments as the heir of last recourse, laden with the responsibilities of seeing to it that the front-line heirs, whether secular or religious, kept to the terms of the testament.[121] Next in popularity came the company of San Domenico at Santa Maria Novella[122] (53) and then, running a distant third, one of the oldest and most venerable companies of the city, Santa Maria Bigallo (15). The appearance of several new societies in the Quattrocento suggests a vitality in Florentine confraternal life not so easily measured by the frequency of pious bequests. The society of San Paolo, attached to the artisan parish of the same name; a new fraternity of clergy; and the society of St. Peter the Martyr, attached to the Dominicans, appeared in these testaments after the turn of the century and immediately began to attract multiple bequests.

Unlike the endowment of hospitals, which followed a rough east/ west contrast in their popularity among cities, the importance of confraternities only adds to the enigma already presented by the tallying of pious bequests. Instead of a monolithic move toward pious recipients that would reflect a new Renaissance ethos, a negative correlation better describes the popularity of those two institutions that provided services for the poor and infirm. Generally, where hospitals were strong (Pisa and Siena), confraternities remained weak, and where confraternal organizations were strong (Arezzo, Assisi, and Perugia), contributions to hospitals were weak or even negligible. Florence was the exception. Moreover, a rough negative correlation between the confraternity and the hospital can be seen in chronological terms. For instance, in the earliest testaments of Assisi, the hospital started at its highest level of success (13 percent of pious bequests), while the confraternity embarked at its lowest (0.02 percent). By the end of the Trecento, the relationship was the opposite: hospitals barely accrued one percent, while contributions to the religious societies constituted 14 percent.

Such a negative correlation perhaps should not come as a surprise. After all, confraternities and hospitals competed for many of the same services. Often companies such as the society of San Paolo in Florence ran their own hospitals or supervised them. For example, the Bigallo supervised as many as nine hospitals by 1400.[123] Nor was this pattern unique to Florence. In Perugia the *disciplinati* of San Giuliano, the *disciplinati* of Sant'Antonio, and the *disciplinati* of San Francesco ran hospitals, and, perhaps most important, the *laici* of Arezzo administered what appears to have been at various times Arezzo's largest hospital.

Could this correlation, then, be a trick of the documentation, resulting from the fact that certain confraternities, at least according to their statutes, forbade their members to accept pious legacies? Such restrictions, if in fact they had continued to be rigorously carried out over the course of my documentation,[124] would bias the trends in just the opposite direction. As James Banker has shown for Borgo San Sepolcro[125] and John Henderson for Florence,[126] after the Black Death, these religious companies increasingly turned for their support, not to the membership fees of their brethren at large, but to a more selective dependence on testamentary legacies from those of middling or greater wealth.

Finally, the confraternities' popularity does not show a clear change in the direction of piety over the course of the Trecento. With the possible exception of Assisi, no rush or gradual transition to civic Christianity emerges from the endowment of these societies. True, in all of these towns except Arezzo, contributions to confraternal life were rare before the 1320s. But, for several of these towns (Arezzo, Florence, Perugia), confraternal popularity peaked in the years immediately preceding the Black Death of 1348 or in those summer months.[127] Afterward, testamentary support either leveled off or declined.[128]

The "Poor of Christ," Dowries, and Servants

As I argued earlier, both handouts of grain to the *pauperes Christi*[129] and dowry funds to poor girls of *buon costume* addressed social problems of the here and now.[130] But the two constituted different approaches to the problem of poor relief. The first, gifts of grain, bread, clothing, or pennies for mourning at the testator's graveside, was a makeshift, one-time solution, more suitable for assuaging the benefactor's conscience than for alleviating the suffering of the poor and infirm. As far as the documents show, testators indiscriminately gave paltry sums to the poor. The funding of dowries for poor girls, by contrast, was neither makeshift nor indiscriminate; instead, the testator's executors, spouse, relatives, or confraternity would scrutinize and then "elect" usually no more than two or three poor girls of *buon costume*. The gift, moreover, buttressed the principal lifetime insurance policy for women of the late medieval and early modern periods—the dowry.[131]

In Siena, the most convincing shift in the choices of piety over six centuries of testaments came in the perception of poor relief. Before the recurrence of pestilence in 1363, dowry funds were rare; handouts to the poor were the principal form of charity that lay outside those institutional channels controlled by parishes, mendicants, hospitals, and confraternities. By the beginning of the Quattrocento, the relationship between these two largely noninstitutionalized forms of charity had reversed. Dowries to poor girls superseded the handouts to the "poor of Christ." And pious legacies never returned to the earlier Trecento pattern; instead, the gap between the two widened through the fifteenth and sixteenth centuries.

Was this pattern peculiar to Siena, or did it constitute a general shift in attitudes toward the poor through large areas of central Italy? As a proportion of all pious bequests, handouts to the poor of Christ were highest in Siena, averaging more than 10 percent from the earliest testaments until 1425. Only Pisa and Perugia approached these proportions (8 percent each). In the other cities these bequests figured less, comprising in Florence only half the Sienese rate and in Assisi only 3 percent of pious bequests. (See table 2.) Nonetheless, the relationship between the two shows that Sienese testators were not acting in isolation. For most of Tuscany and Umbria, the dowry fund was simply not an operative conception for charity in the earliest documents through the opening decades of the Trecento. Here, Siena's development did not lag noticeably behind the others. Few of these dowry funds founded elsewhere antedated the first appearance in the Sienese documents (1318). And of those that did, few took the later form, a foundation to dower a select number of poor virgins.

The earliest dowry fund for these documents comes from Florence. In 1279, the wealthy citizen Saverinus f.q. Iacobi gave 100 lire "to marry and lead into wedlock poor women from the city and *contado* of Florence." This fund, however, bears the traces of the handouts to numerous mouths of the poor of Christ. Instead of providing the entire dowry or a substantial portion of it to a few carefully selected girls, it distributed small funds to numerous women. Saverinus instructed his *fideicommissarii* to give each woman 40 soldi "or no more than 60 soldi" apiece (in fact, notarized dowries were never that small), which would have meant that his fund would have bestowed paltry dowries on from 33 to 50 women.[132] In Pisa, only two pious dowries predated 1318. The first was again hardly a fund in the post–Black Death sense. In 1300, the parish priest of San Desiderio conveyed bedding to one girl upon her marriage.[133] For Perugia, the earliest pious dowry does not originate until 1333, when domina Fina from the village (*castro*) of Monte Fontigiano left 20 lire to marry off an unspecified number of "poor virgin women."[134] And for Arezzo no dowry appears before 1329, when a Ducius f.q. Iacopi left 300 lire both to dress the poor and to provide for the marriage of an unspecified number of poor virgins.[135]

As in Siena, dowry funds were nonexistent or negligible elsewhere until after the recurrence of plague. Only in Perugia did they shoot above 2 percent of all pious bequests in the interval between the first and second plagues. But, after 1363, the percentages of indiscriminate legacies doled out to the poor and of dowry funds began to converge. While pious dowries mounted, legacies to the poor in Florence, Perugia, Assisi, and Pisa reached or approached their highest levels in the period between the plagues; 1362/63 was the turning point. In the last decades of the Trecento, the dowry funds in Florence equaled the number of bequests to the poor, then doubled them in the first years of the Quattrocento. Elsewhere, the shift was not as dramatic; in each of the five towns, however, by the end of the Trecento or the beginning of the Quattrocento, either the forms of poor relief equaled each other for the first time or the dowry funds surpassed the old manner of handouts.[136]

When values are compared for these two forms of social charity, the relative importance of the dowry fund at the end of the Trecento becomes more pronounced. (See table 4.) In Pisa, dowry funds climbed from one-tenth in the interval between the first plagues to double the amount doled out to the poor by the end of the Trecento. In Arezzo, the value of dowry funds exceeded that of handouts to the poor as early as 1348, increasing by the early Quattrocento from two-and-a-half to nearly six times the sums given in bread, clothing, and pennies to the poor. In Perugia, the dowry fund jumped for the same period from a negligible fraction of the gifts to the poor of Christ to almost four times these more traditional means of poor relief. In Assisi, the ratio of dowry values to handouts reversed from about one to ten to nearly five to one by the end of the Trecento. But in Florence, the shift was the most spectacular: legacies to dower poor virgins rose from 0.05 percent of the value of the old dole in 1348 to more than 25 times its value by the early fifteenth century.

A General Assessment

Do the pious choices of ordinary townsmen and villagers confirm recent conclusions about cultural change and piety in the early Renaissance— that there was a turn from the old ascetic forms of devotion and penance toward an interest in resolving social problems of the present, temporal realm? In short, the patterns of piety underpinning the thousands of individual charitable decisions made in these testaments do not show a simple or decisive switch in devotion at the beginning of the Trecento, after the famines of the 1320s, following the Black Death of 1348, or at the opening of the Quattrocento. For one thing, the categories of charity do not divide so easily into two clear directions of cultural choice: the old asceticism or the new social charity. While contributions to nunneries declined through the Trecento in all these societies, the traditional Benedictine monasteries and the parish held their ground. More fundamentally, the mendicant orders founded in the early Duecento generally increased their hold over the souls in each of these six cities through the Trecento and into the early Renaissance. But on which side of the fence should the mendicants be placed? The examples set by the mendicant saints and blessed ones certainly stressed the ascetic life, self-

Table 4.
The Values for Poor Relief

	No. Pious Bequests to "Poor of Christ"	No. Bequests Monetized	Average Price of Bequests (Florins)	Hypothesized Amount of Bequests to Poor (Florins)	No. of all Dowry Bequests	Hypothesized Amount of All Dowry Bequests (Florins)	Ratio of Values of Dowry Bequests to Bequests to Poor
AREZZO							
< 1276							
1275–1300							
1301–25	19	12	12.81	243.39	0	0.00	0.00
1326–47	31	19	51.07	1,583.17	0	0.00	0.00
1348	42	23	11.46	481.32	1	1,240.00	2.58
1349–62	11	5	9.90	108.90	0	0.00	0.00
1363	15	7	12.47	187.05	2	462.00	2.47
1364–75	2	15	12.99	25.98	8	172.64	6.65
1376–1400	30	14	9.82	294.60	8	1,205.05	4.09
1401–25	10	3	6.25	62.50	10	357.50	5.72
ASSISI							
< 1276	6	2	3.85	23.10	0	0.00	0.00
1275–1300	13	7	48.86	635.18	0	0.00	0.00
1301–25	6	4	21.70	130.20	0	0.00	0.00
1326–47	6	3	106.95	641.70	0	0.00	0.00
1348	5	1	106.95	534.75	2	69.76	0.13
1349–62	4	2	8.06	32.24	3	116.25	3.61
1363							
1364–75	0	0	0.00	0.00	1	10.00	0.00
1376–1400	5	1	9.00	45.00	6	212.52	4.72
1401–25	2	1	8.00	16.00	1	0.00	0.00
FLORENCE							
< 1276	1	1	0.17	0.17	0	0.00	0.00
1275–1300	18	10	68.37	1,230.66	0	0.00	0.00
1301–25	24	12	40.52	972.48	0	0.00	0.00
1326–47	23	17	3.55	81.65	0	0.00	0.00
1348	28	19	148.23	4,150.44	1	200.00	0.05
1349–62	15	9	118.04	1,770.60	0	0.00	0.00
1363	24	16	42.32	1,015.68	3	525.00	0.52
1364–75	19	10	37.71	716.49	8	257.68	0.36
1376–1400	15	9	56.58	848.70	16	591.04	0.70
1401–25	11	2	19.80	217.80	20	5,540.40	25.44
PERUGIA							
< 1276							
1275–1300	2	1	216.00	432.00	0	0.00	0.00
1301–25	2	2	0.66	1.32	0	0.00	0.00
1326–47	29	20	12.29	356.41	0	0.00	0.00
1348	30	13	12.07	362.10	6	5.64	0.02
1349–62	11	7	38.99	428.89	3	395.25	0.92
1363	14	4	18.18	254.52	3	46.50	0.18

Table 4.
Continued

	No. Pious Bequests to "Poor of Christ"	No. Bequests Monetized	Average Price of Bequests (Florins)	Hypothesized Amount of Bequests to Poor (Florins)	No. of all Dowry Bequests	Hypothesized Amount of All Dowry Bequests (Florins)	Ratio of Values of Dowry Bequests to Bequests to Poor
PERUGIA *Continued*							
1364–75	19	10	24.21	459.99	6	237.12	0.52
1376–99	62	25	25.50	1,581.00	49	3,874.92	2.45
1400–1425	12	4	37.58	450.96	12	1,756.56	3.90
PISA							
< 1276	12	9	1.56	18.72	0	0.00	0.00
1275–1300	47	38	21.31	1,001.57	0	0.00	0.00
1301–25	230	156	11.57	2,661.10	0	0.00	0.00
1326–47	86	59	26.27	2,259.22	0	0.00	0.00
1348	11	5	13.46	148.06	2	38.76	0.26
1349–61	40	26	136.64	5,465.60	6	688.20	0.13
1362	38	23	29.36	1,115.68	7	254.94	0.23
1363–75	13	11	39.49	513.37	6	76.80	0.15
1376–1400	27	15	29.09	785.43	25	1,619.75	2.06
1401–25	6	4	21.00	126.00	4	70.00	0.56
SIENA							
< 1276	25	14	8.87	221.75	0	0.00	0.00
1275–1300	50	31	144.28	7,214.00	0	0.00	0.00
1301–25	67	40	7.76	519.92	1	0.00	0.00
1326–47	55	33	20.72	1,139.60	1	9.30	0.01
1348	49	24	12.17	596.33	2	186.00	0.31
1349–62	25	20	39.17	979.25	1	6.20	0.01
1363	6	4	3.69	22.14	0	0.00	0.00
1364–75	9	4	31.00	279.00	2	0.00	0.00
1376–1400	23	14	41.19	947.37	11	595.32	0.63
1401–25	14	10	24.22	339.08	18	1,016.28	3.00

denial, and even athletic feats of self-inflicted humiliation.[137] On the other hand, these orders worked directly with the social problems of poverty and human misery in these evolving commercial centers.

For another thing, these cities show no unanimity over time. The differences become no clearer when the other side of piety is examined: last gifts to hospitals, religious confraternities, and the poor. In Siena,

Pisa, and Florence, bequests to hospitals, at least when measured by their values, increased in importance, particularly in the decades preceding the Black Death. These increases arose, however, not from the foundation of a plethora of new establishments, as historians have assumed, but rather from the consolidation of services by earlier established institutions, which, through governmental intervention, succeeded in rationalizing hospital space that had structured such social services in the early communes of the late Middle Ages. This process of monopolization was not an automatic consequence of demographic decline or a consequence of financial disasters following in the wake of the Black Death. The process was set in motion earlier, and it was not universal across the backdrop of plague and population devastation. Here, an east/west division holds. The monopolistic hospital did not emerge in Arezzo, Perugia, or Assisi after the Black Death; in all three cities, contributions to hospitals even declined in the later years of the Trecento.

But that other pillar of early Renaissance spirituality—the religious confraternity—does not corroborate the trends set by the growth of the hospital in the direction of a this-worldly or Renaissance form of piety. Again, the confraternity was a mixed bag of spirituality. It offered solace to the suffering and active engagement for its membership in religious devotion, as well as civic charity in assisting prisoners and those condemned to the gallows, help in confraternal hospitals, and aid to poor virgins. Further, while the confraternity was weak and even nonexistent in the early documentation for all these city-states except Arezzo, cities with strong hospitals did not necessarily support a rich confraternal life or vice versa, at least insofar as the testamentary evidence shows. In fact, the opposite relationship held more often. With the exception of Florence, confraternities and hospitals, instead of representing a unified cultural direction, appear more as competitors for the same social services.

Charity to the poor again creates problems in categorization. While offering aid and solace to the poor and infirm, indiscriminate handouts of bread, clothing, and pennies were in and of themselves acts of devotion not necessarily gauged to change the social realities of suffering and poverty. On the other hand, in all these societies, after the Black Death and especially in the last years of my analysis, another form of poor relief grew at the expense of the old dole—the dowry fund. These bequests were not indiscriminate, one-shot affairs. Instead, by carefully selecting a few poor girls, testators provided the most basic form of social welfare for women over the course of a lifetime. While in all these societies the dowry fund either reached parity with or surpassed the older forms of poor relief, Florence once again proved exceptional by the magnitude of its change; here, dowry funds measured by their values exceeded the momentary handouts by 25 times in the first years of the Quattrocento. Thus, the 21,351 pious bequests studied from these six city-states might corroborate a conception of the Renaissance that is often assumed, even if recently rarely stated in bold letters, and never before argued with systematic comparative support: namely, the exceptional social, political, and cultural development of Florence in the early Renaissance. But, as the beginning of this general assessment stresses, the split in pious choices represented by monasteries, parishes, hospitals, confraternities, and poor relief is questionable, and even by these standards the cultural direction of Florence in the late Trecento and early Quattrocento does not appear to have been all of one piece.

3

The Structure of Pious Bequests

O how stupid and miserable are the men of this world, who risk penalties without end for the slightest earthly delight!

Pride is odious to God and to men; from the very beginning of the world pride was infinitely hateful to God; and He dispised nothing more than the uplifted head. After sin, one must humiliate oneself.

— Jacopo Passavanti, *Specchio della vera penitenzia*

For this reason, it is said that the Christian is humility personified. And as such it is something for which our lord and master Christ has forbidden us any love of the world, and of things which can be lost; and sadness comes from just such love; if adversity is born to him of a thing for which he grieves too much, it is a sign that he loves that thing; and thus he is not a Christian but instead too worldly.

— Domenico Cavalca, "Brani sulla Pazienza"

he quantification of pious choices fails to show a decisive post–Black Death or early Quattrocento shift from the ascetic world of penance and monastic piety toward a "civic Christianity" grounded in a this-worldly ethic of social charity. Bequests to hospitals and religious confraternities did not rise in tandem, which would have reflected a new Renaissance direction of piety. Instead, except in Florence, the two were in competition. And even in Florence, the increase in bequests to hospitals and confraternities, as well as their values, did not mark a counter tendency to give less to the parish and local monasteries, the pillars of religious life in the central Middle Ages. These religious institutions, particularly the five mendicant orders, drew the bulk of pious bequests *grosso modo,* from the earliest documents of the Duecento through the first decades of the Quattrocento. As with my earlier findings on late medieval Siena, the most conspicuous change was a shift in poor relief

away from indiscriminate handouts of bread, clothing, and small sums of money toward dowry funds, which funneled much larger funds to small and select groups of poor virgins. Here, Florence went the farthest, but qualitatively the same trend structured poor relief in all six cities.

In Siena, the structure of pious giving revealed more about changes in attitudes than did the myriad short-term fluctuations registered by pious choices. By the late Duecento, Sienese testators in preparing for their transition to what Petrarch called "that other side of life" strove to do what Saint Catherine of Siena counseled: "to break the earthly cell."[1] The Sienese liquidated their pious holdings, scattering them in paltry allotments from a few pennies to several lire among numerous ecclesiastical organizations, hermits, monks, nuns, and other pious causes strung through the city and the countryside. Such gifts, moreover, rarely came with strings attached—future obligations on the part of the beneficiaries or controls over their use. This mendicant pattern of piety, exemplified by the ascetic ideals and worldly denunciations of the myriad of thirteenth and early fourteenth-century *beati* and *beatae* and spread by the new corps of itinerant preachers, persisted through the horrific events of the Black Death. Only with the recurrence of plague in 1363 did signs of a new system of piety emerge. In the summer months of that year, the number of pious gifts per testator dropped significantly.[2] It was not, however, a secular turning from charitable or ecclesiastical deeds. Indeed, the opposite may have been more the case: the values of pious gifts rose at least by the early years of the Quattrocento, when San Bernardino was preaching in this city's Piazza del Campo. Testators, from humble peasants to humanists, began to rethink their paths to the afterlife by breaking with the long-itemized lists of pious gifts bearing small sums to numerous causes. Testaments that conveyed 25 or more small religious bequests disappeared, and in their place grew a new cult of remembrance in which testators strove to leave a mark on the earthly realm through concrete signs, such as coats of arms carved in religious places or burial plaques, and by perpetual masses requiring constant surveillance on the part of pious and nonpious guarantors. Pious gifts now came more often with conditions and controls placed on universal heirs to perform certain celebrations at precise moments for the spiritual health of testators' souls and those of their ancestors. By the Quattrocento, the Sienese tried more often to determine from the grave the future course of their earthly inheritances. We can now ask whether this new orientation, unveiled through the structure of pious bequests, was peculiar to Siena.

For Siena, the key index of this change was the number of pious bequests per testator. A glance at this index in table 5 at first shows a broad similarity between Siena and the other central Italian towns. In all six cities, the apex in the number of pious bequests came either at the end of the Duecento or in the first decades of the Trecento when, according to Charles de la Roncière, the dual force of a secular clergy and mendicant preachers was successfully persuading the laity of Tuscany to adopt new forms of religious practice and mentality.[3] In Florence, the number rose from fewer than 8 charitable gifts in its earliest documents before 1276 to slightly fewer than 10 in the last years of the Duecento. At the beginning of the Trecento, the number rose insignificantly to its highest level, still a fraction less than 10 gifts. In Arezzo, this high point came at the beginning, the first quarter of the Trecento, and thereafter declined steadily, gradually and consistently.[4] In Pisa, it peaked earlier and soared higher than elsewhere in Tuscany, reaching nearly 14 pious gifts per testator in the 1276–1300 period. In Perugia, as in the other Tuscan towns, the beginning of the Trecento marked the apex of pious giving, when testators gave over 11 gifts per capita. Finally, Assisi, the smallest and poorest of these late medieval towns, with the smallest number of pious entities within its city walls or within its territory, nonetheless exceeded all the others in per capita pious giving. From the earliest testaments preceding 1275 to the last quarter of that century, the number of these gifts more than doubled, from 7 to over 15 gifts per testator—one-and-a-half times the rate of the far wealthier capital of Tuscany, Florence, at its apogee. Afterward, these numbers declined, but on the eve of the Black Death they still remained higher in the city of St. Francis than in the richer cities of Florence, Perugia, and Arezzo.[5]

These differences among the cities' testamentary pious practices cannot be attributed to the sheer number of religious corporations established within a city's walls or in its surrounding countryside ready to benefit from a testator's pious designs. As might be expected from the rich mercantile and ecclesiastical background of late medieval Florence, this city had by far the greatest number of pious institutions reflected in the testamentary choices. Yet, as we have seen, the pious here gave on average to fewer charitable causes than anywhere else,[6] while those in the much smaller Assisi gave on average to more pious causes than did the residents anywhere else.

Moreover, when the number of pious entities from the other cities is considered, the number of ecclesiastical places in no way determined the average number of pious legacies found for these cities. Indeed, the inverse relation was more nearly the case. Florence led with 196 pious entities, followed by Arezzo (123), Pisa (111), Perugia (105), Siena (96), and Assisi (91).[7] If the numbers of pious entities found in the *Rationes Decimarum,* the survey of tithes, are considered, a simple positive correlation between the number of ecclesiastical entities and the number of pious bequests among these six city-states becomes even more doubtful.

For the Tuscan cities (*Tuscie*), several points of comparison are possible from the published tithes—1274–75, 1276–77, 1302–3—while for Perugia only a single record exists, redacted from 1332 to 1334, and for Assisi there are two records from the same period, for 1330 and 1333. From the vantage point of the testamentary evidence, these surveys seriously underrepresent the number of nunneries, and religious confraternities do not appear at all. Nonetheless, if all the religious entities are counted (the Tuscan cities from the 1302–3 tithe), the following rank ordering results:

Perugia	1671 (1332–34)
Arezzo	789
Florence	745
Pisa	382
Assisi	242 (1330), 281 (1333)
Siena	240

The vast majority of these entries were parish, *plebis,* and canonical churches. Since the array of pious legacies pertained more to monasteries, nunneries, and hospitals than to churches beyond one's own parish (at least in the late thirteenth and early fourteenth centuries), it might be argued that a tally of only the former institutions from the *Rationes* would constitute a better sense of the pool of possible religious entities available to the testator's largess. The numbers shrink drastically but the rank ordering remains roughly the same:

Arezzo	91 (1302–3), 54 (1274–75)
Perugia	61 (1332–34)
Florence	45 (1302–3), 42 (1276–77)
Pisa	46 (1302–3), 24 (1276–77)
Assisi	29 (1330)
Siena	14 (1302–3), 6 (1275–76)

Table 5.
The Number of Pious Bequests

Period

	No. Testators	No. Pious Bequests	No. Pious Bequests per Testator
AREZZO			
< 1275			
1276–1300			
1301–25	56	611	10.91
1326–47	92	877	9.53
1348	84	598	7.12
1349–62	63	482	7.65
1363	71	390	5.49
1364–75	88	511	5.81
1376–1400	94	361	3.84
1401–25	100	389	3.89
Total	648	4,219	6.51
ASSISI			
< 1275	18	126	7.00
1276–1300	22	336	15.27
1301–25	19	194	10.21
1326–47	27	225	8.33
1348	27	178	6.59
1349–62	5	81	16.20
1363			
1364–75	14	59	4.21
1376–1400	30	165	5.50
1401–25	128	373	2.91
Total	290	1,737	5.99
FLORENCE			
< 1275	14	107	7.64
1276–1300	43	417	9.70
1301–25	52	516	9.92
1326–47	57	362	6.35
1348	63	491	7.79
1349–62	31	187	6.03
1363	68	420	6.18
1364–75	77	355	4.61
1376–1400	91	358	3.93
1401–25	85	276	3.25
Total	581	3,489	6.01
PERUGIA			
< 1275	2	3	1.50
1276–1300	4	3	0.75
1301–25	10	112	11.20
1326–47	61	301	4.93
1348	79	400	5.06

Table 5.
Continued

Period	No. Testators	No. Pious Bequests	No. Pious Bequests per Testator
PERUGIA *Continued*			
1349–62	20	82	4.10
1363	28	135	4.82
1364–75	51	170	3.33
1376–99	186	732	3.94
1400–1425	73	314	4.30
Total	514	2,252	4.38
PISA			
< 1275	14	123	8.79
1276–1300	42	574	13.67
1301–25	232	2,997	12.92
1326–47	100	905	9.05
1348	15	116	7.73
1349–61	64	513	8.02
1362	39	420	10.77
1363–75	49	239	4.88
1376–1400	110	512	4.65
1401–25	72	167	2.32
Total	737	6,566	8.91
SIENA			
< 1275	35	270	7.71
1276–1300	44	398	9.05
1301–25	50	614	12.28
1326–47	67	628	9.37
1348	55	366	6.65
1349–61	40	251	6.28
1362	24	77	3.21
1363–75	25	104	4.16
1376–1400	61	184	3.02
1401–25	45	196	4.36
Total	446	3,088	6.92

Against what we may have intuited, a negative relationship arises: those city-states where testators spread their pious legacies to fewer charitable organizations and causes were the ones with larger pools of pious entities ready to receive them.[8]

Moreover, in all these cities, the quarter-century preceding the Black Death marked a decline in the number of pious gifts per testator, despite the indications from the *Rationes Decimarum* that the number of religious institutions was on the rise. Between the 1270s and 1302–3, the numbers of these pious organizations more than doubled in Siena and nearly doubled in Arezzo and Pisa.[9] From 1326 to the year of the Black Death, the number of pious bequests ran in the opposite direction: in Siena, they dropped from their apex of just over 12 gifts to just over 9. In Pisa, pious bequests followed the same pattern, falling from almost 13 gifts to 9; in Assisi, although the numbers did turn downward, the decline was insignificant,[10] from around 8 gifts to over 6 per testator. Moreover, the decline in this quarter-century was more dramatic than for any quarter-century in the three cities, Florence, Arezzo, and Perugia. In Florence, the number fell 36 percent; in Arezzo, where all the incremental changes were more gradual than elsewhere, the number dropped by a quarter. In Perugia, these decades of the second quarter of the Trecento were absolutely crucial: the number of pious gifts fell by over half, from more than 11 gifts to under 5.

The plague struck Pisa first in January 1348, carried there by two Genoese galleys returning from Rumania.[11] It then spread to the other cities, reaching Perugia by April.[12] In none of these six cities did the catastrophic mortality of 1348 prompt a decisive break with the past or initiate new directions of piety. In Siena, Pisa, and Assisi, the number of pious bequests continued the slow secular decline begun 25 to 50 years earlier. For the other three towns—Florence, Arezzo, and Perugia—the number of charitable legacies even rebounded in the opposite direction set by the earlier part of the century. The shift, however, was slight and momentary. In the years immediately following the plague until its next recurrence, the numbers everywhere continued to fall, dropping in Florence, Arezzo, and Perugia below their pre-1348 levels.

Finally, after the recurrence of plague in 1362–63,[13] the numbers in all these towns fell to points well below their pre-plague levels and thereafter continued either to fall or at least to level off through the remainder of my period of analysis. After the recurrence of pestilence, no city returned to the long lists of itemized pious gifts, dividing paltry sums among a myriad of religious causes. These changes, moreover, are highly significant after those factors which can readily be demarcated from the documentary evidence are weighted: differences in sex, wealth, social status, town or country residence, whether the document was originally kept by an ecclesiastical archive (a diplomatic scroll) or kept in a notarial protocol housed in a communal archive, whether the testator lay on the deathbed, and whether sons survived to inherit the patrimony.[14] In Siena at the end of the Trecento, testators gave on average only 3 pious bequests, a quarter of the number their ancestors had bequeathed at the beginning of the century. By the Quattrocento, Florentines were giving about the same low numbers of pious last gifts (3.25) as elsewhere, and in Arezzo it was only slightly higher (3.89). Pisa, which at the end of the Duecento gave the most of these Tuscan towns, bequeathed less than any of them by the early Quattrocento (2.32). In Umbria, the trends were the same: by the Quattrocento, the Perugini gave slightly under 4 pious gifts apiece. And in Assisi, where 15 pious legacies had once been the norm, testators gave less than anywhere else except Pisa to charitable causes (2.91).

In summary, the apex in the numbers of pious bequests differed widely at the end of the Duecento—the numbers from the poorest and smallest of these towns (Assisi) vastly surpassed those from the richest (Florence). With the plague of 1362–63 and afterward, these rates of pious legacy began to converge across the wide stretches of Tuscany and Umbria. By the end of the century and into the Quattrocento, the structure of pious giving was almost identical across these Tuscan and Umbrian territories.[15]

A Divergence in the Structure of Piety: Siena, Pisa, and Assisi

Within the frame of these broad similarities of change across Tuscany and Umbria, differences are nonetheless patent. For those cities which possessed substantial samples of testaments before 1276—Pisa, Florence, Siena, and Assisi—the Duecento reflects a broad homogeneity through central Italy. The average value of pious bequests ranged between one and two florins (see table 6), and the variation in the number of these legacies per testator was extraordinarily narrow in comparison to later trends: 7.64 pious bequests on average for Florence; 8.79 for Pisa; 7.00 for Assisi. The last decades of the thirteenth and the first years of the fourteenth centuries radically ruptured the homogeneity of this world of devotion and charity. In Florence, the increase from the late feudal milieu of the early commune went from 7.64 bequests to 9.70 to its apex in 1301–25 of 9.92—an increase of 29 percent over more than 50 years. In contrast, the number of pious bequests per testator in Siena jumped from 7.71 in the earliest documents to 9.05 at the end of the Duecento to its early Trecento apex of 12.28—60 percent and double the Florentine increase. Pious giving in Tuscany's maritime center, Pisa, followed a similar path, from 8.79 to its peak at 13.67 in the last quarter of the thirteenth century—an increase of 56 percent. Testators from

Assisi, the bastion of Franciscan piety, registered the most extraordinary change: pious bequests more than doubled, from 7 in the days of St. Francis and his immediate entourage to 15.27 between 1276 and 1300, when the order was spreading most vigorously throughout the Western world.[16]

A second broad difference in pious giving in these city-states stems from this first fundamental historical difference that arose with the advent of mendicant piety at the end of the thirteenth century. Two patterns of change emerge over the Trecento. In one, the Sienese model, the average number of pious bequests per testator tapered off gradually through the first two-thirds of the Trecento, then fell abruptly by half with the recurrence of pestilence. It tumbled largely because of the total disappearance of those long lists of 25 or more itemized bequests that earlier had characterized the wills not only of the rich but also of modest artisans and others without family names or large landed estates.[17]

The drop for the latter half of the Trecento was even more dramatic in Pisa and Assisi than in Siena. The summer months of the plague's recurrence, however, cannot be designated the turning point in these towns as precisely as in Siena. First, the plague returned to Pisa a year earlier (1362) than elsewhere in Tuscany and Umbria. Pisans reacted to this relived trauma in just the opposite direction from their Tuscan neighbors to the southwest. Instead of turning their backs on the mendicant practice of liquidating estates into tiny parcels directed to numerous pious causes, they embraced it with a last gasp of renewed vigor: the number of pious gifts sprang back to its highest level since the opening quarter of the Trecento, just under 11 pious gifts per testator.[18]

The change, moreover, was occasioned not by a general rise in pious bequests but by a return to testaments bearing the old stamp, dispersing large numbers of pious gifts of paltry sums. Of the 40 testaments redacted during the year of the plague's second assault, six bequeathed 20 or more pious gifts, and three distributed paltry sums to more than 35. For instance, in May of that year, a widow of a rural notary from the Arno village of Pontedera made 36 pious grants ranging from her gown, coat, and best brownish cloth (*panni persi meliores*) offered "to Our Lady" (presumably a painting or a wooden statue) existing next to the crucifix at the altar of Saint Thomas Becket (Cintuberio) in the cathedral of Pisa to her residual properties dispersed to the poor of the hospital of Santa Chiara. Hence the fragmentation and dispersion of her patrimony even exceeded that suggested by the high number of her itemized bequests. One of those grants conveyed the relatively large sum of 100 lire to the

"Poor of Christ," each to receive between 10 and 30 soldi, so that as many as 200 *pauperes Christi* would benefit from this single but dispersed gift alone. Another legacy dispersed 15 lire to all prisoners incarcerated in Pisa's communal prison, none to receive more than 10 soldi.[19]

Another woman in this plague year, this time still married, fragmented her pious contributions even further, spreading them among 38 pious causes. Again, the actual number of itemized gifts understates the extent of this splintering of property. One bequest allotted 20 soldi to 15 poor friars in each of the monastic orders of Pisa; another gave 10 soldi to each hermit in the via di San Pietro a Grado (near the sea); still another extended 3 lire for the health of her soul to all those derelicts who "paced the streets [*facendas vias consuetas*]" near the churches of San Pietro a Grado and San Jacopo ad Podio.[20] Another married woman, a Dominican tertiary (*pinzochera*) and the daughter of a notary, distributed her pious goods among 43 different causes—a number that easily rivaled the long-listed testaments of the late Duecento. Her gifts ranged, moreover, from tiny sums to hermits' cells in various streets of the city and suburbs and to those "who made the streets" of the city's cathedral to her largest legacy, a 25-lire commemorative meal to be consumed by the Dominican congregation for the health of her soul.[21]

The Pisan reaction and return to the mendicant solution to salvation proved, however, short-lived.[22] In the following year, when the plague spread to other parts of central Italy, the Pisans made the most abrupt about-face found over this series of documents, exceeding even the Sienese turn of 1363. The number of pious gifts fell from 10.77 to about 2 per testator in 1363.[23] Nor was this collapse an aberration of the small sample provided by that post-plague year. Over the interval 1363–75, Pisans gave annually less than half of what they had bequeathed in 1362, and the numbers continued to dwindle through the end of my period of analysis, reaching by the end the lowest level for any of these towns.

After 1362, only one Pisan testament itemized 25 or more pious bequests. In 1392, domina Tema, the widow of the knight (*miles*) Lord Grinnzelli, of the magnate Sismundi family, made 30 pious bequests. But while this noble lady made numerous gifts to churches in the territory of Pisa, her will was far more varied and intricate than the usual late Duecento or early Trecento will composed simply of the names of religious institutions and the amounts donated to them. Lady Tema bequeathed, for instance, 30 florins to the Franciscans in Pisa but demanded in return the celebration of a thousand masses for the health of her soul. She gave various strips of landed property "to dower" the

Table 6.
The Values of Pious Bequests

Period	No. Pious Bequests Monetized	Proportion of Pious Bequests Monetized	Average Value of Pious Bequests	Hypothesized Amount of Pious Bequests	Pious Sums per Testator	No. Pious Bequests	Pious Bequests per Testator
AREZZO							
< 1275							
1276–1300							
1301–25	515	0.84	1.83	1,118.13	19.97	611	10.91
1326–47	714	0.81	4.2	3,683.40	40.04	877	9.53
1348	374	0.63	19.84	11,864.32	141.24	598	7.12
1349–62	388	0.80	5.39	2,597.98	41.24	482	7.65
1363	286	0.73	10.64	4,149.60	58.45	390	5.49
1364–75	357	0.70	8.89	4,542.79	51.62	511	5.81
1376–1400	248	0.69	11.38	4,108.18	43.70	361	3.84
1401–25	240	0.62	14.02	5,453.78	54.54	389	3.89
Total 1					56.35		
Total 2	3,122	0.74	8.28	34,933.32	53.91	4,219	6.51
ASSISI							
< 1275	111	0.88	1.68	211.68	11.76	126	7.00
1276–1300	305	0.91	3.14	1,055.04	47.96	336	15.27
1301–25	162	0.84	2.56	496.64	26.14	194	10.21
1326–47	191	0.85	4.42	994.50	36.83	225	8.33
1348	124	0.70	6.41	1,140.98	42.26	178	6.59
1349–62	53	0.65	10.44	845.64	169.13	81	16.20
1363							
1364–75	50	0.85	3.11	183.49	13.11	59	4.21
1376–1400	107	0.65	4.88	805.20	26.84	165	5.50
1401–25	205	0.55	3.95	1,473.35	11.51	373	2.91
Total 1					42.84		
Total 2	1,308	0.75	4.01	6,965.37	24.02	1,737	5.99
FLORENCE							
< 1275	71	0.66	1.01	108.07	7.72	107	7.64
1276–1300	377	0.90	30.96	12,910.32	300.24	417	9.70
1301–25	443	0.86	6.86	3,539.76	68.07	516	9.92
1326–47	269	0.74	11.70	4,235.40	74.31	362	6.35
1348	403	0.82	34.61	16,993.51	269.74	491	7.79
1349–62	111	0.59	48.15	9,004.05	290.45	187	6.03
1363	306	0.73	25.09	10,537.80	154.97	420	6.18
1364–75	235	0.66	21.56	7,653.80	99.40	355	4.61
1376–1400	228	0.64	18.33	6,562.14	72.11	358	3.93
1401–25	174	0.63	83.37	23,010.12	270.71	276	3.25
Total 1					160.77		
Total 2	2,617	0.75	26.23	91,516.47	157.52	3,489	6.01

Total 1: Calculated as the sum of hypothesized amounts of pious bequests divided by the total number of testators.

Total 2: Calculated as the sum of each period's pious sums per testator divided by the number of periods (for columns 3 and 5).

Table 6.
Continued

Period	No. Pious Bequests Monetized	Proportion of Pious Bequests Monetized	Average Value of Pious Bequests	Hypothesized Amount of Pious Bequests	Pious Sums per Testator	No. Pious Bequests	Pious Bequests per Testator
PERUGIA							
< 1275	1	0.33	1.00	3.00	1.50	3	1.50
1276–1300	2	0.67	123.25	369.75	92.44	4	0.75
1301–25	94	0.84	2.53	283.36	28.34	112	11.20
1326–47	262	0.87	5.97	1,796.97	29.46	301	4.93
1348	310	0.78	6.65	2,660.00	33.67	400	5.06
1349–62	62	0.76	26.92	2,207.44	110.37	82	4.10
1363	96	0.71	9.91	1,337.85	47.78	135	4.82
1364–75	140	0.82	9.81	1,667.70	32.70	170	3.33
1376–99	425	0.58	20.03	14,661.96	78.83	732	3.94
1400–1425	133	0.42	29.44	9,244.16	126.63	314	4.30
Total 1					58.17		
Total 2	1,525	0.68	13.46	30,311.92	58.97	2,252	4.38
PISA							
< 1275	107	0.87	1.59	195.57	13.97	123	8.79
1276–1300	527	0.92	4.43	2,542.82	60.54	574	13.67
1301–25	2,637	0.88	3.05	9,140.85	39.40	2,997	12.92
1326–47	730	0.81	13.57	12,280.85	122.81	905	9.05
1348	83	0.72	4.99	578.84	38.59	116	7.73
1349–61	352	0.69	22.97	11,783.61	184.12	513	8.02
1362	327	0.78	7.22	3,032.40	77.75	420	10.77
1363–75	136	0.57	11.22	2,681.58	54.73	239	4.88
1376–1400	264	0.52	19.00	9,728.00	88.44	512	4.65
1401–25	80	0.48	9.69	1,618.23	22.48	167	2.32
Total 1					70.28		
Total 2	5,243	0.80	7.37	48,391.42	65.66	6,566	8.91
SIENA							
< 1275	233	0.86	9.72	2,624.40	74.98	270	7.71
1276–1300	344	0.86	19.68	7,832.64	178.01	398	9.05
1301–25	530	0.86	3.31	2,032.34	40.65	614	12.28
1326–47	516	0.82	14.22	8,930.16	133.29	628	9.37
1348	280	0.77	8.25	3,019.50	54.90	366	6.65
1349–62	217	0.86	7.23	1,814.73	45.37	251	6.28
1363	64	0.83	13.60	1,047.20	43.63	77	3.21
1364–75	79	0.76	9.83	1,022.32	40.89	104	4.16
1376–1400	103	0.56	42.28	7,779.52	127.53	184	3.02
1401–25	138	0.70	24.44	4,790.24	106.45	196	4.36
Total 1					84.57		
Total 2	2,504	0.81	15.26	47,110.53	105.63	3,088	6.92

Total 1: Calculated as the sum of hypothesized amounts of pious bequests divided by the total number of testators.

Total 2: Calculated as the sum of each period's pious sums per testator divided by the number of periods (for columns 3 and 5).

altar of Saint Basil in the church of Santa Cecilia, directing that part of
the revenues (40 florins) finance the commission of "a beautiful panel
painting well ornamented and painted with the figure of Saint Basil and
other saints," that another part purchase a large altarcloth with two
serviettes "to be elaborately stitched" for the health of her own and
her relatives' souls. To furnish the altar of Saint Basil further, she
instructed her executors to sell off all her household tools to commission another large altarcloth for the major altar of the Franciscan
church. To the infirmary of the Dominican monastery of Santa Caterina
she gave the remainder of her inheritance but not in the old fashion
as an unencumbered bequest; instead, she added the condition that
these pious heirs never sell or in any way alienate her "inheritance";
otherwise, the properties would pass to the principal hospital of Pisa,
the Misericordia.[24]

At the end of the Duecento, the extraordinarily high numbers of
pious bequests distributed from the smallest and poorest of these cities—
Assisi—declined steadily to the Black Death in 1348. The interval
between plagues marked, however, a sharp reversal: the number of pious
bequests momentarily climbed to the highest point found for any time
period and for any of the six cities, 21.16 gifts per testator. Yet, because
of the small number of testaments found for these years (six), this
reversal must be taken only as suggestive. One testament that pushed
these figures upward was that of the unusually wealthy merchant Jacobus
quondam Vannis alias Zuccha, who provided funds, not only to endow
a family chapel in the cathedral and to construct a hospital for his
religious confraternity (see Chapter 2), but for 45 other pious causes.[25]
Another testament from 1362, that of Maragoncellus f.q. Andrutii Ciccarelli Maragonis, topped the wealthy alias Zuccha's count by one and
was filled by numerous grants of only 20 soldi to numbers of flagellant
societies, nunneries, and hospitals in Assisi and the surrounding countryside.[26] But even without Zuccha's munificence and Maragoncellus's
fragmentations, the average number remains high for this interval—8.5
gifts—and suggests a momentary reversal of the secular decline in the
number of pious grants.

Then, for the crucial year of the plague's return in 1363, only one
testament survives in the archives systematically surveyed for this study—
the notarial books housed in the Biblioteca Comunale, the *pergamene*
"Instrumenta" collection preserved in the Sacro Convento of the Franciscan basilica, and the Capitolare archives of the cathedral. This testatrix,
a widow from the countryside, Castro Podii Morici,[27] certainly reflects

the pattern of pious giving that would become the standard in these documents to the end of my survey. It was a radical break with the previous long lists of itemized bequests. Beyond the customary five soldi to the commune's hospital, this widow made only two pious bequests: one set aside five soldi for her burial in the parish church of her native village; the other left her residual properties to the custodian of the altar at the Sacro Convento.[28]

An archival darkness not found for the other cities studied unfortunately clouds attempts at statistical analysis for Assisi in the year of the plague's return, 1363.[29] In his survey of all the archives in Assisi and its hinterland, Cesare Cenci lists another testament for this plague year found in busta Z of the Franciscan archives, and I have found a third one in this same "envelope" of scattered documents.[30] This meager sample nonetheless suggests that 1363 was as decisive for Assisi as it proved for Siena. None of the testaments specified more than five pious bequests, and together they averaged a mere three and a quarter. Nor did this abrupt fall in pious bequests result from destitute testators; instead, these legacies bear the marks of another strategy for the afterlife—a cult of remembrance. Friar Johannes Lolli left funds for his burial and a sculpted tombstone (lapide sculto).[31] Of the five pious bequests of Ser Daniel domini Francisci Ciccoli, four were commissions for concrete works to endure beyond the ephemeral moments of his funeral masses. He left 100 lire "or more" for his grave, which he elected "near the door [prope hostium]" of the Franciscan church. To demarcate further his earthly remains he commissioned a painting for that spot (in dicto pilo) with a precision unprecedented for testaments from Assisi, demanding that "Our Lord, Jesus Christ" be painted on the cross, with the Virgin "to the right," Saint John the Evangelist "to the left," and the blessed Francis and Mary Magdalene at the foot of the cross. He then ordered his vault to be covered. (Et voluit et mandavit quod supra dictum pilum fiat quaedam trasanda.) Although these were Ser Daniel's principal commissions, he also left sizable ones to build water wells for the church of San Damiano (25 lire) and for the disciplinarii of the confraternity of Santo Stefano (the amount to be determined by its rector).[32]

Finally, Bernardus domini Guidonis, of porta di San Francesco, delved into the future affairs of his contingent heirs with a specificity not found for the Sienese documents until the sixteenth century. Remarkably, he left his three legitimate sons, along with his "natural" (i.e., illegitimate) son, Stefanus, with equal parts as his universal heirs. If these sons died, Bernardus's three brothers and then their descendants would assume the inheritance. In this case, the dowries of Bernardus's daughters, the already married Iacoba and Chaltutia, whose 200-lire dowry was earmarked exclusively for the entrance fee to the convent of her choice, would increase to match that given to his third daughter, the only one previously granted an *ultra dos*. He then provided Iacoba another 100 florins, if she should ever become separated from her current husband, Bartolomeus (*quod seperaretur de matrimonialis inter eam et dictum Bartolomeum*). Bernardus then turned to his household servant, Finella, to whom he had granted 50 lire. If this *famula* should be pregnant and bear a son, this child should become an heir and assume one-quarter of all the testator's goods communally, along with the above-mentioned Stefanus (which may cause one to wonder about the testator's recent relations with his domestic). But if Finella should bear a daughter, the testator's efforts to fix the future went a step farther: he demanded that his illegitimate son, Stefanus, marry her to collect his part of the patrimony (*Stefanus debeat eam maritare de parte sibi tangente*). The testator's last demand forbade any of his sons or heirs to divide or sell any part of the estate without "the expressed permission" of his executors.[33]

By the 1370s, reasonable numbers of testaments can once again be unearthed for Assisi, in part from the charters preserved in the "Instrumenta" of the Franciscan basilica but mostly from the earliest surviving protocols of Assisan public notaries. These sources show a devotional world of ordinary townsmen and villagers completely transformed from the times preceding the second strike of pestilence. The long lists of small itemized gifts to numerous Franciscan monasteries in the city and the surrounding countryside, to nunneries, and to the poor have now disappeared, and the average number of pious gifts dropped to less than one-third of the late Duecento levels and even less when compared with the years separating the first and second strike of pestilence. By the end of the period of my analysis, the numbers fell still farther, to less than three gifts per testator: one-fifth the average bequeathed a century earlier. Thus, the three cities with the highest numbers of pious bequests in the late Duecento and early Trecento ended up with the lowest numbers in the last decades of the Trecento and the early Quattrocento. Not only was this fall more drastic for Assisi, Pisa, and Siena, it also came more abruptly. For these cities, the most dramatic collapse in the number of pious legacies and hence in the patterns of piety (to be elaborated later) came either with the recurrence of plague in 1362–63 or in the year immediately thereafter.

The Second Pattern

The other three cities—Florence, Arezzo, and Perugia—at no period reached the average numbers of pious bequests seen for Siena, Pisa, and Assisi. Of these latter three cities, Perugia scored highest: over 11 pious bequests on average between 1301 and 1325,[34] followed closely by the Aretines (10.91) and lastly by those possessing the most, the Florentines (9.92). Perugia then experienced the most abrupt decline registered by any of these cities before the Black Death: between 1326 and 1347, its number collapsed by more than half, to just under 5 bequests per testator. The subsequent history of pious giving in the city known for its Duecento flagellant movements and religious enthusiasm then sketched the most unified, consistent, and stable pattern of pious testamentary giving for any of these cities.[35] In the summer months of 1348, nothing changed in terms of individual giving; the number of pious bequests even rose insignificantly, from 4.93 gifts to 5.06.[36] Over the hundred-year period 1326–1425, the most substantial change came immediately after the recurrence of pestilence in 1363, when last gifts fell significantly by one-and-a-half, from 4.82 to 3.33.[37] By the early Quattrocento, Perugini, who in the early Trecento gave the least of the six cities to pious causes, were now giving the most, 4.30—a level that was not significantly different from that of a hundred years earlier.[38]

The richest of these cities, Florence, reached the lowest maximum for the number of pious bequests of any of the six cities. From its high point in the opening years of the Trecento, that number gradually declined through the early decades of the Quattrocento, rising slightly upward only with the outbreaks of pestilence in 1348 and 1363. Unlike the trends found for Siena, Pisa, and Assisi, no sudden change in this structure of piety occurred over the two centuries analyzed. The largest decline came on the heels of the Black Death. In the ensuing 15 years between the successive strikes of pestilence, the number of pious gifts fell from 7.79 to just over 6 gifts per testator.[39]

Reactions in Florence to the pestilence were the opposite of those in Siena or Assisi. A close look at these years however, shows that the average number of bequests masks a divergence in the Florentine re-actions, especially in 1348. While most had limited their pious gifts to no more than 6 beneficiaries, a larger number than in the previous two decades parceled out their pious donations to numerous pious recipients. From 1325 to 1347, only two testators made over 25 pious bequests; in the year of the Black Death, more than five testators thus splintered their pious contributions. One of these Black Death testators, a notary and son of a notary, Gullielmus from Castro Fiorentino but living in the Florentine parish of San Lorenzo,[40] left 64 itemized pious bequests, the third largest number found for any period in the Florentine testaments. The only earlier Florentine testament with more pious bequests came from the fabulously wealthy Contessa Beatrice, the daughter of Count Ridulfo da Cappaja and the widow of Count Marcovaldo, who possessed extensive landed estates in the districts of Florence, Pistoia, Lucca, and Pisa. She distributed her vast properties over 70 different pious causes.[41] And the only Florentine testament with more pious bequests than this one came from another Black Death victim, this time when the plague returned to Tuscany in 1363. The widow of Michele di Uberto de Albizzi, who lay on her deathbed in June of that year, left 78 itemized pious bequests, which included 22 different nunneries located within the walls and in the suburbs of Florence as well as eight hospitals.[42]

Arezzo closely followed the pattern seen for Florence. A gradual decline in per capita pious giving was momentarily reversed with the summer months of pestilence in 1348. Reactions in Arezzo were also the opposite of those in Siena and Assisi. Instead of casting aside the models of piety adopted from the mendicant preachers and practiced by ordinary citizens and villagers over the previous 50 to 70 years, some Aretine testators returned to the pattern of dividing their pious patrimonies and spreading them over numerous pious beneficiaries. Six testators each gave over 25 pious gifts in their wills of 1348. The nobleman and scion of the signorial rulers of Arezzo stretching back to Bishop Guido, the *Nobilis, Sapiens, et Potens Vir Dominus* Tarlatus Miles natus quondam Nobilis et potentis viri Angeli domini Tarlati, from Pietramala, gave the most of these Black Death testators in Arezzo: 47 pious bequests. The values of those monetized gifts exceeded all but one other testament found for any city in my samples, amounting to 5,937 florins.[43] As we shall see later, Tarlatus's benevolence did not, however, simply follow mendicant dictates of disseminating one's worldly estate into tiny slivers with no thought of leaving future traces of his memory.

Yet, not all of these Black Death testators were so rich and powerful. The surgeon *Magister* Angelus, son of another guild master, Benincasa, gave almost as many pious gifts as the powerful Tarlatus (41 pious bequests). Instead of dowry funds of 4,000 lire or a 4,000-florin gift to construct the major chapel at the Franciscan mountain shrine of La

Verna,[44] the surgeon's bequests included contributions that would have been tiny even by the standards of the late Duecento. One item dispersed no more than 12 pennies to all the nuns of Arezzo and those within a one-mile radius of the city. Another gave 12 pennies for prayers to all regular priests in the five mendicant friaries. Angelus further ordered the confraternity of clerics to distribute two *staii*[45] of baked bread among the poor and sick (*pauperibus medicantibus*). Finally, in contrast to the notary and son of a notary Symoneus, who in 1338 provided for building locked book cages to preserve for future generations his vast library of 156 titles and who established stringent safeguards against their sale, loan, or theft, the surgeon ordered the sale of his books (priced individually) in order to disperse his pious offerings in packets of pennies and shillings.[46]

When the plague returned to Arezzo in 1363, the testament of a married woman from neighboring Borgo San Sepolcro even exceeded the number of pious bequests conveyed in the testament of the noble and powerful Tarlatus. Before embarking on her pilgrimage to St. Francis's birthplace, domina Ceccha, the wife of Bartolus, called Pazo, made 50 itemized pious bequests. As in the testament of the surgeon, these were for the most part tiny monetary offerings: 40 soldi to the Augustinians of Borgo San Sepolcro, 10 soldi to the *laudesi* fraternity of the Albizia, 10 soldi to the Aretine nunneries of Sant'Elisabetta, the sisters of Agnus Dei, the Ursulines, and so on.[47]

In summary, the numbers of pious gifts divide these six cities into two groups, which were not demarcated by any geographical east versus west or Tuscan versus Umbrian line, as some of the indices of pious choices may have earlier suggested. Nor was the difference one of prehistoric, antique, or even medieval origins corresponding to earlier tribal or lingual boundaries or the later influence of Lombard settlement and law. In the earliest documents until 1275, the six had not yet diverged from one another in the average numbers of pious bequests or their choices of beneficiaries. (See table 5.) Instead, the differences originated in the last decades of the Duecento and persisted for nearly a century. But after the recurrence of pestilence in 1363, these societies with widely differing histories and political and economic systems began once again to resemble one another. By the late Duecento, the first group, Assisani, Pisans, and Sienese, had bequeathed more gifts to pious causes than had testators in the other three territories. But beginning with the period of famines in the 1320s, the number of gifts from the first group gradually began to decline; the most significant jolt in the direction of giving, however, came in the summer months of the plague's return (or for Pisa, the year afterward).

The other three towns—Arezzo, Florence, and Perugia—never reached the same heights in fragmenting their pious contributions. Moreover, except in Perugia, where pious giving collapsed to between four and five gifts per testator in the quarter-century preceding the Black Death, pious giving declined gradually and steadily through the Trecento and early Quattrocento. For none of these towns did the recurrence of plague in 1363 or immediately thereafter register traumatic shock waves quite as powerful as in the first three towns. But even in these cities and their territories, the recurrence of pestilence *did* mark a definitive turning point. After 1363 (and after a momentary reversal in pious giving in Florence), these testators, as in the other three city-states, finally cast aside once and for all the older mendicant pattern of piety and its stratagem for salvation.

Wealth and Piety

To what extent did differences in wealth determine the different trends in pious giving among these six city-states? In reaching conclusions about changes over time and space, the various multiple regression models controlled for the individual wealth of testators by calculating wealth as the average sums of the values of itemized pious and nonpious gifts. Wealth was the most significant of the dependent variables found in the general model. According to its beta coefficient, a testator's wealth determined over a quarter of the standard deviation in the number of pious legacies.[48] When the cities were analyzed singly, the effect of wealth on piety ranged from determining nearly 50 percent of the standard deviation in Pisa (+ .496) to one-sixth of it in Assisi (+ .149).[49]

Estimating the wealth of the pious donors from their testaments, however roughly, is fraught with difficulties. First, a host of problems characteristic of medieval coinage and monies of account hamper even the evaluation of individual itemized bequests—such as differences in coinage, types of florins, and places of minting.[50] Second, testators rarely estimated the residual properties left to their universal heirs, whether those heirs were ecclesiastical bodies, close relatives, or persons who bore no obvious relation to the testator.[51] Those residual properties were often the testator's prized properties such as land and the family's principal residence, often mixed with residual mobile property—tools, clothing, textiles, and other household goods. Obviously, these possessions represented a far larger portion of the estate for the rich and powerful than they did for the poor. On the other hand, some testaments leave clues suggesting that these universal heirs may not have always been so lucky. The residual properties, on occasion, could be awash with debts and obligations, and only out of charity might the chosen heir assume the financial burdens of becoming the "universal heir." As Maria Serena Mazzi and Sergio Raveggi report from their study of inventories in Quattrocento Florence, peasants frequently renounced their paternal inheritances, judging them as *"potius damnosam quam lucrosam."*[52] Such testators, moreover, were not confined to the poor and destitute; even a figure as rich and prominent as Pope John XXIII (reputed to have had more than a million florins deposited in Florentine banks in 1415) could leave his executors with financial problems in securing the funds to carry out charitable and artistic works.[53]

Third, not all the itemized properties were liquidated into coin or estimated monetarily, and those least often monetized, similar to a testator's residual properties, were landed properties and houses— usually the most valuable possessions. Fourth, as seen for Siena, testators and their notaries tended in all six cities to liquidate less property into monetary gifts as the years progressed. (See table 6.) In fact, for the other five cities the decline was steeper, starting as high as 92 percent of all pious bequests for Pisa in the last years of the Duecento and falling to only 48 percent there by the end of my analysis. These tendencies suggest that the values of pious contributions become progressively more understated as we pass through the latter half of the Trecento and the early Quattrocento. Testators were holding on to their prized landed properties, refusing to alienate them or allow their heirs to alienate them. As Alberto Tenenti has argued from literary and artistic evidence and as I discuss in greater detail in Chapter 5, testators increasingly attached their self-esteem to worldly possessions, wishing to hold onto them to the grave and beyond.[54]

Despite the problems in determining the monetary value of testamentary gifts, the data show trends and comparisons across the city-states that are in line with what we might have suspected from the general economic histories of the towns. Although testators on average gave fewer pious bequests in Florence than in the other cities, the values of their pious legacies towered over the rest. Florentines gave on average 118.16 florins to pious causes over the time span of roughly two centuries and were followed by those from the older banking center and second-ranking city in population, Siena (91.69 florins), then by the maritime republic, Pisa (65.66 florins), then Perugia (58.97 florins)[55] and Arezzo (53.91 florins). Finally, Assisi, the smallest of these commercial cities but the one which by far contributed the most numerous pious bequests at its height, trailed the others at a considerable distance; the average of its pious legacies amounted to 24.05 florins, one-fifth that of the much more prosperous Florence. These results follow the general correlation between size of town and per capita wealth that David Herlihy has drawn from the Catasto tax records for the Tuscan towns under the rule of Florence in 1427.[56]

The trends over time in the values of pious gifts for the individual cities corroborate our general knowledge of economic change in central Italy during the late Middle Ages. These values declined most sharply in Assisi, where testators gave on average 11.51 florins in pious gifts during the early decades of the Quattrocento—only one-eighth the value at the heyday of Assisi's religious efflorescence in the last decades of the Duecento, despite an inflationary spiral that continued through the third quarter of the Trecento. The increases in pious giving toward the end of my period were most pronounced in Florence, which became the hub of a Tuscan regional economy in the late Trecento and early Quattrocento.[57] Here, in the first years of the Quattrocento, the values returned to near their early Trecento heights—270.71 florins, or twenty-three-and-a-half times as much as in Assisi. Thus, Florence, which from the number of pious bequests appeared the most miserly of cities, from the valuation of these gifts appears as the most generous. How much did the differences across the various city-states and over time depend on the financial wherewithal of the testator? For this evaluation, the nonpious gifts can serve to control for differences and changes in the amounts testators gave to charities, both over time and across geography.

The value of these nonpious gifts, combined with the pious ones, forms a slightly different hierarchy of wealth. Florence remains the wealthiest (754.04 florins per capita) and Assisi the poorest (118.45 florins). (See table 7.) Indeed, by these calculations Florence was perched even higher above the rest; its nearest competitor then becomes the second regional capital, Perugia (402.03 florins), followed by Siena (384.78 florins), Arezzo (368.81 florins), and then in fifth position, surprisingly, Pisa (203.11 florins), most probably the wealthiest of these cities during its commercial reign in the Duecento.

The economic straits of testators may have been more dire in Pisa than elsewhere in Tuscany, first from the disastrous trade agreement with the Florentines in 1369 that crippled indigenous Pisan industries; then the political turmoil, famine, and economic crisis of the 1390s;[58] then Florence's devastating war undertaken to incorporate the maritime province (1406); and finally the dual effects of plague and malaria, which possibly were more devastating in the territory of Pisa than elsewhere.[59] At least one testament points to these troubles. A rural notary Johannes, the son of the former notary Alammani, from Palaia, then living in the urban parish of San Frediano, redacted his will in the year of the Florentine conquest of Pisa. One of his principal gifts was his "large farm house," "mostly burnt to the ground," in the neighboring village of Calci. The gift was made to a Tomeo, the son of Coli Cavalli, and to Tomeo's nephew Lorenzo on the condition that, within six months after the testator's death, the two would build a new roof (*coperire vel coperiri facere dictum casalanum*) and thereafter "live always in the house with their families and their household belongings."[60] In the first quarter of the fifteenth century, the value of testamentary gifts in Pisa was less than one-third the value of what Pisans had left immediately following the Black Death (1349–61).[61] Similarly, fortunes in Assisi had turned downward following the resurgence of plague in the 1360s. By the end of my period of analysis, the real values of its testamentary gifts had fallen by more than half their value at the beginning of the Trecento.[62]

The other four cities show the opposite trend. Indeed, the return of riches in these city-states appears to bear out contemporary chroniclers such as Matteo Villani of Florence and Agnolo di Tura del Grasso of Siena, as well as numerous mendicant preachers, who pointed with regret to the abundance of wealth and the new opportunities after the Black Death that so freely awaited the *gente nuova* and eased their influx into power and prosperity.[63] In Florence, testators gave more at the beginning of the Quattrocento than at any other time since the late Duecento, bequeathing one-and-a-half times more in constant florins than their ancestors had at the beginning of the Trecento. And these figures most likely undervalue the rise of testamentary wealth at the end of the Trecento and in the early Quattrocento for two reasons: as stated above, testators tended to liquidate fewer of their more valuable properties over time; and the calculation of constant florins is based on grain prices, which fluctuated more radically than the bulk of property conveyed by testators, such as houses and land, hence dampening the estimates for the early fifteenth century. Testators from Perugia more than doubled the values of their legacies in constant florins from the beginning of the Trecento to the advent of the Quattrocento. From 165.68 florins, the

Table 7.
The Values of Nonpious Bequests

Period	No. Testators	No. Nonpious Bequests	No. Nonpious Bequests Monetized	Proportion of Nonpious Bequests Monetized	Average Value of Nonpious Bequests	Hypothesized Amount of Nonpious Bequests	Nonpious Sums per Testator	No. Nonpious Bequests per Testator	Value of Nonpious Bequests per Testator	Ratio of Pious to Nonpious Bequests	Ratio of Values of Pious to Nonpious Bequests	Value of All Itemized Bequests per Testator (Florins)	Constant Florins	Value of All Itemized Bequests per Testator (Constant Florins)
AREZZO														
< 1276														
1276–1300														
1301–25	56	314	168	0.54	16.28	5,111.92	91.28	5.61	91.28	1.95	0.22	111.25	1.00	111.25
1326–47	92	548	211	0.39	59.15	32,414.20	352.33	5.96	352.33	1.60	0.11	392.37	1.41	278.27
1348	84	459	217	0.47	29.77	13,664.43	162.67	5.46	162.67	1.30	0.87	303.91	1.41	215.54
1349–62	63	320	104	0.33	50.17	16,054.40	254.83	5.08	254.83	1.51	0.16	296.07	1.52	194.78
1363	71	390	176	0.45	43.98	17,152.20	241.58	5.49	241.58	1.00	0.24	300.03	1.52	197.39
1364–75	88	505	173	0.34	80.20	40,501.00	460.24	5.74	460.24	1.01	0.11	511.86	2.13	240.31
1376–1400	94	405	114	0.28	67.70	27,418.50	291.69	4.31	291.69	0.89	0.15	335.39	2.12	158.20
1401–25	100	473	117	0.25	109.39	51,741.47	517.41	4.73	517.41	0.82	0.11	571.95	1.64	348.75
Total	648	3,414	1,280	0.37		204,058.10	314.90			1.24	0.18	352.85		
ASSISI														
< 1276	18	69	35	0.51	1.85	127.65	7.09	3.83	7.09	1.83	1.66	18.85	0.00	0.00
1276–1300	22	107	68	0.64	10.17	1,088.19	49.46	4.86	49.46	3.14	0.97	97.42	0.00	0.00
1301–25	19	84	48	0.57	15.75	1,323.00	69.63	4.42	69.63	2.31	0.38	95.77	1.00	95.77
1326–47	27	117	55	0.47	16.24	1,900.08	70.37	4.33	70.37	1.92	0.52	107.21	1.41	76.03
1348	27	111	49	0.44	7.21	800.31	29.64	4.11	29.64	1.60	1.43	71.90	1.41	50.99

	5	32	12	0.38	125.00	4,000.00	800.00	6.40	800.00	2.53	0.21	969.13	1.52	637.58
1349–62	5	32	12	0.38	125.00	4,000.00	800.00	6.40	800.00	2.53	0.21	969.13	1.52	637.58
1363														
1364–75	14	80	29	0.36	6.27	501.60	35.83	5.71	35.83	0.74	0.37	48.94	2.13	22.97
1376–1400	30	215	62	0.29	15.72	3,379.80	112.66	7.17	112.66	0.77	0.24	139.50	2.12	65.80
1401–25	128	542	131	0.24	14.52	7,869.84	61.48	4.23	61.48	0.69	0.19	72.99	1.64	44.51
Total	290	1,357	489	0.36		20,990.47	72.38	4.68		1.28	0.34	180.19		
FLORENCE														
< 1276	14	51	22	0.43	20.12	1,026.12	73.29	3.64	73.29	2.10	0.11	81.01	0.00	0.00
1275–1300	43	297	165	0.56	113.33	33,659.01	782.77	6.91	782.77	1.40	0.38	1,083.01	0.00	0.00
1301–25	52	337	190	0.56	65.28	21,999.36	423.06	6.48	423.06	1.53	0.16	491.14	1.00	491.14
1325–47	57	266	115	0.43	79.73	21,208.18	372.07	4.67	372.07	1.36	0.20	446.38	1.41	316.58
1348	63	321	162	0.50	110.87	35,589.27	564.91	5.10	564.91	1.53	0.48	834.65	1.41	591.95
1349–62	31	149	73	0.49	145.71	21,710.79	700.35	4.81	700.35	1.26	0.41	990.80	1.52	651.84
1363	68	479	243	0.51	103.31	49,485.49	727.73	7.04	727.73	0.88	0.21	882.70	1.52	580.72
1364–75	77	414	172	0.42	134.09	55,513.26	720.95	5.38	720.95	0.86	0.14	820.35	2.13	385.14
1376–1400	91	505	222	0.44	102.33	51,676.65	567.88	5.55	567.88	0.71	0.13	639.99	2.12	301.88
1401–25	85	384	127	0.33	202.03	77,579.52	912.70	4.52	912.70	0.72	0.30	1,183.41	1.64	721.59
Total	581	3,203	1,491	0.47		369,447.60	635.88			1.09	0.26	745.34		
PERUGIA														
< 1276	2	14	9	0.64	15.71	219.94	109.97	7.00	109.97	0.21	0.01	111.47	0.00	0.00
1276–1300	4	28	12	0.43	163.66	4,582.48	1,145.62	7.00	1,145.62	0.11	0.08	1,238.06	0.00	0.00
1301–25	10	64	38	0.59	21.46	1,373.44	137.34	6.40	137.34	1.75	0.21	165.68	1.00	165.68
1326–47	61	404	223	0.55	8.61	3,478.44	57.02	6.62	57.02	0.75	0.52	86.48	1.41	61.33
1348	79	537	289	0.54	15.51	8,328.87	105.43	6.80	105.43	0.74	0.32	139.10	1.41	98.65
1349–62	20	153	88	0.58	90.59	13,860.27	693.01	7.65	693.01	0.54	0.16	803.39	1.52	528.54
1363	28	185	84	0.45	31.31	5,792.35	206.87	6.61	206.87	0.73	0.23	254.65	1.52	167.53
1364–75	51	300	137	0.46	50.42	15,126.00	296.59	5.88	296.59	0.57	0.11	329.29	2.13	154.60
1376–99	186	1,160	505	0.44	74.61	86,547.60	465.31	6.24	465.31	0.63	0.17	544.14	2.12	256.67
1400–1425	73	382	132	0.35	96.92	37,023.44	507.17	5.23	507.17	0.82	0.25	633.80	1.64	386.47
Total	514	3,227	1,517	0.47		176,332.80	343.06			0.70	0.19	430.61		
PISA														
< 1276	14	78	58	0.74	1.34	104.52	7.47	5.57	7.47	1.58	1.87	21.44	0.00	0.00
1276–1300	42	290	171	0.59	19.11	5,541.90	131.95	6.90	131.95	1.98	0.46	192.49	0.00	0.00

Table 7.
Continued

Period	No. Testators	No. Nonpious Bequests	No. Nonpious Bequests Monetized	Proportion of Nonpious Bequests Monetized	Average Value of Nonpious Bequests	Hypothesized Amount of Nonpious Bequests	Nonpious Sums per Testator	No. Nonpious Bequests per Testator	Value of Nonpious Bequests per Testator	Ratio of Pious to Nonpious Bequests	Ratio of Values of Pious to Nonpious Bequests	Value of All Itemized Bequests per Testator (Florins)	Constant Florins	Value of All Itemized Bequests per Testator (Constant Florins)
1301–25	232	1,391	865	0.62	13.55	18,848.05	81.24	6.00	81.24	2.15	0.48	120.64	1.00	120.64
1326–47	100	540	325	0.60	31.12	16,804.80	168.05	5.40	168.05	1.68	0.73	290.86	1.41	206.28
1348	15	73	34	0.47	11.98	874.54	58.30	4.87	58.30	1.59	0.66	96.89	1.41	68.72
1349–61	64	318	162	0.51	44.27	14,077.86	219.97	4.97	219.97	1.61	0.84	404.09	1.52	265.85
1362	39	208	131	0.63	28.95	6,021.60	154.40	5.33	154.40	2.02	0.50	232.15	1.52	152.73
1363–75	49	254	116	0.46	29.20	7,416.80	151.36	5.18	151.36	0.94	0.36	206.09	2.13	96.76
1376–1400	110	429	191	0.45	54.13	23,221.77	211.11	3.90	211.11	1.19	0.42	299.54	2.12	141.29
1401–25	72	211	73	0.35	39.76	8,389.36	116.52	2.93	116.52	0.79	0.19	138.99	2.12	84.75
Total	737	3,792	2,126	0.56		101,301.20	137.45			1.73	0.53	200.32	1.64	
SIENA														
< 1276	35	222	109	0.49	61.24	13,595.28	388.44	6.34	388.44	1.22	44.99	17,865.07		
1276–1300	44	311	182	0.59	54.70	17,011.70	386.63	7.07	386.63	1.28	158.39	61,624.72		
1301–25	50	361	186	0.52	37.19	13,425.59	268.51	7.22	268.51	1.70	80.15	21,790.56	1.00	21,790.56
1326–47	67	446	204	0.46	20.63	9,200.98	137.33	6.66	137.33	1.41	500.72	68,900.61	1.41	48,865.68
1348	55	192	112	0.58	62.50	12,000.00	218.18	3.49	218.18	1.91	70.48	15,594.97	1.41	11,060.26
1349–62	40	170	78	0.46	46.96	7,983.20	199.58	4.25	199.58	1.48	49.31	10,041.29	1.52	6,606.11
1363	24	123	71	0.58	20.11	2,473.53	103.06	5.13	103.06	0.63	27.09	2,894.92	1.52	1,904.55
1364–75	25	155	65	0.42	32.19	4,989.45	199.58	6.20	199.58	0.67	16.19	3,430.13	2.13	1,610.39
1376–1400	61	276	94	0.34	24.42	6,739.92	110.49	4.52	110.49	0.67	19.44	13,307.30	2.12	6,277.03
1401–25	45	215	82	0.38	53.58	11,519.70	255.99	4.78	255.99	0.91	57.40	14,948.89	1.64	9,115.18
Total	446	2,471	1,183	0.48		98,939.35	221.84	5.54	221.84	1.25	119.70	26,775.08		

value of legacies in constant florins reached 386.47 at the beginning of the Quattrocento. Similarly, these values doubled over the Trecento in Siena.[64] And Arezzo, unlike impoverished Pisa, appears to have prospered under Florentine suzerainty. From the opening of the fourteenth century to the early decades of the fifteenth, the values of legacies per testator trebled from 111.25 constant florins to 348.75.

Although wealth certainly did affect the number of pious legacies a testator might make within a certain society and at a particular moment in time (as the multiple regression models have shown), the data on testamentary wealth show no ironclad correlation between wealth and the number of pious gifts when the cities are compared. At the end of the thirteenth century, Florentines on average gave fewer pious bequests than anywhere else, while the value of their legacies, both pious and nonpious, had reached their peak of 1083.01 florins. In contrast, Assisani were then granting the greatest average number of charitable bequests, more than one-and-a-half times that of the Florentines, when the average value of their total itemized properties amounted to 97.42, less than one-tenth the wherewithal possessed by those in the emerging commercial hub of Tuscany.

Nor did the economic fortunes of testators in the wake of the Black Death determine the general decline in the number of pious bequests in each of these city-states. As we have seen, the Black Death of 1348 and its subsequent tremors did not produce, universally and consistently, the same economic consequences across this restricted geography.[65] The plagues (after an initial period of dislocation) may have created a relatively uniform supply and demand nexus, where wages rose and grain prices fell.[66] Yet the experiences, particularly of that middling group which regularly redacted notarized wills, were variable, along with the rise and fall of fortunes found for individual cities and their territories. After the Black Death, a small town such as Assisi, like those smaller towns that fell into the political and economic ambit of Florence, most likely lost its commercial and industrial independence in the face of stiffer competition from neighboring Perugia.[67] Perugia, on the other hand, gained at the expense of Assisi and other towns and villages within its growing economic sphere, as indeed the population trends suggest (see Chapter 1). Pisa had its own particular history. It lost its economic hegemony first in competition with Genoa on the seas of the western Mediterranean with the defeat at Meloria in 1284 and then in the early Trecento in Tuscany in competition with the Florentines.[68] Moreover, these data indicate that, unlike other places, after a period of 20 to 25 years, Pisa does not seem to have risen from the Black Death's devastation and dislocation with a "more rational" or "dynamic" economy[69] or a better standard of living for those who survived.[70] Instead, warfare and malaria overdetermined that late Trecento and early Quattrocento economic history.

The economic history sketched through the testamentary legacies of Arezzo is, however, the most surprising trend. The little work that has thus far been devoted to the economic history of this cultural and university center has focused largely on its late Duecento and early Trecento misfortunes, when according to this historiography, Arezzo, like so many other places in Tuscany, had already entered a period of steady and irreversible decline, which then accelerated with its devastation and incorporation into the Florentine state in 1384.[71] Perhaps the Aretines, or at least those of middling wealth, as Judith Brown has argued for late Quattrocento and Cinquecento Pescia,[72] and Michael Mallett for late Quattrocento Pisa,[73] benefited from symbiotic ties with the dominant power, Florence. Indeed, Federigo Melis makes such an argument for the Aretine economy, claiming that trade routes changed and the Casentino town became the linchpin connecting the Tyrrhenian with the Adriatic Sea in a new regional and international economy.[74] Evidence for this new Aretine prosperity, however, rests on a few mercantile success stories—Ubertino di Simo (d. 1361), his son Simo d'Umberto (d. 1393),[75] Agnolo di Biagio, Feo di Lando, Giusto di Bartolomeo, Lazzaro di Giovanni di Feo Bracci (d. 1425), and his son-in-law—Baccio di Magio. Some of these fortunes (Umberto di Simo died in 1361) were in fact accumulated before Arezzo's submission to Florentine control.[76] Perhaps the city's recovery was partially a matter of economic opportunities arising in the wake of the Black Death's destruction, though, as the comparison of cities suggests, such a simple economistic explanation by itself will not suffice. Moreover, other historians have seriously questioned the extent of Aretine recovery, especially by the first decades of the Quattrocento.[77]

At any rate, we can certainly argue that the decline in the number of pious bequests, which characterized all of these six cities following the recurrence of pestilence in the 1360s, did not result from general impoverishment or a decline in the fortunes of individual testators. While in Arezzo, Siena, Perugia, and Florence economic fortunes appear to have improved in the last decades of the Trecento, the numbers of their pious bequests came tumbling down just as with those cities that fared less well.

The number of pious bequests per testator, although a key statistic for uncovering changes in patterns and attitudes toward charity and the afterlife, is not, as we saw earlier in the case of Siena, a reliable key for understanding levels of pious giving either for the individual or the society. What, then, can be said quantitatively of the relative weight of these city-states' outlays to pious institutions? Since economic power and standards of living varied radically from place to place as well as over time, the ratio of pious to nonpious gifts and the ratio of their values might serve as an index of differences in pious expenditure relative to wealth. Unlike the patterns seen in my earlier work on Siena (particularly for the period immediately after 1425), these ratios show a general trend toward a greater secularization of bequests by the last decades of the Trecento. The recurrence of pestilence in the 1360s was the watershed. Before, the number of pious bequests consistently exceeded gifts to friends and kin everywhere except in Perugia. Afterward, nonpious outnumbered pious bequests everywhere except Pisa.

In Florence, from the earliest documents until 1275, testators gave over twice as many pious as nonpious gifts. (See table 8.) From that high point, these ratios declined steadily for the next 125 years. Similarly, in Arezzo, pious nearly doubled nonpious gifts in their earliest records (1305–25) and slid steadily from then on. The Pisan trend was more complex: the ratio of pious to nonpious gifts also peaked in the first quarter of the Trecento and then declined. With the recurrence of pestilence in 1362, however, Pisans, more than those from the other cities, returned to matters of the soul as pious gifts doubled the others. But immediately afterward they abruptly reversed these momentary impulses, giving as elsewhere more to friends and kin than to the pious.

This ratio of bequests was highest in Siena during the plague of 1348, testators there giving nearly two pious gifts for every nonpious one. But when the plague returned, the ratio reversed itself; for every pious gift, the Sienese gave nearly two nonpious ones. It was at the birthplace of St. Francis, however, that piety measured by these ratios reigned supreme; at the end of the Duecento, Assisani were giving three times as many legacies to the church as to relatives and friends. But even here, this practice changed after the second occasion of pestilence; as elsewhere, testators inverted their habits, passing property more often to nonpious ends than to the pious.

The ratio of the values of these two sorts of gifts yields, at first glance, a different image of pious spending in these six cities. While the numbers of pious bequests may have regularly outstripped the nonpious ones

Table 8.

The Ratio of Pious to Nonpious Bequests

Period	Ratio of Pious to Nonpious Bequests	Ratio of Values of Pious to Nonpious Bequests	Ratio of Pious to Nonpious Bequests	Ratio of Values of Pious to Nonpious Bequests	Ratio of Pious to Nonpious Bequests	Ratio of Values of Pious to Nonpious Bequests
	AREZZO		ASSISI		FLORENCE	
< 1276			1.83	1.66	2.10	0.11
1276–1300			3.14	0.97	1.40	0.38
1301–25	1.95	0.22	2.31	0.38	1.53	0.16
1326–47	1.60	0.11	1.92	0.52	1.36	0.20
1348	1.30	0.87	1.60	1.43	1.53	0.48
1349–62	1.51	0.16	2.53	0.21	1.26	0.41
1363	1.00	0.24			0.88	0.21
1364–75	1.01	0.11	0.74	0.37	0.86	0.14
1376–1400	0.89	0.15	0.77	0.24	0.71	0.13
1401–25	0.82	0.11	0.69	0.19	0.72	0.30
Total 1	1.24	0.18	1.28	0.34	1.09	0.26
Total 2	1.26	0.25	1.73	0.66	1.23	0.25

Period	Ratio of Pious to Nonpious Bequests	Ratio of Values of Pious to Nonpious Bequests	Ratio of Pious to Nonpious Bequests	Ratio of Values of Pious to Nonpious Bequests	Ratio of Pious to Nonpious Bequests	Ratio of Values of Pious to Nonpious Bequests
	PERUGIA		PISA		SIENA	
< 1276	0.21	0.01	1.58	1.87	1.68	0.49
1276–1300	0.11	0.08	1.98	0.46	1.28	0.46
1301–25	1.75	0.21	2.15	0.48	1.70	0.14
1326–47	0.75	0.52	1.68	0.73	1.41	0.69
1348	0.74	0.32	1.59	0.66	1.91	0.18
1349–62	0.54	0.16	1.61	0.84	1.47	0.15
1363	0.73	0.23	2.02	0.50	0.63	0.28
1364–75	0.57	0.11	0.94	0.36	0.67	0.10
1376–1400	0.63	0.17	1.19	0.42	0.67	0.31
1401–25	0.82	0.25	0.79	0.19	0.91	0.10
Total 1	0.70	0.19	1.73	0.53	1.25	0.32
Total 2	0.68	0.21	1.55	0.65	1.23	0.29

Total 1: Calculated as the sums divided by the total number of bequests.
Total 2: Calculated as the sum of each period divided by the number of periods.

before the 1360s, rarely did their values do so as much. It happened only with the earliest documents in Pisa and Assisi. Although not as tidily as the trends set by the frequencies of legacies, the ratios of values, nonetheless, follow roughly the same patterns: testators spent more on pious as against nonpious causes before the recurrence of pestilence than afterward. The transformation in piety thus measured was not, however, as radical as when measured in numbers of bequests. In Florence and Perugia, the relative values of pious as against nonpious gifts even began to turn upward by the early years of the Quattrocento.

Behind these broad similarities, however, the values of gifts reveal once again sharp differences among these societies. Perhaps surprisingly, the two communities that were the closest geographically were the farthest apart in their testamentary budgets. Perugia allotted less than any other city-state to pious causes over the course of these documents, with pious bequests at only 19 percent of the nonpious in value, while in the Franciscan mecca it was the highest, amounting to 67 percent. Before the second plague in Umbria, these differences were even more accentuated; afterward, Assisani gave about the same proportions of their estates to the pious as the Perugini, and at the beginning of the Quattrocento even less.

Relative to their wealth, the Pisans gave about the same as the Assisani: about two-thirds as much for pious as for nonpious bequests. In Arezzo and Florence, on the other hand, pious gifts were worth only a quarter of the nonpious—almost as little as in Perugia—while the Sienese ratio was closer to those found in Assisi and Pisa. Once again, these statistics on the structure of giving uncover the same division of these city-states into two triads.

Thus, wealth was not the overriding determinant of the number or value of pious bequests. Those societies which spent the most on pious last gifts (Assisi, Pisa, and Siena) also followed most closely the mendicant dictates before the recurrence of pestilence by fragmenting their pious donations into numerous pieces. These societies were not, however, the richest; indeed, they were more nearly the poorest. Nor was wealth the overwhelming factor determining the decline in the values of pious giving or the even sharper fall in the number of pious bequests. Testators in four of the six city-states clearly benefited from economic opportunities that began to grow by the 1370s; yet all these societies, regardless of economic fortunes, gave less in number and in value to the church and charity.

A Mixture of Pious Intentions

These statistics make it clear that while a society like Florence may have willed less to pious causes relative to its economic well-being, it gave nonetheless more *in absolute terms*. At the same time, Florentines were giving fewer pious bequests than elsewhere. Does this paradox reveal something crucial about piety and attitudes toward property during the heyday of mendicant preaching, when these societies differed from one another more radically than in the Duecento or later after the second Black Death? Certainly, Florence before the plague had testators who, in good mendicant fashion, sprinkled their pious sums over a vast landscape of ecclesiastical and charitable beneficiaries. We have already encountered the fabulously wealthy Contessa Beatrice, whose 1279 testament granted 70 separate and itemized gifts to pious causes. The largest of these was a 300-lire endowment to the nunnery of San Pietro a Monticelli—to be sure, a grand expense by late Duecento standards, but not so overwhelming in relation to the countess's landed properties that stretched through the territories of four city-states: Florence, Pistoia, Lucca, and Pisa. Most of her gifts were far smaller, several amounting to legacies a peasant might bestow—5 lire to the female recluses of Maiano, 5 lire to the poor of the Ospedale di San Piero Gattolino, 10 soldi to a nun at the abbey of Pratovecchio.[78]

Less affluent Florentines also scattered their alms among similarly large arrays of pious beneficiaries. In the same year Saverinus, a citizen of Florence otherwise identified only by a patronymic, made 46 pious bequests. Many were deemed in shillings—100 soldi for the minor friars of Figlino (Valdarno), 100 soldi for the Franciscans at Barberino (the Mugello), 100 soldi for the minor friars at Castro Fiorentino, 100 soldi for the minor friars at Borgo San Lorenzo, and so on.[79] Several of his, however, were not simple, straightforward sums of money, but substantial funds earmarked for specific purchases and purposes. His opening itemized gift was his largest, 200 lire to the Franciscans at Santa Croce. And, unlike so many donors of one-line itemized legacies that fill testamentary ledgers of central Italy in the late Duecento, Saverinus placed specific obligations on his holy recipients: that 50 lire of this gift were to be given to the sacristy to purchase "a book, that is an *antifonario* or a *letionario* or a missal or any other book of great necessity," and that another 50 lire should go to the *opera* of the chapel in its infirmary "for the ornamentation and furnishings of its altars."

In 1301 Ermellina, a widow of the nobleman from the Malispini lineage, made 45 separate pious bequests. Her estate was not nearly so enormous as the properties of the Contessa Beatrice, and the monetized parcels that she sprinkled across the ecclesiastical landscape were on average considerably smaller. Most amounted only to 10 soldi (which would not have even provided the cheapest cloak for one of the poor of Christ). Some conveyed even less: for instance, 2 soldi to the friars at Santa Croce for two masses; 2 soldi to the Cathedral of Santa Reparata, again for two masses; and 5 soldi to the nuns tied to the parish church of San Iacopo tra le fosse.[80]

Earlier the same year, the Lord Schiatta f.q. domini Bocche f.q. domini Rayneri Rustici, of the Abbati family, gave an even larger number of pious bequests (55). Although he was considerably richer than the noble lady, Ermellina, many of his gifts were amounts calculated in shillings— 40 soldi for the hospital of the Bigallo, 20 soldi for a hospital in the rural town of San Casciano, 20 soldi for the nuns of San Matteo Arcetri, 20 soldi for the nuns of Torre in the Valdipesa, 20 soldi for the recluses of Santa Maria Urbana, and so on. Not all the nobleman's property conveyances, however, were so straightforward and simple; nor, when facing death and the dispersion of property, did he leave behind all worldly and future considerations of his lineage. He earmarked "one-eighth part of 30 parts" of all his palaces, houses, lands, and buildings in the Florentine parishes of Orsanmichele, San Bartolommeo al Corso, and San Martino al Vescovo to his *consortes* and blood relatives (*suis consortibus et consanguineis*) of the lineage of the Abbati (*de stirpe Abbatorum*). The nobleman then painstakingly and in complex detail filled a considerable portion of his long will by specifying more precisely what he meant, *"scidelicet"*: to Domino Guerrerio Domini Renzi and Picchino f.q. domini Raneri Rustici, "two parts of eight parts of the said eighth part," and to Feltruccio f.q. domini Durantis f.q. domini Raneri de Abbatibus, Bocchino, et Niccolò, et Jacomino, et Nero, et Teruccio f.q. Terucci f.q. domini Durantis f.q. domini Raneri, one part, that is, half a part to Feltruccio and the other half to the others; and the other part to Bettino f.q. domini Batis f.q. Rustici de Abbatibus. And the list of relatives and their respective shares and parts of shares goes on. Moreover, Schiatta placed on these heirs the charitable obligation of first granting 50 lire to "the poor in need" before assuming any of the "rents or accommodations" from these properties. The list of shares in the patrimony was followed by another gift to one of the above-listed *"consortes et consanguines"* of the houses and lands in the Castro Cappiani, including the *"jus patronatus"* the testator possessed in the church of San Michele de Morniano in the plebatus of San Vito in Incisa, provided that this relative pay off within six months a debt of 300 florins.[81]

On first impression, the fragmentation of these property rights into fractions of already divided fractions might appear to underscore the mendicant perspective. But, in comparison to testaments such as the one from the widow Ermellina, described above, or the dozens of noble wills redacted in Siena or Pisa during the early years of the Trecento, Schiatta's secular concern to map in mathematical detail the precise property portions and the incumbent charitable obligations of his heirs is striking. In Siena and Pisa during the early Trecento, even the nobility devised long lists of simple, straightforward legacies and refrained from spinning such complex webs. At the close of their testaments they simply named their universal heirs, giving them equal rights to the patrimony. Or in cases (as is clear from Schiatta's will) where no direct heirs survived, they most often left the estate to a hospital or some other ecclesiastical institution without further elaboration.

Lord Schiatta's long lists of legacies, moreover, differed in a second respect from those found for the merchant elite of early Trecento Siena or Pisa. While directions for how the body was to be honored in funerals during the first half of the Trecento are rare, Schiatta gave "for the love of God" the honorary scarlet and fur, which his Franciscan pallbearers were to wear to glorify his burial; one of the three to don these honorary furs of nobility was to be a member of the Abbati *stirpe*.[82]

In a 1312 testament, a commoner (*discretus vir*), Ricchuccius f.q. Pucci, who lived in the parish of Santa Maria Novella, gave 42 separate pious gifts. A number of these conveyed paltry sums — 3 soldi for masses to the friars of Santa Maria degli Angeli; another 6 soldi for candles; 6 soldi apiece to 12 nunneries of the city and suburbs; 15 soldi to the hospital of San Bartolommeo de Mugnone; 17 soldi to the preaching friars of Cortona, another 17 soldi to the Dominicans at Pistoia, and so on. But again, not all of these pious bequests were such single-line direct conveyances of pious sums; other matters, such as earthly memory, were clearly at stake. One of Ricchuccius's first bequests was of considerable sum, given that he was a nonmagnate citizen of the early Trecento — 700 lire to the Capitans of the *laudesi* confraternity of Santa Maria Novella. Moreover, he obliged these friars to use it to purchase landed property and from this property's yearly rents to distribute 100 lire in perpetuity to the poor. But the testament's relatively small bequests were the most remarkable. Five lire were to go yearly for two ounces of oil — one ounce for the "continuous" illumination of a lamp in front of the crucifix in the church of Santa Maria Novella "painted by the distinguished painter named Giottus Bondonis from the parish of Santa Maria Novella" and located near a lantern constructed of bones, which the testator had earlier purchased for that Dominican church (*coram quo crucifixo est laterna ossea empta per ipsum testatorem*). The other ounce associated this testator's perpetual memory with one of the most important art objects from

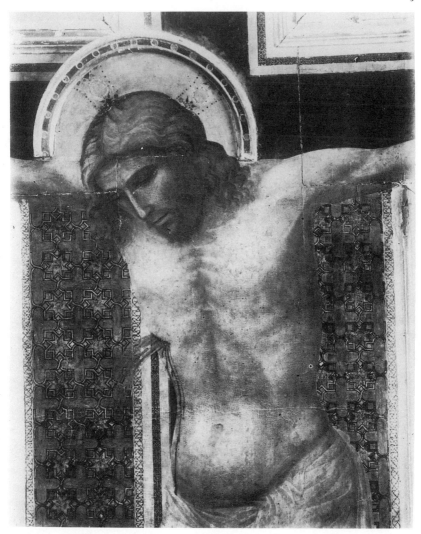

1. Giotto, *Painted Cross* (detail). Sacristy of Santa Maria Novella, Florence (Courtesy Soprintendenza alle gallerie-Firenze, no. 25405).

Tuscany of the latter Middle Ages: it was to illuminate a large panel painting (*magna tabula*) of the blessed Virgin—which was none other than Duccio's *Rucellai Madonna*, commissioned by the *laudesi* of Santa Maria Novella in 1285.[83] Nor did Ricchuccius's schemes for remembrance end here. Again, he invoked the name of an artist to enhance his own reputation and lasting memory—an act unprecedented in the nearly thirty-four hundred testaments sampled for this study—by bequeathing a mere 20 soldi to the Dominicans at Prato, adding that it was to be burnt "for the illumination of the beautiful panel painting existing in the church of this monastery which he, this Ricchuccius, had earlier commissioned to be painted by the excellent painter named Giotto Bondone of Florence."[84]

Another of Ricchuccius's pious bequests endowed the friars of Santa Maria Novella with 12 lire "for a modest and honest meal [pro una moderata et honesta refectione sive pitantia] to be given to the monastery on the feast day of the blessed Juliana, the Virgin and Martyr, which occurs on the 16th day of February." This day, he then added, was also the day of the "felicitous memory of the man Ricchus, called the miller from the parish of Santa Maria Novella, whose loss," the testator exclaimed in his will, "was a debt to the human condition." (Ricchus was the testator's beloved uncle for whose salvation he had already given pious gifts.) To honor his own and his deceased uncle's souls at the meal, the testator further demanded the presence of the captain and the treasurer of the confraternity of Santa Maria Novella, who happened to be his blood relative Lippus Bonagratie, and his father-in-law, Baldus Venture Borghi, both parishioners of Santa Maria Novella. In this assembly congregated to enjoy the testator's feast, the prior of Santa Maria Novella was to celebrate a solemn office for the dead and for the salvation of the testator, his late uncle, and all his relatives, the living as well as the dead. Ricchuccius here made no overtures toward mendicant humility, nor did he evoke the ephemeral world of human memory and action. Instead, he commanded the prior to commemorate the testator and his uncle and afterward, when preaching to the assembled parish congregation in the church of Santa Maria Novella, to proclaim this testator's munificence.

Ricchuccius continued this long will with another small gift, which again went well beyond the purview of the typical simple, one-line legacy of the early Trecento. He left 20 soldi to the minor friars of Santa Croce—8 soldi for bread, wine, and candles, to be dispensed when Ricchuccius died, and the remaining 12 soldi to purchase candles of soft wax (cera humida) at Christmas "to illuminate the night of this birth," while three masses were to be celebrated in Santa Croce "for the reverent benediction of the infant child this night born in the manger to the Virgin Mary." Nor did Ricchuccius's solemn demands for the rights of his benefaction end here. He further insisted that the guardian of the Franciscans at Santa Croce solemnly commemorate his own and his late uncle's souls, again calling attention to their earthly deeds by insisting that the guardian mention in his sermons to his "assembled congregations" that both the testator and his uncle had served as captains of the *laudesi* confraternity of Santa Maria Novella. The Franciscan guardian, moreover, was further to praise and "restore to memory" the time when the testator had been the executor of the testament of this uncle, the testator claiming that in this role he "had brought honor to the friary and to the entire province" through his administration of "his [uncle's] charitable largess"—that is, "through works, buildings and the money" that remained from selling off the properties "liberally bequeathed" by his beloved uncle.[85] In the testaments from Siena, Assisi, and Pisa, no self-proclamation or stress on earthly memory at any time comes close to that of this Florentine commoner at the beginning of the Trecento, whose testamentary efforts at self-promotion went so strongly against the current of mendicant ideology.

Like the other towns, Arezzo before the second outbreak of pestilence possessed wills with long lists of single-line legacies conveying small sums and asking little in return. One of the earliest was the 1305 will of the knight in the Order of the Blessed Mary, Iacobus f.q. Benecente, who left 50 pious gifts, mostly of 20-soldi allotments to the hospital of Brune for sheets, to the hospital in the communal piazza for sheets, to the hermits of Lignano, and so on. In 1308, Margarita, the widow of Gavardi Aldobrandini, left 35 pious bequests, which splintered her estate into even thinner shards: 12 pennies to the bishop, 5 soldi to the confraternity of the Franciscans, 40 soldi to be dispersed among all those within the city of Arezzo who had walled themselves in (*muratis et carceratis*), 3 soldi to the nuns of Santa Margarita, 5 soldi to the hermits of Sanpolo, etc. In a fashion that recalls the anguish and disgust of the contemporaneous poet Cecco Angiolieri of Siena, who angrily derided the mendicant hypocrisy of his parents and the consequent loss of his inheritance,[86] the widow left a token 20 soldi to her secular son, Bindo, instituting him as an heir with the formulaic condition that he remain quiet and content and ask for no more. Against the tradition of preserving and passing her estate down successive generations, the widow left as her universal heir her other son, Dominus Alexius, a monk living in the hills of Camaldoli.[87]

The 1310 testament of another woman, domina Adelascia, the widow of Bruni f.q. Completti de Volpis, of Arezzo's *plebis* church, evoked the same religious ideology. Not a single one of her pious sums dispersed over 33 pious causes constituted a significant gift by which the beneficiary might have had cause to remember her, and none placed any conditions or demands on the recipients of her largess. All were conveyances in coin except three for small weights of wax and negligible measures of bread. Further, monetary sums of up to a paltry 10 shillings constituted more than two-thirds of these itemized legacies to confraternities, parish churches, nunneries, and hermitages. The largest of her gifts was for 50 lire, but it was not to be spent on a single religious person or entity; rather, her executors were to purchase clothing and to disperse it to the "poor and destitute." Clearly, this testator, like so many men and women before the plague of 1363, was intent, at least when on her deathbed, on banishing any thought of earthly remembrance or attachment to earthly property. Along with many other Tuscan and Umbrian testators, she acted out the antimaterialism that Petrarch eloquently expressed at the very end of this tradition: "Now I come to the disposal of those things which men call goods, although frequently they are rather impediments to the soul,"[88] or what Saint Catherine more simply labeled, along with children and other relatives, as matters "on loan,"[89] and what earlier had been a common topos in mendicant preaching. Jacopo Passavanti decried throughout his writings "the stubbornness and misery" of "men of the world." For Domenico Cavalca, a Pisan Dominican, the essence of Christianity was humility, and worldliness was the worst of sins.[90] Even the pragmatic peacemaker, the Dominican Giordano da Pisa, who, Daniel Lesnick has argued, supplied the oligarchic patrons of Santa Maria Novella with an ideology suitable to their social and political dominance,[91] saw earthly gain and worldly pride as the cardinal sins to be combated first and foremost: "I find one fault in this world," said Giordano, "and it is general to all peoples. It is an evil love of the world."[92]

But in Arezzo, unlike Pisa, Siena, and Assisi, no single ideological pattern so thoroughly dominated testators' passions and strategies for salvation. Alongside testaments like those of the widows Margarita and Adelascia, whose scattering of earthly remains so well bespoke the ideals of mendicant piety, others, such as Lord Symoneus, the son of Ser Benvenuti, certainly had other ideas than what Saint Catherine would later instruct as the need to be "forgetful of self" to become "utterly consumed in the fire of divine Charity."[93] While the wealthy Symoneus did make a few small bequests—a 15-soldi gift to the nuns at Santa Maria di Plonta and 10 soldi to those of the Poor Clares at Monte Calvi—even these came with demands for remembrance. In both cases, the nuns had to earn these paltry sums through chanting in unison 50 paternostre with Ave Marie and a Posalterum for the salvation of his soul.

More importantly, this long will was not devoted to splintering and dispersing the testator's patrimony over a wide array of churches, confraternities, hospitals, and hermitages. Instead, its bulk concentrated on the opposite: how to preserve for posterity his massive library, whose volumes and titles he individually enumerated and painstakingly divided between the Dominicans and Franciscans—works by Cicero, Pliny, Thomas Aquinas, Cassidorus, Isodore of Seville, Boethius, Seneca, Livy, Clement, Paul; the fables of Aesop; books on prayer, consolation, music, history, and agronomy. After the long lists of authors, titles, and the volumes in which they were bound, Lord Symoneus placed conditions on his generous gift. Both religious orders were to keep these volumes locked within their monasteries in closets secured with iron chains (sub catena ferrea); "no prior, friar, conversus or any other person" should ever "remove or alienate from this room or monastery for any reason or by any right or by any kind of alienation—exchange, accommodation, loan, deposit, sale, trade or by any right whatsoever of removal or theft—any book from these chambers; otherwise, the books would pass to the custody of the other friary."[94]

Nor was this his only gift that placed demands on his beneficiaries and would later tie his name to a foundation to be preserved after his death. Symoneus's opening gift "assigned" 200 lire of annual income from his landed estates to the Dominican friars, who in return were to build an altar "in a place which his executors deemed decent." With this income the friars were "to celebrate masses at the altar continuously, that is every day, and on Mondays and Fridays they were to chant a mass for the dead, for the souls of the testator, his relatives, his brothers, sisters, and other blood relations [consanguineorum], his business associates [sotiorum], servants and benefactors." On the other days masses were to be said with prayers for the testator and for the souls of all the above-mentioned categories of relations and associates.

This testator founded yet another altar, this one in Arezzo's cathedral. Here, he pried much further into the affairs of the church by "electing" through the instrument of his will the first priest for his chapel, Orlandus Umveli, who was to officiate divine masses "unless impeded by illness." Symoneus, moreover, required this priest to participate every day in the celebration of masses in the cathedral along with the other canons and clerics. He then set out the rules for the chaplain's successors: they were to be priests "of good and honest life, condition and fame" and descendants defined "through both sexes" of the former Ser Benvenuti, the testator's father. And if at the time of succession more than one of his descendants should be living and also happened to be "a sacerdos of honest life and good condition and fame," then the post should devolve on the first-born of these relatives. And if none of his descendants at that time happened to be priests, then the priests of the cathedral should elect "in concord" a man "of good merit and fame, truly constituted in the sacerdotal rank and at least 30 years old." Such demands for the succession of chaplains at private altars and especially for familial sinecures that ran down male bloodlines cannot be found in Sienese samples until well into the Cinquecento.[95]

The childless Symoneus named his sister, a nun at Santa Maria de Plonta in Arezzo, and this convent as his universal heirs. But his efforts at self-memorialization and concern for the physical well-being of his future relations did not rest here. He gave his residual properties to the convent de Plonta on condition that it construct a house "de novo" within its walls with 30 cells for 30 virgin girls born in Arezzo who would assume the rule and habit of the convent. Moreover, he provided once again for his unborn descendants by insisting that the convent accept into these cells any daughters of his sister Beatrice and the daughters of his deceased brother Vanni if they should wish to become nuns. Finally, these nuns, in exchange for the testator's largess, were to pray for the souls of "his relatives, brothers, sisters, business associates and benefactors."[96]

Altarpieces

Monumental gifts commissioned in wills to remind the lay and the holy of testators' earthly glory and to assist in the future salvation of their own souls and those of their ancestors did not necessarily depend on such enormous outlays or building funds as Lord Symoneus's 30-cell monastery or his 156-book library with its specially constructed cabinets, locks, and keys. The testaments of Arezzo, Perugia, and Florence were rich in a form of memorialization almost altogether missing from testaments of the late medieval art center, Siena—commissions for sacred and funerary art. As I shall argue later, testators from Arezzo—a place that hardly ranks in art history above its neighbor to the southwest, Siena—commissioned more works of art per capita in testaments than anywhere else. In these commissions, unlike the offerings of small mon-

etary sums, testators asserted their personalities and desires and expressed their aesthetic values and devotional passions through specific
demands regarding composition, subject matter, and placement within
particular churches, monasteries, and confraternities.

Some of the earliest commissions for altarpieces and other panel
paintings in these documents came from Arezzo. Against the Trecento
trend of dispersing gifts widely over the ecclesiastical and sacred horizons,
domina Iacopa, the widow of Vanni Bonsi, in her 1321 testament concentrated her initial pious gifts on her parish, the *plebis* church of Arezzo:
first, two large candles valued at 6 lire; next, 25 lire for ecclesiastical
objects and furnishings to be used in the church. She then "demanded
and wanted the image of the Virgin Mary" and, next to her, the images
of St. John the Evangelist and Saint Michael painted in this *plebis*. Her
next itemized bequest demanded another painting "at the will of her
executors"—the image of Saint Barbara. For the execution of both
paintings she offered 20 lire—a small sum when measured against known
contracts for monumental works of the period, such as the *Rucellai
Madonna,* which fetched 150 lire in 1285,[97] but which would have been
hefty by the standards of the shilling contributions common to early
Trecento pious gifts. The testatrix, moreover, added a phrase that comes
as close as any in these laconic testamentary demands to the "proto-
humanist" sentiments of her contemporaries Duccio, Giotto, and Simone
Martini: she asked that the images be painted "beautifully and with
lively faces [*vive facce*]."

Unlike the founding of a hospital or an endowment for a chapel,
testamentary art commissions were not so exclusively the domain of
the rich and powerful. As we saw earlier, the son of a blacksmith from
Bibbiena devoted a large section of his modest will to commissioning a
painting, which called for the donor and his deceased father to be shown
genuflecting on each side of the Virgin and to bear the self-commemoration, "Here is Montagne the Blacksmith; here is Pasquino [the son
of] Montagne."[98] Deathbed commissions for sacred paintings could originate from even more humble social levels than that of a blacksmith's
son. Ten-lire altarpieces were not uncommon. In 1331, Martinus Bernardi, from the Perugian village of Villa Plancarpinis, most likely a peasant
or even a rural laborer—his wife's dowry amounted to a mere 25 lire—
donated the bulk of his pious sums (10 lire out of 15 lire 10 soldi,
including his funeral expenses) for the painting of *"una magesta"* to be
placed in his parish church of San Giovanni.[99] In 1348, a Nallus f.q. Pepi
Salomonis, from the village of Castro Casallalte, just across the border

of Perugia in the district of Todi, left 10 lire for a *Maestà* (*pro una maiestate fienda*) in the church where Nallus was to be buried, Santa Maria in Castro Leone, which lay just on the other side of the border in the *contado* of Perugia.[100] Another Perugian testator, *"Magister"* Fillipus Ciutii Ciampantini (most probably a master artisan), this time from the city, and again in the year of the Black Death, donated 10 lire for a painting to beautify (*in reactatione*) the altar of his religious confraternity, the *disciplinati* of San Domenico. Here the testator's instructions were less demanding: his pious sums were to be "converted" into "painted figures."[101] Finally, an ironmonger, Donatus f.q. Ciani, from Arezzo, in 1348 gave eight lire to his parish church and place of burial, Sant'Adriano, to finish making a chasuble (*una planeta*) on which he ordered the painting of "the Blessed Glorious Virgin Mary with her child Jesus Christ" as well as for other "beautifications and ornamentations" in this church.[102] As will be seen in chapters 6 and 7, three cities distinguished themselves in the quantity of art commissioned both before and after the Black Death. These were the three that most resisted a total adoption of the mendicant zeal for piety and instead practiced early on a mixture of self-denial and self-commemoration and promotion not to be found in significant portions or with such explicit proclamations in the other towns until after the return of pestilence in 1363.

The Donoratico and the Tarlati

In contrast to Florence, Arezzo, and Perugia, the largest number of testaments of the mendicant stamp—wills that liquidated a testator's property and then dispersed it in paltry sums over numerous pious causes—is found in late Duecento and Trecento Pisa. Over one hundred Pisan testaments, just under one in seven from all levels of Pisan society, conveyed 20 or more itemized gifts each to charities and religious institutions.[103] Sixteen testaments conveyed 40 or more pious legacies; all of these preceded 1363. The records, nonetheless, do show that even in Pisa the mendicant sway was not completely monolithic, especially in records before the Trecento. In fact, the earliest notices of sacred art and the earliest testamentary commissions found in the samples drawn for all six cities come from Pisa. In 1264, Lazarus f.q. Talliapanis, formerly from the Borgo of San Genesio, then living in the Pisan parish of San Cristoforo in the quarter of Chinzica, left, among his numerous bequests, four lire for oil to be burnt "every day and night in a lamp in front of the figure of the Virgin Mary and the Lord Jesus Christ in honor of the Virgin." Another lamp was to be kept lit in front of the figure of the Holy Cross, again located in his parish church. Twenty years later, the long-distance trader Angelus Spina f.q. Ruggeri Spine, of Messina (Sicily), who claimed to have been living in Pisa "now for years," expressed cosmopolitan and eastern proclivities by ordering an icon (una chonia) with gold gilding (deaurata) and depicting Saint Nicholas. The work was to be made and painted and the materials purchased in Pisa but placed "above the great chapel [supra cappellam grossam]" in the church of Saint Nicholas in the Sicilian village of Monivento.[104]

One of the most remarkable of these early commissions certainly eschewed any notions of mendicant self-deprecation, but again it involved a testator with international horizons. In 1284, the merchant Palmierus f.q. Vicini, from the Pisan parish of San Martino, bequeathed the then extraordinary sum of 160 Pisan lire[105] to the church of Mary Magdalene in the village called Alabialma (Le Balme), located in the district of Marseilles, to produce out of wax an ex voto figure of himself.[106]

But toward the end of the Duecento through the Trecento until the 1370s, such commissions fade away almost entirely from the massive number of testaments whose parchments became crammed with numerous single-line charitable bequests of negligible sums. One of the most extraordinary of all these "mendicant" testaments found for any of the six cities came from a Pisan—in fact, a nobleman of the ancient Gherardesca feudal lineage and the founder of the short-lived Signoria of Pisa, which ended with his death in 1341.[107] Despite his achievements and the concrete works initiated in his lifetime—the completion of the celebrated leaning tower, builder of the Palazzo degli Anziani,[108] founder of the University of Pisa, and celebrated by historians for bringing about Pisa's last "golden age"—Bonifacius Novellus, Count Donoratico, when faced with death did little to perpetuate his fame and glory. Instead, his 1337 testament dispersed the estate richest in the sum of its monetized legacies of the thirty-four hundred testaments selected for this study into a multitude of itemized slivers. His 167 separate itemized bequests totaled 13,172.57 florins (not including the certainly more valuable landed properties left to his universal heirs). Nearly 90 percent (148) of those bequests worth approximately 6,671.84 florins went to pious causes. Many did not even exceed three lire, such as those gifts to the sacristy of the Carmelite church, to the infirmary of the monastery of San Donnino, to the infirmaries at the convent of San Bernardo, Santa Clara, Sant'Anna, Ognissanti, and Sant'Agostino.

The average of the count's monetized pious bequests was 45.08 florins—hardly modest by early Trecento standards. Yet a number of large bequests drew this average upward. These were, moreover, for the most part unlike the chapel foundations or the commands for hospital or monastic constructions, which dotted the early Trecento testaments from Arezzo, Perugia, and Florence. With one or two exceptions, even Bonifacius's larger legacies carefully circumvented any mundane desire to leave a concrete presence for the veneration or even association of the testator's name with a pious institution, a new foundation, or a new construction. To atone for his illicit gains, the count gave 400 lire to the poor of Pisa; for the health of the souls of his relatives and his son, his executors were to distribute 200 lire to the poor; 400 lire were to go to the poor in the lands of the Gherardesca; 400 lire to the "poor and destitute" in the villa Conese and the villa Massargia as well as for marrying off poor girls; 1,000 lire—again, a gift spawned by guilt over earthly endeavors—were to be distributed to those whom the count had "damaged" or caused to go into debt. Finally, the largest of the count's pious gifts was also the vaguest: if his son should die without heirs, 1,000 florins should go to the poor.

Of his 148 pious gifts, only two failed to circumvent self-commemoration. The first was a gift at the end of this lengthy testament that was again contingent on the death of his son and universal heir. In this case, the count's enormously valuable properties were to be fragmented and distributed to numerous pious and nonpious parties. But of these, one called for the construction "in our place, Collis Sallecti, and in our house in this place" a nunnery of the order of Santa Clara that would receive for "its endowment and perpetual charity" all the "possessions, farms [poderi] and real estate [bona stabile]" in that locality. The second ordered his executors to buy landed property worth 600 lire to endow the high altar in the count's ancestral parish of San Martino Chinzica[109] and to support the altar's chaplain, whose rights of election would be the property and responsibility of the count's heirs. If the male line of heirs should become extinct, the rights of election would "devolve" on the abbess of the convent of San Martino, attached to the parish, and the abbess of the convent of All Saints, near Pisa. Another 400 lire was then given to help complete the construction of the choir of this parish and to finish its altar.[110]

To put the designs and sentiments opaquely expressed in this enormously rich testament into perspective, we need to cross the map of Tuscany and look at this count's peer and contemporary, "the noble, wise and powerful man" Dominus Tarlatus miles natus f.q. Nobilis et potentis viri Angeli domini Tarlati, from Pietramala, citizen of Arezzo, whose family ruled the territory of Arezzo from the opening years of the Trecento to 1336. His was the only will found in my samples to approximate that of the Donoratico in its total of monetized bequests, 11,957 florins, 5,937 florins of which went to pious causes. This grandiose sum, however, filled less than a third as many itemized pious bequests as found in the testament of Count Bonifacius: 47 as against 148. Of the monetized gifts, Tarlatus's were on average six times the value of those bequeathed by the Pisan Donoratico. To be sure, Tarlatus, like his counterpart to the west, made bequests of relatively small sums. But the smallest of these were personal gifts and went, not to the nameless poor or to nuns and monks in a myriad of orders scattered throughout the city and countryside, but to individually enumerated and named household servants — maids, cooks, *"familiares,"* and "boys."

It was the big gifts, however, that sharply distinguished the two men's religious ideologies and divergent passions for salvation. Tarlatus gave the largest single religious bequest found in these documents for any city at any time. At the center of this fabulous gift lay quite literally Tarlatus himself. "For the praise, reverence and honor of the Omnipotent God, the Blessed Virgin Mary his mother, the Blessed Michelangelo, Blessed Francis and the entire celestial court," 4,000 florins were "to be spent for the work, construction and completion" of the Franciscan church, which he claimed "now to have begun and founded in the sacred place at La Verna" — the mountaintop wilderness, which constituted the minor friars' first undisputed possession, acquired in 1213. He then specified that the money was to be spent on a chapel so grand that he called it both a church and a chapel, located in the middle of the church (of La Verna) where the testator had elected the sepulcher for his body. Tarlatus demanded that his grave lie "before and immediately next to the predella of the altar in this chapel, that is in the middle of the church."[111] The church still preserves his memory, bearing his arms and those of his wife on the pilaster of the third bay of the nave and in the sacristy, with this inscription under the portico of the church:

A.D. MCCCXLVIII. Nobilis. Miles. dominus. Tarlatus. de Petra Mala. et domina. comitissa. Johanna. de. Sancta. Flora. uxor. eius. edificari. fecerunt. istam. ecclesiam. ad. honorem. Beatae. Mariae. semper. Virginis.[112]

Anticipating a trend in poor relief which would not fully materialize in these towns until the very end of the Trecento, Tarlatus distributed his poor relief to specially elected poor virgins rather than in small allotments doled out indiscriminately to the poor of Christ (or for dowries) like the largest bequests bestowed by his peer to the west, Count Fazio. Tarlatus's second largest pious bequest established an extraordinarily prized dowry fund of 4,000 lire to enable 40 virgin girls to marry. Unlike indiscriminate handouts, this sum would have provided substantial dowries even by the standards of master artisans or shopkeepers of the mid-Trecento (100 lire for each girl). Moreover, Tarlatus's rules for selection were geographically specific: 20 were to be "found" (*prout reperiantur*) in the city of Arezzo, 4 were to come from the *castro* of Bibbiena and its curia, 2 from Pietramala, 2 from Montaguto Stalla, 2 from Montecchio and Vignale, 4 from Chiusi, and 1 each from Giampareto, Serra, Villa Ama, Roccha Verano, and Castro Sieci.

Further, Tarlatus supplemented the earlier endowment by his wife, the Nobile et Sapiens domina, Domina Contessa Johanna, of Santa Fiore, for a chapel under construction and ordained in the cathedral of Arezzo. His construction plans touched less grandiose projects as well—100 lire for the building of a single hermit's cell at the hermitage of Camaldoli. Finally, his small bequests to churches, monasteries, and nunneries differed from those of the Pisan ruler. Instead of coin, Tarlatus also gave at this level something concrete—silver chalices (valued at 12 florins apiece) for the altars of 13 different churches in the territory of Arezzo.

In conclusion, the message of mendicant preachers sank deeper roots into the psychology of testators from Assisi, Pisa, and Siena than is apparent from testaments redacted in the other three cities. Even the wealthy and well-born in these territories carefully shunned the hubris of earthly memory in their plans for salvation. Aretines, Florentines, and Perugians differed from the other three city-states, not only in the number, but also in the character of their pious bequests. While they too sought salvation by spreading their pious wealth over a number of charitable causes, they did not at the same time circumvent all desires for earthly memory before the recurrence of plague in the 1360s. Within monotonous lists of pious contributions fragmented into small amounts of coin, those from Arezzo, Florence, and Perugia often embraced the contradictory ideals of self and lineage to be commemorated through perpetual masses, meals, altarpiece commissions, and burial tombs emblazoned with coats of arms plastered in sacred places.

The differences between these cities, as I shall illustrate more fully

in subsequent chapters, became less pronounced after the second occurrence of plague in the 1360s, regardless of the differing economic
fortunes that ran in the wake of the Black Death and through the early
Quattrocento. The convergence in the patterns of piety and the structure
of testamentary giving in the six city-states was even more striking than
that portrayed by the earlier differences. Nor can these changes in pious
giving be attributed simply to a shrinking pool of pious beneficiaries after
the demographic incursions of the Black Death (as might well have been
hypothesized from a view of the Sienese testaments seen in isolation).
As we saw in Chapter 2, not everywhere did hospitals, such as Siena's
Santa Maria della Scala, gobble up smaller institutions through the
Trecento, thus forming a near-monopolistic megahospital. Nor did the
nunneries in all these places all but disappear, as seems to have been
the case in Siena, where the female convents remained few in number,
at least as the recipients of pious legacies during the second half of the
Trecento.[113] Despite such institutional and organizational differences
from place to place, the six cities show a common trajectory in the
patterns of pious bequests for the late Trecento and early Quattrocento.

Here, 1348 was not the watershed. In fact, for that date or the interval
separating the two outbreaks of pestilence, the number of pious gifts
and the extent of the parcelization shot upward, at least momentarily,
in Florence, Arezzo, Perugia, and Assisi. After 1363, the trend was
different: the old mendicant-inspired wills, in which testators tried to
relinquish all ties to earthly possessions by liquidating their worldly
goods and then parceling them out to numerous churches and pious
causes, all but disappeared. After controlling for differences in wealth,
the status of the testators, the type and origin of the documents, whether
the testator lay on the deathbed, residency in a city or the countryside,
and whether the testator had surviving sons to inherit the patrimony,
the testaments reveal a global change in attitudes toward charity and
the afterlife that swept through large swaths of central Italy. We need
now to turn to the ways testators expressed this new consciousness in
what they demanded for their bodies, their property, and their artistic
commemorations.

II

Directions from the Grave

4

The Body

Everywhere I turn my terrified eyes funeral rites disturb me; filled with caskets, the temples resonate with mourning, and the cadavers of nobles and plebs alike lie about without honor.

—Petrarch, "Ad seipsum"

he numbers of pious gifts per testator and the qualitative data on testamentary commissions for art, chapel foundations, and dowry funds separate the six cities into two broad camps: Florence, Arezzo, and Perugia, on the one hand; Assisi, Pisa, and Siena, on the other. In the late Duecento and early Trecento, testators from the first group took on, less decisively than those from the second group, the mendicant strategies of diffusing their pious designs over the ecclesiastical landscape and thereby shunning signs of earthly hubris. To be sure, the wealthiest from Florence, Arezzo, and Perugia did disperse their pious bequests over large numbers of charitable causes. Their testaments, however, were often split between these mendicant ideals and the desire to be remembered on earth. Even lowly artisans and peasants from these city-states might stake a claim on earthly agencies to further their temporal memory, while, by contrast, those from the ruling elites in the other three city-states, powerful men such as the early Trecento Donoratico of Pisa, in spite of enormous wealth, made few legacies that left concrete signs for earthly remembrance or demanded specific tasks from future heirs or pious beneficiaries.

We need to press this investigation further, to go beyond the systematic but sometimes arid statistics on the values and numbers of pious bequests, their ratios, and their trendlines over time to try to incorporate the flesh and blood of actual individual aspirations that can be gleaned as well from the testaments. The contrast between the two wealthiest testators found in my samples—the Aretine Tarlati and the Pisan Donoratico—shows not only a structural difference measured quantitatively and abstractly by the size, value, and number of pious gifts. At the center of the most valuable pious bequest found in any of these documents lay quite literally the body of the "noble and powerful man" Tarlatus. It provided the endowment to build "the middle chapel" of La Verna, which was to enshrine the body and sepulcher of the noble testator. The equally powerful and possibly even wealthier Count Donoratico was certainly not oblivious to the last rites in regard to his own body. He elected to be buried in the sepulcher of his father and uncle, located in the Franciscan church of Pisa; and one of his most valuable gifts, 800 lire, was to be dispersed for his burial, wax and candles, masses, and sums to the poor to be distributed on the day of his death and on the seventh and thirtieth days afterward.

The difference was not merely quantitative—that Tarlatus spent nearly ten times as much as his contemporary for the perpetual commemoration of his body. Rather, it was the difference in the character of these two allocations of money. While Count Donoratico's charity would vanish after "the thirtieth day" (unlike some others in Pisa, he did not even make provisions for the anniversary of his death day), Tarlatus made the largest single pious contribution to preserve and commemorate his body for perpetuity by means of a lasting work of sacred art and architecture. The French anthropologist Robert Hertz once said that to understand a society, look to see what happens to the body.[1] Did these testamentary provisions change over time or vary systematically from region to region in regard to the last rites and final resting places, and if so, what do they tell us?

Funerals

PISA   Not until the late sixteenth century, after the Council of Trent and the Counter Reformation had fully penetrated Siena, did testators regularly orchestrate the movements of their funeral processions; the weights of the candles and torches; the groups responsible for carrying the coffin; and the numbers, ranks, and religious orders of those who would accompany the corpse from the residence to the parish church to the burial grounds. In fact, the Sienese wills before the end of the Quattrocento hardly mention the funeral—the number of masses; the allotments of wax, candles, bread, wine, or clothing for the poor. On this score the Sienese notaries and testators were, however, the odd ones out. Their wills only referred to burial expenses, which may or may not have included the funerary preparations. Of course, these matters may have been routinely administered by the parish or the religious confraternity (as indeed was the case in the Florentine company of Orsanmichele).[2]

In contrast to Sienese testamentary practice, Pisan notaries and their clients specified their funerary expenses in the routine, formulaic phraseologies almost from the earliest records. The 1263 will of Adalasia, the widow of Alberto from Vecchiano, then living in the urban parish of San Piero a Vinculo, elected to be buried in the monastic church of San Michele of the Discalciatori and gave eight lire to be spent on the day of her death and the seventh and thirtieth days.[3] Other early documents specified more precisely to what ends these sums were to be spent. A Lazarus, formerly of San Genesio, then living in the Pisan parish of San Martino, labeled as "funeral expenses" the sums for the days of his death, the seventh and thirtieth, and the anniversary.

Clearly, the funeral in Pisa was not seen as a single ceremony at a single moment in time; rather, it could drag out over the course of an entire year. Unlike most of these Pisans, Lazarus made specific monetary allocations for each of the various moments in his funeral. On the day of his death, his *fideicommissiari* were to pay six lire for "offices" at altars, for clerics, for his shroud (*cilicium campannorum*), for bread to be given to the poor and for his burial. On the seventh day, another six lire were to be donated to the poor and to clerics for bread and for the health of the testator's soul, and, on the thirtieth, another six lire would go for the same. Finally, he allocated two lire for bread to be doled out to the poor on the anniversary of his death.[4]

On occasion, testators and their notaries separated the burial expenses from the other funeral costs. An Ugo sive Federigo, from the parish of San Lorenzo, paid the Franciscans of Pisa 3 lire to be buried in their church, but donated over five times that amount for his funeral: 15 lire for masses to be sung on his death day; 10 soldi for masses "and other things" on "the seventh" and another 10 soldi for the same on "the thirtieth."⁵ Funeral and burial expenses in Pisa varied from several lire to as much as the 800 lire left for Count Donoratico's three-day celebration. The notary and son of a notary Guido f.q. Petri, from the village of Calcinaria, who at the time of his 1313 testament was living in Pisa's new hospital, then called the Misericordia of Santo Spirito, must have fallen on hard times. His will conveyed only two bequests: his bed, valued at a meager 3 lire, was to go to the Pisan hospital, and his burial expenses. He elected his place of burial at (apud) the hospital of the Misericordia and left only two lire to be distributed for funerary and burial costs on the day of his death plus "the seventh" and "the thirtieth."⁶

These sums contrast with the more lavish plans of the Pisan citizen Petrus f.q. Celli de Gaytanis, who in 1360 elected to be buried in the Cathedral of Pisa at the foot of the steps to the main portal. He was to be clothed in a suit (una rauba), which he specified as "his best cloak and hat [mantello et caputio de melioribus]." If he were to die at his country estate, in the village of Cascina, he asked that he be buried in the choir of the village's plebis church, "that is behind the major altar" of this church. For his death day, "the seventh," and "the thirtieth," he ordered that 300 lire be spent: first, to dress each of his nephews in a gown and a coat; then, to pay the priest Johannes f.q. Cionis, this priest's brothers, Gerradus and Iacobus, and the priest's niece domina Lippa (presumably for his funeral procession, though this is not specified). Second, the major allocation was to buy a gravestone (quandam lapidem) to be placed on top of his sepulcher, where the testator's name and his coat of arms were to be sculpted.⁷

The most extraordinary of these Pisan funeral expenses comes, however, from someone who instructed his executors "not to make his funeralia pompous, but rather honest and discreet as [they] should find fitting." Johannes, archbishop of Pisa, died shortly after redacting a will in February 1362, leaving 500 florins for a chapel in the cathedral of Pisa, which would provide a stipend for the "continuous" services of a sacerdos to sing masses for the archbishop's soul. This altar was to be Johannes's burial chapel:⁸ "under the stone and marble steps on the right hand side of this church [the cathedral] above a certain marble sarcophagus (arca) then under construction [ibi fienda et ponenda]," the archbishop "desired and demanded" that it be sculpted "in the form and image of the archbishop" and that he be buried in that place. If "any obstacle" should block his burial in the "major church," he ordered the transfer of these monies to endow an altar and to sculpt his sarcophagus in the monastic church and parish of San Paolo Riperarno. And were this impossible, the massive funerary legacy would devolve on the monastic church outside Pisa, Saint Jerome at Agnano.[9]

A month later, the archbishop's executors commissioned *Magister Ninus f.q. Magistri Andree de Pontehere*, from the parish of San Lorenzo de Rivolta, "goldsmith, master and sculptor of stone" (known to art historians simply as Nino Pisano), to execute the tomb and funerary sculpture (*facere, fabricare, sculpere, ponere, ordinare, laborare et murare ac solidare*) in the Pisan cathedral at the precise place first desired by the former archbishop. The commission expanded on the archbishop's cursory designs for his self-preservation. The sepulcher where "the body of the Lord Archbishop was to be placed" should be built, the executors specified, with marble from Carrara.[10] Above "this tomb and sepulcher," Nino was to sculpt in relief (*sculpta relevata*) the image of the Lord Archbishop in "archepiscopal form" with a marble pillow under his head (*cum plumaccio de marmore sculpto subtus capite*) and a marble angel on each side. Above the tomb, there should be a marble sarcophagus (*arca*) with "kneeling arches" (*archettis inginocchiatis*); on the "face of the tomb," he should sculpt a "pietà" in the middle with an angel on each side. On one side of this sepulcher, the image of the Virgin Mary with two angels should appear; on another, the image of the blessed John the Evangelist, again with two angels; on the third side, the image of Saint Peter; and on the fourth, Saint Paul. All these figures were to be carved in marble. Under the tomb, the archbishop's sarcophagus repeated the decorative scheme of three bracketed arches and, on both sides, his sculpted coat of arms. The archbishop's *fideicommissarii* were to pay Master Nino 210 gold florins within 15 months of the date of this contract for all the sculpture and his expenses.[11]

If we think of the funeral not as the Pisan notaries would have it— the ensemble of events from the burial to the masses and bread doled out to the poor, which might last a year after death—but as the procession of the body to its final resting ground, then the Pisan testaments before the second half of the Quattrocento were not so different from the Sienese ones. Few alluded to the candles, the weights of wax, and who should carry or accompany the body to the grave. Quite unlike the elaborate plans and complex movements that those on their deathbeds schemed in Siena by the late sixteenth century, these funeral plans were at best laconic outlines. Nonetheless, more of these arrangements can be found for the maritime city than for the other towns examined in this study. The earliest, dated 1322, comes from a widow who elected

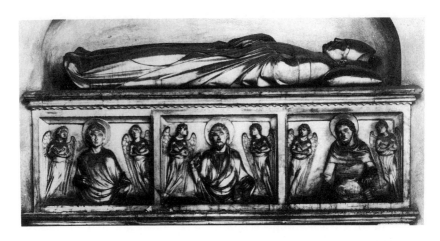

2. Nino Pisano, Sarcophagus and Reclining Effigy of Archbishop Giovanni (Scherlatti),
   d. 1362. Camposanto, Pisa.

burial in the parish and monastic church of San Paolo Riperarno. She
specified for the day of her death and funeral that all the monks of this
monastery should participate, along with 12 priests (*sacerdotes*), and that
each should carry a candle weighing nine ounces.[12]

In 1345, a villager from Calcinaria left 200 lire for his funeral to be
distributed to "prelates and clerics to intercede at his grave."[13] In 1346,
the judge and *operarius* at the Opera di Santa Maria Maggiore ordered
his body "to be honored" when carried to his grave by the intercession
of the cathedral canons, the friars who served in that major church as
well as those who served "minor churches," plus 40 Franciscan friars
and 40 Dominicans of Santa Caterina.[14] In 1347, the widow of a notary
from Campanilo presently married to another notary from Pisa left 40
lire for her burial and *"exequiis."* For this sum, she asked that she be
dressed in canonical robes and buried in the cathedral of Pisa, and that
her body be accompanied (*ad sociandum corpus*) by the Franciscan friars
and the cathedral canons and all their chaplains.[15] In 1364, Henricus of
Serena (Serengo, near Milan) asked that his body be carried to the grave
with the intercession of the Franciscan friars, each bearing one candle
weighing a half pound.[16]

In 1380 the druggist Stephanus was the first in these wills to request
a lay confraternity to accompany his body to the grave, asking for the
intervention of the *disciplinati* of San Simone and giving each lay brother
who "will accompany my body well" the customary allotment of one

candle weighing a half pound.[17] Less than three years later, another Pisan testator requested the spiritual assistance of his confraternity, ordering them to clothe his body in the vestments of the *disciplinati* of Sant'Antonio de Spassavento and to carry him "humbly and devoutly" to his grave in the monastic church of San Paolo Riperarno.[18] In 1397, the wife of a knight (*miles*) from the Lanfranchi family ordered the chaplains of the cathedral to accompany her body to its holy grounds in the Campo Santo. Each chaplain was to carry two torches.[19] In 1416, a nobleman from the Ripafratta family failed to specify exactly who was to carry his body to the monastic church of San Paolo in their ancestral village, but insisted that it be accompanied with "at least" two torches of wax "and no more."[20] In 1418, the widow of the notary from the village of Marti made only one itemized bequest: it instructed her heirs to bury her "honorably and decently" in the tomb of her former husband in the Pisan church of San Viviano and demanded the intercession of the Franciscan friars "up to but not exceeding 20 brothers" plus six to eight chaplains from the Opera del Duomo, each to be given ten soldi.[21]

Among the notaries in these six cities, the Pisans alone began the lists of testamentary bequests with the testator's itemized expenditures for the funeral and burial. These vague allotments for wax, masses, and bread, grain, and coins for the poor, however, rarely specified the burial arrangements or the procession to the grave. Curiously, these clauses became less concrete over time. Particularly after the recurrence of pestilence in 1362, Pisans left these matters — the numbers and expenses for burial masses and the exact monetary sums or measurements of grain to go to the poor — increasingly to their executors' discretion. Paradoxically, this decline of testators' interest in precise funeral costs paralleled, as we have seen from the spotty evidence above, an increase in attention to arranging one's own funerals. More importantly, the decline correlates with the increasing care testators took to specify the location of the bodily remains and to memorialize them with tombstones (*lapis*), inscriptions, monuments, altars, and chapels. Before trying to resolve these enigmas over corporeal concerns and funerals, let us examine the funerary remains left by the testaments of the other four cities.

AREZZO   The notaries in Pisa most consistently indicated their clients' choice of burial (96 percent of the testaments), and those in Arezzo provided it the least often (49 percent of the cases). (See table 9.) While this comparative fact might suggest something about the importance of

Table 9.
Burials

Period	No. Testators	No. Burials	Proportion of Burials
AREZZO			
< 1276			
1275–1300			
1301–25	56	29	0.52
1326–47	93	46	0.49
1348	88	29	0.33
1349–62	66	21	0.32
1363	72	15	0.21
1364–75	87	39	0.45
1376–1400	96	56	0.58
1401–25	101	85	0.84
Total	659	320	0.49
ASSISI			
< 1276	18	4	0.22
1275–1300	22	12	0.55
1301–25	19	18	0.95
1326–47	27	25	0.93
1348	27	25	0.93
1349–62	5	5	1.00
1363			
1364–75	14	14	1.00
1376–1400	30	30	1.00
1401–25	128	125	0.98
Total	290	258	0.89
FLORENCE			
< 1276	14	3	0.21
1275–1300	42	10	0.24
1301–25	54	24	0.44
1326–47	61	43	0.70
1348	73	54	0.74
1349–62	39	28	0.72
1363	74	64	0.86
1364–75	91	70	0.77
1376–1400	113	83	0.73
1401–25	92	80	0.87
Total	653	459	0.70
PERUGIA			
< 1276	2	2	1.00
1275–1300	4	2	0.50
1301–25	10	7	0.70

Table 9.
Continued

Period	No. Testators	No. Burials	Proportion of Burials
PERUGIA			
Continued			
1326–47	61	40	0.66
1348	79	73	0.92
1349–62	20	20	1.00
1363	28	27	0.96
1364–75	51	51	1.00
1376–99	196	179	0.91
1400–1425	73	70	0.96
Total	514	471	0.92
PISA			
< 1276	14	9	0.64
1275–1300	42	42	1.00
1301–25	233	221	0.95
1326–47	98	96	0.98
1348	14	13	0.93
1349–62	66	64	0.97
1363	40	40	1.00
1364–75	50	47	0.94
1376–1400	112	109	0.97
1401–25	72	70	0.97
Total	741	714	0.96
SIENA			
< 1276	35	14	0.40
1275–1300	44	25	0.57
1301–25	50	38	0.76
1326–47	67	57	0.85
1348	55	49	0.89
1349–62	40	29	0.73
1363	24	14	0.58
1364–75	25	24	0.96
1376–1400	61	50	0.82
1401–25	45	40	0.89
Total	446	340	0.76

memorializing the body in these two cultures, I would argue from evidence on specific burials, tombstones, and burial altars (to be reported later) that these statistics are misleading. They instead reflect differences in notarial formula and custom. In Pisa, the notary automatically began his template of questions with the "election" of the place of burial and the expenses for the *die obitii,* the "seventh," and "the thirtieth" days. If the testator did not have a ready answer, he or she (or perhaps the notary) would answer with the formula *videlicet videbintur fidecommissarii.* In contrast, Aretine notaries did not begin their questioning with the body or the soul. Instead, they usually led the testator immediately into the individual itemized bequests, pious or nonpious. When the "elected" place of burial did appear, it did not necessarily come formulaicly at the top of the itemized bequests as was the case with testaments from the other towns. For instance, Angelus f.q. Rossi de Catenaccis's selection of his burial in 1359 came in the middle of his will and was not followed with the formulaic phraseologies found elsewhere, such as *Et Iubeo ac relinquo corpus meum sepelliendum tempore mortis mee apud Ecclesiam . . .* Instead, the Aretine left 150 lire "or more if his executors saw fit" for his funeral and sepulcher and for the anniversary of his death. He demanded that his body be buried in the new church of the Franciscans "in that place in the church towards the portal where the women entered the church."[22]

The Aretine testators said little more about their funeral processions than the Sienese. The only suggestion of a procession comes early in these documents, earlier than in Pisa, and is linked to the earlier and more significant activity of the religious confraternities. In 1308, a man from the village of Torre Classeris (Chiassa), after several nonpious bequests (not the first itemized allocation as it would have been in Pisa), donated 10 lire for the expenses of his burial in the confraternity of the Clerics of the *Plebis* of Classe (Chiusi) and "for their assembly at the time of his death."[23]

Funerals are mentioned in other Aretine testaments, but their expenses were usually clumped together with the burial. One exception to this notarial practice was the testament of domina Druda f.q. Iacobi Conti, from the Sassoli family and the widow of an Aretine notary. At the very end of her testament (even after the appointment of her universal heirs), she elected her grave with the Franciscans and spent 16 lire for the construction of her grave (*monumentum*), which "was to be walled in [*muratum*] and covered well and decently to enclose it completely." She then allotted nearly twice that sum (30 lire) for her other burial expenses and the funeral—wax, her burial clothing (*pannis mortualibus*), and for the clerics to accompany her to the grave.[24] The ironmonger Niccolaus f.q. Uguccii pleaded for modesty in his funerary arrangements in 1361, leaving 25 lire for the *opera* of the Augustinians so that he could be buried at the foot of the pulpit in their church (*in pede leggii*) and dressed "with devotion" in the habit of his lay confraternity of the blessed Trinity. He further wished to be buried underground "without any monument or tomb or casket or funerary pomp." Only four double candles should burn at his funeral, one in his parish of Sant'Adriano and the other three in the Augustinian church.[25] But from this paucity of information, the historian should not assume that the Aretines were oblivious to the outcome and final preservation of their bodily remains. As we shall see, these corporeal matters were of foremost importance in their minds, especially from the late Trecento on.

FLORENCE   Like the Aretine notaries, those from Florence rarely alluded to funeral processions and their costs. Again, the earliest provisions for funerals came from a testator's association with a religious confraternity. In his 1320 testament, the well-known Florentine notary,[26] administrator (*familiaris*) of the confraternal hospital of the Florentine clerics, and cleric (*clericus*) Ser Grimaldus f.q. Campagni, from Pesciola, chose his grave in this hospital and desired the participation of the confraternity's priests, along with the Servites and the monks of San Marco, to attend his burial and mourn for him on the seventh day. For their services, each was to be given two-and-a-half soldi.[27] In 1378, a testator from Vicchio in the Mugello chose his parish of San Lorenzo as the site of his grave and demanded the presence of his kin (*consortes*) "to honor his corpse."[28]

    The most specific of the funerary plans found in these Trecento and early Quattrocento testaments was only slightly more elaborate than the laconic requests cited above and certainly could not hold a candle to baroque Counter Reformation extravaganzas. As in Aretine testaments, the 1396 funerary instructions of the "merchant in the city of Paris" Iacobus de Juochis did not immediately follow the formulaic phrases that opened the itemized bequests—in Iacobus's case, *In primo tamquam bonus catholicus et verus Christianus quia anima est dignior . . .* Instead, they came in the middle of this lengthy document. "If the light of day should pass from his body while in the city of Paris," his executors should see that it be transported back to Florence and buried in the minor friars' church in a chapel, which he had recently (*quam noviter*) ordered to be built. On the day of his death, he instructed the four mendicant orders of Florence—the Carmelites, the Augustinians, the Dominicans, and the Franciscans—to sing vigils for his death "over his body" in the Franciscan church and to celebrate one solemn mass for the health of his soul and his kin. Such an "international" funeral illustrates not only the long-distance relations common to Florentine merchants of the late Trecento but also those of the mendicant orders.[29]

Again, we should not infer from this lack of attention to the body's last passage that Florentines were unconcerned with the preservation of their bones or with the links between bodily remains and earthly memory. Moreover, those with concrete plans to extend their earthly memory and that of their lineages need not have come from the nobility or merchant elite in late Trecento Florence. To take one example: Domina Mante, the widow of Ser Antonio (probably a notary) and the daughter of a parishioner from San Lorenzo, who did not bear a family name, said nothing in her 1369 testament about her funerary preparations or processions; yet, the entire document revolved around a single pious bequest—300 florins for the foundation and endowment of a chapel in the church of San Lorenzo that was to house and exhibit the monument bearing her earthly remains. Within one month, the prior of San Lorenzo was "to institute" in her chapel, then being constructed in San Lorenzo under the name of the blessed Bernardo and Antonio, a chaplain "of mature age, of praiseworthy conscience and reputation and who did not possess a benefice from any other church." This chaplain and his successors were to celebrate "continuously and daily, solemn masses perpetually for the praise of God and for the souls of her daughter, her former husband, her kin and herself." Moreover, each year in perpetuity on the feast days of the blessed Bernard and Antony the chaplain should celebrate "honorably" solemn masses and divine offices, and the prior was obliged to perform each year in perpetuity on the seventh of January an anniversary mass consuming ten pounds of candles made with new wax.

The widow Mante went beyond the ephemeral materials of masses and consumed wax to buttress her earthly memory. She required a stone plaque (*quidam lapis*) "to be placed, sculpted and designed" in this chapel where her coat of arms and that of her former husband "were to be cut in stone for their perpetual memory [*intagliato ad perpetuam memoriam*]." Hers was to have a white background with black lilies; that of her deceased husband, a blue field with two lilies, their stems intersecting across the background. Next, the prior and congregation of San Lorenzo were to construct and "to ornament respectfully . . . next to and facing this chapel" a sepulcher where she was to be buried and the bones of her former husband and her children translated. Finally, the testator prohibited any sale, alienation, or rental of her houses, along with their wells and passageways (volte), in the parish of San Lorenzo; these properties were to "remain in perpetuity, to persist to the end [in perpetuum remanere, persistere ad hoc maximum]" to provide the revenues for the construction of her chapel and the celebration of masses for her soul and that of her husband.[30]

UMBRIA   Like the notaries in Pisa, those in Perugia early on almost invariably provided a slot in their formula, immediately following the election of the burial site, to specify the testator's funeral expenses. Usually it was clumped with the burial, wax for candles, masses, funeral clothes, and, where relevant, the widow's mourning robes and "other expenses." Rarely was the price for the pilum separate from the other expenses, and often these phrases were followed by another formula, which left these decisions to the executors' discretion. Of the 564 testaments, fragments, and codicils selected for Perugia and its territory, not a single one specified who was to fill the ranks and movements of the funeral procession, even though the Perugini in these samples commissioned more paintings destined for burial vaults than did residents of any other city.

In Assisi, the notaries also provided a space for their clients to specify their funeral costs; these could include a sum for wine as well as money for clerics, the poor, wax, and construction of the tomb. The "honorable religious man" and priest dominus Consulus Victorius, rector of Saint Stephen in Assisi, directed in 1348 that one salumen (or soma) of wine,[31] two canisters of bread, and two torches be carried behind the corpse on the way to his grave in the Basilica of San Francesco.[32] Nonetheless, as in Siena and Perugia, details of the funeral—burial masses, donations to the poor, the clergy and family members that were to accompany the body's final procession, and the funeral costs—hardly appear in these documents.

Burial

A first glance at testators' attention in their wills to their bodies and their burial does not corroborate the division of the six city-states into the two large groupings discovered earlier. As mentioned then, the Pisan testators most consistently began their formulaic outlines by prompting the testator to "elect" a church for burial, followed by the sums to be expended on the body's physical and spiritual preparation for the grave and thereafter. Ninety-six percent of them selected their burial grounds.[33] Only in the earliest documents before 1276 did the notaries and their clients fail to supply this information: fewer than two-thirds of the testators indicated their future graves. But this figure compares favorably with that of the other cities during these early years, when only a fifth of the testators in Florence and Assisi elected their burial places, while in Siena the percentage was negligible.[34]

By contrast, Arezzo ranked lowest in testators' selection of graves, followed by Siena (76 percent), Florence (79 percent), and Perugia (92 percent). But these figures, as suggested earlier, appear to have depended heavily on the notarial formula followed in these different civic communities. In Arezzo, Siena, and Florence, particularly in the testaments for the earliest documents through the first half of the Trecento, notaries did not invariably take up these matters immediately after the clichés about the hour of death, the fragility of humanity, or the uncertainty of earthly existence. Instead, as with domina Druda from Arezzo, whose elaborate construction plans for burial came at the end of her testament, or as with the Florentine merchant of Paris, whose instructions came in the middle, these matters of the body could arise anywhere in the testament.

More suggestive is the frequency with which testators specified concretely where their bones were ultimately to lie instead of giving the vague formulaic response of *apud ecclesiam*. This information might indicate location without large outlays of money or new chapel constructions. For example, an Aretine priest in 1348 requested burial in the church of San Vito "next to the portal [*hostium*] through which one could pass into the cemetery of this church."[35] More dramatic was the Aretine condottiere's desire to leave all his armament to the fraternity of the Misericordia, *except* his helmet, which was to rest along with his other insignia on top of his grave in the church of the Servites.[36] At the other extreme were the large-scale construction projects of monuments enshrined with newly built chapels possessing perpetual endowments for masses and a chaplain, as seen in the testaments of the Aretine widow Mante and the *potens vir* Tarlatus.

Of course, consistent notarial prompting of the testator to name his desired place of burial would most likely create higher percentages in the reporting of more precise locations, especially of the former sort that required words more than expenditures. In those earlier times and in cities such as Arezzo, where the notaries left it more to the testators to specify their place of burial, such desires and plans might have been lost among the myriad of preoccupations swarming in the dying testator's head and left as yet another of the unstated chores to be arranged by the heirs or executors. Perhaps these choices were more often left blank in Arezzo because of the importance of lay religious confraternities. Thus, merely by being a member of one of these devotional societies, the testator might simply assume that the religious company would handle the burial arrangements. (As we have seen, the Aretines left a greater share of their pious bequests to these lay groups than elsewhere.) Yet, no clear correlation runs through these cities between confraternal participation and the frequency of burial choices. The percentages for Siena and Florence were about the same (76 percent and 79 percent, respectively), whereas their sponsoring of confraternities was on the opposite ends of the spectrum for these six towns.

When the more specific level of information is examined—that is, when testators went beyond the notarial formula of "electing" the church by the simple but imprecise phrases of "apud" or "in ecclesia" and instead specified the particular spot where their bones were to rest[37]— the hierarchy of these six city-states shifts. From being the least concerned about burials, Aretines even in absolute terms emerge, after the Florentines, as the most preoccupied with them. And, as we shall see, with regard to new constructions that concretely individuated the testator and his lineage, the Aretines were the most obsessed with the memorialization of their bodies. Conversely, with these more specific locations and especially with efforts to preserve earthly remembrance through tombstones, monuments, and chapels, Assisi, which ranked near the top in terms of the frequency of formulaic burial choices, falls to the bottom, far beneath those three cities—Arezzo, Florence, and Perugia— which were less zealous in adopting the mendicant strictures against the hubris of earthly memory. In Assisi, only 18 testators went beyond their notaries' prompting to specify their bodies' location or set aside monies to commission concrete markers. The earliest such command goes back only to the year of the Black Death, 1348, when two testators specified more than the notarial formula would have required: one desired to be buried next to the *pilum* where the prior of the lepers' hospital was entombed;[38] the other demanded his body be interred in the chapel of San Biagio in Santa Maria del Vescovo.[39] The next testament specifically to demarcate a grave came in 1360: Vangnutius Francisci ordered his burial in the church of San Francesco in the chapel of Sant'Antonio de Vienna then under construction. Furthermore, 80 florins were to be spent for paintings and other ornamentation for this chapel, as well as for the testator's tomb (*pro uno pilo*), "to be built above ground in that chapel where his body was to be buried."[40]

The next example of a burial site construction in Assisi must await the end of the century. One of the few noblemen to appear in the Assisi testaments, Nobilis venerabilis vir ac Egregius decretorum doctor, Nerius f.q. Guidonis, a canon lawyer, was not, however, a native of Assisi but came from the Tuscan village of Chianciano in the diocese of Arezzo. He directed work not on his first choice of burial (in the Holy Basilica of Assisi, where the friars might bury him wherever they pleased) but in the sepulcher where his father lay in the Franciscan house of his native town. If he were to be buried in Chianciano, these friars were "to sculpt and incise" a stone plaque bearing his family coat of arms and his own name and title memorialized by the inscription "Sepulcrum domini Nerii Guidonis de Nicoloctis de Chianciano decretorum doctoris et olim vicarii generalis domini Episcopi Assisinatis." This noble immigrant further supplemented the dowry and the building fund for a chapel with an altar then under construction that was to encase this burial shrine, where his uncle as well as his father lay. Twenty-five florins were to be spent for the *"fabrica"* of this chapel, which was to be named (*sub vocabulo*) Sancte Marie et festo Assumptionis, and another 25 florins for a chalice, a missal, a chasuble of chamois (*una planeta camisia*), and other altar furnishings. Lord Nerius then established the electoral procedures for the altar's chaplain, who would be required to say daily masses for the testator's own and his ancestors' souls. He did not privatize these rights or channel them down the *vinculi* of his male heirs, unlike the vast majority of those stating electoral rights and conditions for chapel foundations in Arezzo, Florence, and Perugia, especially by the late Trecento. Instead, he left them with the community of his native town, *pro comune Chianciani.* If the chaplain proved deficient in his tasks, another was to be chosen "in this way by the said commune with the Bishop of Chiusi always represented in these elections according to the letter of the law."[41]

In a new testament in the following year, 1400, the former vicar general dropped his more modest first choice of burial, that is, "wherever the friars pleased" in the Franciscan basilica of Assisi and set out from the beginning that his sepulcher was to be placed within the Franciscan church of San Giovanni, located in Chianciano. This time around he specified even more precisely the position of his tomb: "within this church in the wall [*in muro parietis*] which is opposite the chapel of San Martino." He further supplemented the possessions for the clerics delegated to this altar by bequeathing them all his books on canon law, which he then enumerated individually.[42] But this noble immigrant's attention to matters of memorializing bodily remains was for Assisi the exception and suggests that the ecclesiastical institutions available within a territory, their unwritten customs and sentiments, may have strongly conditioned testators' expectations and desires for memorialization.

Other Assisian references to places of burial which went beyond the simple choice of church usually identified the grave only vaguely as that of the testator's ancestors (*suorum antecessorum*) or as the place where a relative was buried, usually the father or the husband. On rare occasions, the husband might even follow his wife to a conjugal grave, as in the 1362 testament of Iacobus f.q. Vannis alias Zuccha, who elected his sepulcher *"in quam requiescit corpus domine Francesche quondam uxoris mee."*[43]

Only in Siena did testators approximate such indifference to the body. While in Assisi 6 percent of testators and 7 percent of those who "elected" burial places identified their graves beyond the church, the Sienese went beyond the formulas in 7 and 10 percent of the testaments, respectively. (See table 10.) But, in Siena, this indifference was more striking than the statistics suggest. Even those from the old lineages — the Tolomei, Salimbeni, and Piccolomini — did not order their names inscribed, coats of arms sculpted, or tombstones erected above their graves until the latter part of the Quattrocento.[44] The only Trecento example of tomb constructions found in these samples comes in a 1340 testament of the Salimbeni. The body was not his own but rather his son's, which he ordered the Franciscans to exhume from one place in their church and bury afresh (*mortuario novo*) within the father's chapel beneath the vaults of the son's former burial place.[45]

FLORENCE   The history of tombstones, sepulcher constructions, and chapels once again separates Florence, Arezzo, and Perugia from the other three cities. In the sheer numbers of specifically demarcated graves, the Florentines led the list. Nearly one-quarter of all these testators specified or demanded from clerics the location of their graves by going beyond the formulaic phrases — *apud, in ecclesia,* or *in cimiterio.* The earliest do not antedate those drawn from Siena or Assisi but appear only in the quarter-century preceding the Black Death. In Florence, however, they were at the outset monumental affairs. In his 1334 testament,

Table 10.
Specified Burials

Period	Specified Graves	Burial Chapels	Monumental Sepulchers	Burial Chapel with Monuments	Burial in Ancestral Graves	Total	Proportion of Testators
AREZZO							
< 1276							
1275–1300							
1301–25	0	3	0	1	0	4	0.07
1326–47	1	5	2	1	0	9	0.10
1348	1	2	4	4	0	11	0.13
1349–62	2	3	1	3	0	9	0.14
1363	1	2	1	2	0	6	0.08
1364–75	0	11	1	3	1	16	0.18
1376–1400	2	9	0	1	2	14	0.15
1401–25	1	12	1	2	14	30	0.30
Total	8	47	10	17	17	99	0.15
ASSISI							
< 1276							
1275–1300							
1301–25							
1326–47	0	0	0	0	1	1	0.04
1348	2	1	0	0	0	3	0.11
1349–62	0	0	0	1	1	2	0.40
1363							
1364–75							
1376–1400	2	1	1	0	1	5	0.17
1401–25	0	2	0	0	5	7	0.05
Total	4	4	1	1	8	18	0.06
FLORENCE							
< 1276							
1275–1300							
1301–25							
1326–47	1	2	1	1	1	6	0.10
1348	1	3	3	1	3	11	0.15
1349–62	1	4	0	0	4	9	0.23
1363	3	2	3	1	4	13	0.18
1364–75	1	6	3	3	2	15	0.16
1376–1400	3	6	5	1	13	28	0.25
1401–25	2	1	3	1	45	52	0.57
Total	12	24	18	8	72	134	0.21

Table 10.
Continued

Period	Specified Graves	Burial Chapels	Monumental Sepulchers	Burial Chapel with Monuments	Burial in Ancestral Graves	Total	Proportion of Testators
PERUGIA							
< 1276							
1275–1300							
1301–25	2	1	0	0	0	3	0.30
1326–47	0	1	1	0	0	2	0.03
1348	0	0	3	1	0	4	0.05
1349–62	0	1	3	0	0	4	0.20
1363	0	1	0	0	0	1	0.04
1364–75	1	4	3	0	0	8	0.16
1376–99	2	14	5	3	10	34	0.17
1400–1425	2	2	1	0	14	19	0.26
Total	7	24	16	4	24	75	0.15
PISA							
< 1276							
1275–1300							
1301–25	2	1	3	0	2	8	0.03
1326–47	1	2	2	0	4	9	0.09
1348	1	0	0	0	2	3	0.21
1349–62	2	0	3	1	4	10	0.15
1363	1	0	0	0	0	1	0.03
1364–75	1	2	2	0	4	9	0.18
1376–1400	1	2	3	0	13	19	0.17
1401–25	4	1	2	0	24	31	0.43
Total	13	8	15	1	53	90	0.12
SIENA							
< 1276							
1275–1300							
1301–25	0	1	0	0	0	1	0.02
1326–47	0	0	0	1	1	2	0.03
1348	0	0	0	0	1	1	0.02
1349–62	0	0	0	0	3	3	0.08
1363	0	0	0	0	3	3	0.13
1364–75	0	0	0	0	3	3	0.12
1376–1400	0	0	0	0	7	7	0.11
1401–25	0	2	0	0	11	13	0.29
Total	0	3	0	1	29	33	0.07

Albizius f.q. Nardi Gentis, from the parish of San Pancrazio, specified with remarkable detail for these documents the exact place of his burial: the Dominican church of Santa Maria Novella, "opposite the chapel of All Saints, which was situated in the bell tower of this church and just outside the portal [*hostium*], at the foot of the bell tower door." The friars at this spot were to construct *de novo* a "beautiful sepulcher" and other ornamentations. Specifically, "the altar existing in this chapel" was to be adorned with panel paintings (*tabolis picturis*), vestments, altarcloths and other ornaments, a chalice, and other decorative "necessities." For these expenses, along with the stipend to employ a friar to celebrate masses, the testator offered the hefty sum (by early fourteenth-century standards) of 160 florins.[46] Already by 1340 the first plaque memorializing a grave appears in these documents. Curiously, it did not advertise the testator's own bones but his son-in-law's. The notary and nephew of the earlier mentioned notary Grimaldus, Landus f.q. Ubaldini Compagni, from Pesciola, wished to be buried in a tomb (*avello*) located in the cloister of his parish church of San Frediano (Florence), which he had purchased and where his son-in-law was buried. So as to avoid any mistake, the notary specified that a marble plaque "should describe" the grave — "*sepulcrum Cennii Canterini.*"[47]

In Florence, the plague of 1348 spawned a bumper crop of new tomb constructions, chapels, and other means of demarcating individual graves, perhaps as a result of the threat of mass burials coupled with the fear of abandonment, which we have already encountered in the case of Franco Sacchetti's character, Basso, who left an annual feast for flies because, unlike his wife, brothers, and children, they had not abandoned him in his final illness. Literati and chroniclers alike — Graziani from Perugia, Ranieri Sardo from Pisa, Boccaccio and Petrarch — repeated similar stories of brothers abandoning sisters, husbands abandoning wives, fathers and mothers abandoning sons and daughters, and claimed that these experiences were widespread through the horrific summer months of 1348.[48] In that year, one-fifth of those who "elected" their burial places went beyond the notaries' formula to identify more precisely the locations of their bones. The plague-ridden months of June and July spurred all of these, and four devised plans for new tomb construction to ensure that their bodies would be individually interred and properly memorialized.

The most modest plan came from Filippus f.q. Roselli de Bacherellis, who spent only 5 florins for the construction of his tomb (*avellum*) in his parish church of Santa Cecilia, along with another 5 florins for the *avellum* of his deceased father, Rosellus (perhaps also a victim of the 1348 scourge) in the suburban hill church of Santa Maria de Marignolla.[49] A similar zeal spread through the countryside. In July, a domina Niccholosa, the widow of Franciscus Sacchetti of Florence (not the famous writer of the end of the century) and the daughter of the former Andrea Petri de Maglis then living in the fortified village of Vico, left 25 florins to her parish of Sant'Andrea to "execute a well ornamented tomb," where she desired her body "to be put and placed."[50]

The most elaborate and expensive of these monumental burials came, as might be expected, from the top of Florentine society. In the first itemized bequest in his July testament, Albertus f.q. Lapi de Albertis, from the Alberti parish of Sant'Iacopo (in the neighborhood of Santa Croce), ordered the construction of a chapel in Santa Croce to house the bones of "the testator, his children and his future descendants" in a place to be chosen not by the friars but by the tutors Albertus appointed for his children. This construction, to be completed within three years, was not to exceed the colossal sum (by mid-Trecento standards) of 500 florins. Albertus then introduced the possibility of the only clan-sponsored chapel to be found in these documents for any of these cities at any time by stipulating that if his consortes wished to "participate" in this spiritual-familial venture, he would put up one-fifth the costs.[51] Despite incursions into these burial grounds by Vasari and Cosimo I, a plaque and remains from 13 tombs show that Albertus's plans to preserve the memory of his line were carried out without the assistance of his "consortes": "Albertacci et Dom. Lapi de Albertis et filiorum cuius anime requiescant in Pace. an. Dom. MCCCXXXXVIII."[52]

The tendency in Florence to individuate and specify one's own grave was not, however, a one-time aberration provoked by the outbreak of plague and its threat of possible mass burial. In the years separating the first and second occurrences of pestilence, the percentage of those stip-ulating precise locations or wishing to build tombs de novo increased from one-fifth to one-third of those specifying the place of burial. With the recurrence of plague in 1363, the percentage momentarily dropped to the level reached in 1348, but the number of new constructions, whether of burial chapels or tombs without altars, continued to increase. This second plague initiated the expensive burial chapel complex of Franciscus f.q. Masi de Alferris, who gave the Dominicans of Santa Maria Novella four years from the day of his death to build "a beautiful and respectful" chapel to honor the Omnipotent Lord, the Virgin Mary, and Saint Francis. It was to be constructed above the "ground" where

Francesco's bones were to lie—in the church of Santa Maria Novella or "around" it, to be decided by the prior, friar Agnolo Lippi de Adimaribus. But Francescus named the chapel himself, in fact after himself, the chapel of Saint Francis—a hard pill for the Dominicans to swallow and the source of future litigation.[53] The testator left 400 florins for this project, or if his heirs in any way impeded the payment, the friars could demand 500 florins.[54]

Another will drawn up in 1363 attests to the increasing importance that burial grounds and lineage played in the formation of Florentine identity during the latter half of the Trecento. A parishioner of Santo Stefano al Ponte desired to be interred in the sepulcher he was constructing at the foot of the steps leading to the chapel of Sant'Andrea in his parish, and "every single bone [*omnia et singula hossa*] of his ancestors [*mortuorum predecessorum*] existing in a certain vault [*avello*]" in the cloister of this church was to be removed and placed in the testator's new sepulcher. The responsibility for this tomb and its expenses was left to the testator's executors.[55]

A parishioner of San Iacopo tra le fosse who was undistinguished by either a noble title or a family name, and who redacted a will in the year of the plague's return, shows that desires for corporeal memorialization, construction of an individuated burial place, and the pursuit of memory through lineage were not exclusive to the great families. Johannes f.q. Bartoli Martelli looked to the future through his progeny with a five-lire donation to his parish church and a promise from the abbot of the monastery of San Salvi, who was also his parish rector. Johannes ordered a vault (*avellum*) constructed there to house the bodies of his children and their descendants.[56] Finally, a tomb planned in June of that plague year by the nobleman Nepus f.q. domini Pauli domini Nepi della Tosa spelled out even more emphatically the urges for a consortial and dynastic piety. He ordered his burial with the Dominicans of Santa Maria Novella, opposite the chapel of San Marco, where two of his kinsmen, dominus Pinus and dominus Ciampus, both knights (*milites*) and members of the Florentine della Tosa family, had been buried. Above this sepulcher, he ordered the friars to make a marble plaque bearing the testator's familial coat of arms and "the letters expressing the proper names and the family names (*cognominia*) of the said dominus Pinus, dominus Ciampus and Nepus."[57]

The increasing importance of familial burial places is associated with the recurrence of pestilence in 1363 and parallels the growing importance of lineage in the lives and strategies for the afterlife of Florentines across social class. From the earliest specifications through the year of the Black Death (1348), references to familial burial grounds (whether the place of burial of a son, wife, husband, father, or more vaguely the ancestors) occurred in the testaments of less than 5 percent of those who "elected" their burials and in the wills of less than one-fourth of those who specified more precisely the location for their bones. Only after 1363 did these ancestral grounds characterized by phrases such as *suorum antecessorum, antiquorum, ascentium premortuorum,* or *suorum mortuorum* begin to predominate over new burial constructions or other means of locating a future site for testators' bones. By the last quarter of the Trecento, nearly half of all such burial specifications referred to ancestral graves. In the first years of the Quattrocento, the percentage jumped higher: over half of all Florentine testators chose an ancestral burial ground, and 87 percent of all sites specified beyond the ecclesiastical institution were graves that had already been founded by a previous member of the family.

This trend paralleled the more general tendency of Florentines who identified with precision their place of burial. By the last quarter of the Trecento, this proportion jumped from a fifth to over one-third of all burial places. Then, in the early Quattrocento, the rate increased more dramatically, doubling from one-third to two-thirds. If testators from the rural villages of the Florentine *contado* are separated out, the rate was even higher: three-fourths of Florentine testators in these years individuated the locations of their final resting grounds within churches and monasteries.[58]

While the testaments show the increase of familial vaults and th is a declining need to build new monuments to individuate and memorialize corporeal remains, plans to construct grandiose monuments and tomb-chapel complexes continued to dot these documents. By the late Trecento, moreover, efforts to add on to projects initiated previously by relatives and ancestors enter the records. In 1371, Dominus Niccolaus f.q. Senucci Benucci de Benucciis, rector of Santa Cecilia, chose to be buried in this church "in front of and next to the chapel opposite the new bell tower of the church." The chapel had been built earlier by an ancestor (*ancestor testatoris*), a certain Ser Orlandus, but it is not clear whether it had been a burial chapel. At any rate, by the time of this will, the priest claimed that the chapel had no endowment and lacked the proper furnishings. He then proceeded to dedicate the major portion of his long and complex will to completing this single task—specifying the endowment, furnishings, paintings, *ius patronatus,* and the electoral proceedings of the chaplains and their obligation to perform cycles of perpetual masses in his renewed burial complex.[59]

A burial chapel commissioned in 1375 by a married woman, domina Zanobia f.q. Bancini Ranucci, required the friars of Santa Maria Novella to dig up the bones of her former husband Iacobus and those of her deceased son Johannes and rebury them along with her own bones in a sepulcher in the chapel dedicated to the namesake of her former husband, San Jacopo. The friars were to celebrate yearly masses for her own, her deceased son's, and her former husband's souls. (Curiously, her present husband, Andrea Ciani, was not mentioned.)[60]

The burial designs of a citizen and merchant of Florence, Antonio f.q. Lapacci Cini, illustrate how, by the Quattrocento, burial projects could expand into complex ornamental schemes affecting large spaces within the churches that were to host the bodies. During his lifetime, the 1411 testator had already built his own burial "tomb and monument" in his parish church, the monastery of San Pancrazio. A large portion of his will was devoted to ensuring that the chapel surrounding this monument would be built and decorated according to his stipulations. He demanded that it be built "under the title and name of Saint Nicolas of Bari" and that the expenses needed to bring it to completion should come from his holdings in the Florentine communal debt, the Monte.[61] He further ordered that the chapel be "ornamented and painted" with the narrative (*cum storia*) of Nicholas of Bari. To begin the chapel construction, he insisted that first a stained-glass window be constructed and all the other necessities for the honorable use and completion of the chapel be provided.[62] For these necessities, the new construction, and the chapel's endowment, the testator donated the hefty sum of 750 florins. The fees, however, were not to be paid out in one lump sum but in yearly installments provided during the course of construction and during the time it took to finish painting Saint Nicholas's life. Once the work was completed, the chaplain was to perform a feast for Saint Nicholas each year, burning four large candles weighing a pound each at the chapel's altar, singing a high mass (*missa magna*) along with low masses (*misse parve*), and spending three-and-a-half florins for a commemorative meal (*pietanza*) to be consumed by the abbot and the monks. In addition, the abbot and monks were to celebrate *in perpetuum* an anniversary feast for the soul of the testator and his ancestors in which 20 pounds of wax were to be burnt, 30 masses celebrated, and four-and-a-half florins spent on bread, wine, and incidentals.[63]

The most expensive of the burial complexes found in these documents for Florence came in the first years of the Quattrocento. Filippus f.q. domini Castellani, from the aristocratic Frescobaldi family, spent one thousand florins for a burial tomb to glorify his corpse and those of his descendants at the foot of the predella of the altar in the new chapel located in the Augustinian church of Santo Spirito. This large endowment indicates that by the early Quattrocento there were signs of competition for available dynastic space in the prestigious Florentine churches and heightened obsessions over the symbols of lineage.[64] The endowment was given on condition that no coat of arms other than that of the Frescobaldi be placed on his sepulcher. To secure this promise from the friars and for *"bona cautela,"* the testator deposited those thousand florins for 10 years with the wool guild of Florence, which was required to parcel out the sums for the work on his chapel and grave. Filippus then gave yet another hundred florins for the chapel's "ornamentation and beautification." If work on his burial complex did not begin within those 10 years, the legacy would be annulled and the monies distributed to the poor of Christ.[65]

Such worries over the infringement of alien bodies and symbols on one's family burial chapel may well have become justified by the early Quattrocento. Signs of limited chapel space and concerns over protecting these spaces for posterity appear in other testaments. In 1423, the vintner Johannes f.q. Landi della Malvagia, a citizen of Florence, elected his burial in his ancestral vault in the church of Santa Trinità. In a separate itemized act made later on in his will, he gave his children, both male and female, as well as their descendants, the right to bury their bodies (*ius interendi et seppelliendi corpora defunctorum*) in this sepulcher, on condition that they never "sell, trade or in any way alienate" the tomb.[66] Others in the last years of my investigation made gifts of burial rights (as though they were property rights) to more distant kin. Thus, in 1417, the "provident man" Augustinus f.q. Francesci Ser Johannis gave "to the sons and descendants" of his deceased nephew Ugolini Vieri the right to bury their bodies (*ius inferendi corpora*) in the sepulcher of the testator, his father, and his ancestors, located in the cloister of Santo Spirito.[67]

Although the projects of the early Quattrocento did become more complex and expensive, as the previous examples have illustrated, new burial projects of more modest dimensions had certainly not yet disappeared. In 1417, the "provident" Arrigus f.q. Bandini de Falconeriis donated between 10 and 12 florins to the Servite church of Santissima Annuziata for the "new construction of his tomb," to be placed in the chapel of his ancestors.[68] Farther down the social scale, Junta f.q. Migloris Gadocti, a wool producer (*ritagliator*), desired to be buried in the then Benedictine church of San Marco and left a mere 30 florins to construct his burial tomb in that church.[69]

AREZZO   To judge by the percentages of specified graves, the Aretines appear to have been less preoccupied with the ultimate fate of their bodies than were the Florentines. In Arezzo, 15 percent, as opposed to 21 percent in Florence, made such extraformulaic demands for where their bodies were to rest. We have already seen, however, that notarial practice in regard to the election of the grave differed in Arezzo from the other city-states. If only those testators who actually elected their burial church in these documents are taken for the denominator, the comparative statistics look different: the Aretines jump to the top of the list, as intent as the Florentines on individuating their graves. Thirty-one percent placed demands on churches to inter their bodies in specific graves, in comparison to 29 percent for the Florentines.

Aretines further surpassed their richer neighbors to the northwest in the extent to which they used the resources of their patrimonies to construct new graves and funerary monuments. In Florence, more than half of the specified sepulchers were places already planned and constructed by deceased kin or more distant ancestors.[70] Only 62 wills (drawn up by 14 percent of those who selected graves) in Florence set out plans to construct new burial tombs or future family vaults. The Aretines,[71] in contrast, relied less than the Florentines on the previous plans of the dead and instead, more often than anywhere else, used their testaments to finance the construction of new tombs.

The first of these plans to memorialize the body may have appeared in the Aretine documents well before they surfaced in Florence. In 1308, Acursus f.q. Ridofini, from the Casentine town of Torre Classeris (Chiassa), devoted his entire will to one end—the endowment of a chapel in his *plebis* church. After arranging for his funeral procession to this church, where he would be buried, he donated all of his property to support a "suitable" priest (*ydoneus presbiter*) as chaplain (*capellanus sive mansionarius*) to reside in this church and "continuously" to chant masses and holy offices for his soul and the souls of his kin. In addition, he was obliged to celebrate an anniversary mass at the altar "in honor and in reverence" of the blessed Mary Magdalene. This priest was allowed no other benefice than the care of this chapel, and if he should ever accept another, his enjoyment of the *usufructus* to Acursus's property would be annulled.

Acursus then used his testament to elect the first chaplain, the priest Vannius f. Orlandi Ugolini, from this *plebis*. After the death of this priest, the rights of election would pass to the testator's brothers, Bandinus and Finus.[72] Although the testator founded this chapel in the church where he elected his grave, it is not altogether certain from the will that it was in fact to be a burial chapel.

The first testament unmistakably to associate a chapel construction and foundation with the site of burial came later, in 1325, but still early by the standards of Florence or, for that matter, any of the city-states here examined. The nobleman Farinata f.q. Gualterii de Ubertinis, from Fogna (perhaps a descendant and namesake of the infamous Ghibelline leader whom Dante consigned to the depths of the Inferno),[73] devoted nearly his entire testament to his burial and the foundation of his chapel. He first donated 10 lire to the Opera Maioris of the cathedral to construct his grave and to bury him "humbly." He further provided 100 florins (large by early Trecento standards) for his funeral expenses, which would include graveside masses (*exequiis*) and handouts to the poor and the shamefaced poor (*vecundis*) of the city. He then founded a chapel in the cathedral with various landed properties and perpetual rents that together would provide the chaplain with a yearly subsidy of 101 *staia* of grain. The nobleman prohibited "any long-term rental or *emphiteosis* [a perpetual lease][74] or any other contract or alienation" and required the sacerdotes of this chapel to celebrate masses and vespers on the feast day of the birth of the "glorious Virgin" in September and to administer "a good and sufficient" feast (*prandium*) for all the canons and chaplains of the cathedral, who would offer prayers to God for himself, his dead son Bindinus, and all the dead of his family. The chaplains, moreover, were to offer every year in perpetuity one *sestario* of baked bread to each of the religious orders and charities in Arezzo: the Dominicans; the Augustinian hermits; the Servites; the nuns of Montiscalci, of Santo Spirito, of Santa Maria Novella, and of Santo Sperandio, and 30 *sestarii* of grain to the shamefaced poor at the cathedral. The rights of election (*ius patronatus ex fondatione*) were given to the abbess and nuns of Santa Clara, who were entrusted with the appointments of "chaplains of good comportment and fame, born of legitimate matrimonies and at least 36 years of age, who professed no wayward or apostate sect [*et quo non sit alicuius religionis apostela vel egressus*] and who had never given birth to a child."[75]

Indeed, more chapels were founded per testator, and more burial monuments enshrined in chapels in Arezzo, than in any other of these cities. In 1345, the citizen Johannes f.q. Cionis Detavive left 500 lire for the endowment, furnishing (*fulcimentis et paramentis*), and construction of a chapel in the Dominican church "next to" the testator's sepulcher.[76] Another testament drafted in 1348 by the same testator repeated these burial demands, but increased the funds to 600 lire.[77] In the same year, the judge dominus Johannes f.q. Baroncini spent 70 florins to construct a chapel "next to his grave" in the Dominican church and required the friars to tear down an old wall so that the chapel would come into the vault that lay above the cloisters.[78] As we have seen, the year of the Black Death brought the most elaborate and expensive of the burial complexes found at any time for any city in these documents: the 4,000-florin burial monument of the *potens vir* Tarlatus to compose "the middle church" of the Franciscan mountain shrine at La Verna.[79] In 1359, Angelus f.q. Rossi de Catenaccis provided another hefty fund, from 500 lire to 200 florins, to Arezzo's minor friars to construct "a beautiful and honorable" chapel and to furnish it with chalices of gold and silver, a missal, and vestments for the altar. He next bequeathed 150 lire for his funeral, an anniversary mass, and the construction of his burial "monument" to be located "in that spot" in the new church "towards the door where the women entered the church."[80]

In 1362, Ser Nicholaus f.q. Ser Lanani de Grassis made more elaborate demands on these minor friars for the memorialization of his corporeal remains, ordering the construction of a chapel, to be named Saint Nicholas, in a place in their church chosen by his brother, a friar, and a merchant. For gold and silver chalices, a missal, and other furnishings for the altar, he left 200 florins and the silk robes that belonged to his wife. On the feast day of Saint Nicholas, the friars were to make offerings (*fiat elimosina*) to the walled-in hermits (*muratis*) and to the poor of the city—four *staii* of "baked bread" and four of wheat bread. The friars were to celebrate daily masses in the chapel in honor of the Lord and the blessed Nicholas for the souls of the testator and his relatives, and a record of these recitations (*signum vel litere*) was to be kept in this chapel. Next, Ser Nicholas returned to the matters of his body, demanding that in front of the altar of this chapel a walled sepulcher (*sepulcrum muratum*) be built with a tombstone. Apparently this Aretine must have made frequent business trips to Pisa and made provisions for his body should he die there. In this case, he was to be buried in the Pisan monastic church of San Michele in Borgo, where he called for the intercession of the Franciscans, the Dominicans, the Augustinians, and all the monks of the Camaldolite order. His body, however, was to rest in Pisa only temporarily—in the time, that is, it took for his body to decompose (*usque ad tempus quo eius corpus fuerit consumptum*). Afterward, "his bones" were to be translated to Arezzo to be buried in his tomb, which was to lie in front of the altar of the chapel whose construction his testament had initiated.[81]

By the plague's return (1363), the call of the ancestors, as in Florence, also began to be heard in Arezzo. In that year, the daughter of a rural notary who had subsequently moved to Arezzo, domina Gora f.q. Ser Acolti notarii f.q. Acolti de Falcona, ordered a chapel built in the Dominican church of Arezzo for the health of her own and her dead predecessors' souls. The chapel was to be constructed above the "body" of her deceased brother, *Magister* Gregorius, "thus to preserve the perpetual memory of the said *Magister* Gregorius [*ad hoc ut sit perpetua memoria*]*.*" For this construction and for its paintings she left 150 florins and, beyond these fees, whatever her executors deemed just to furnish the altar and to bury the testatrix there "at the altar."[82]

The third recurrence of plague, in 1374, stimulated a flurry of chapel constructions and funerary decoration in Arezzo. No fewer than 10 testators ordered chapels in the same church where they elected to be buried. At least four of these were unmistakably burial chapels. The "egregious doctor" of both laws (canon and Roman law), dominus Francescus Johannis de Acceptatibus, in his first testamentary act demanded that his burial "monument" be constructed with a stone plaque sculpted with his coat of arms in Santa Maria della Pieve, next to the baptismal font.[83] He further required that his patrimony pay for a chapel under the name of Saint Francis to be built in the same place, and he commissioned a painting for that chapel showing "when the blessed Francis received from Our Lord Jesus the stigmata" and the narrative "ystoria" of Francis's life. Further, his estate was to provide an annual stipend of 150 *staii* of grain, three *congios*[84] of wine, and one *quartum*[85] of olive oil to support the chapel's chaplain. The *ius patronatus*, or right to elect the chaplain, instead of reverting to the Franciscan friars or to some other religious group, was channeled to the doctor's universal heir, to that heir's son, and then to "the other males of his lineage born of legitimate marriage [*maschulos de domo sua legiptios et de legiptimi matrimoni natos*]." The elected chaplain was to be at least 25 years old, "constituted as a sacerdos, a man of good condition, life and family." He was "to reside continuously in this benefice" to recite masses and other divine offices for the souls of the testator and his deceased kin. The doctor then ordered the chapel to be built honorably and with the best materials and, if possible, completed within eight months of his death. He next expressed a worldly pride not to be found in the documents from the Sienese, Assisani, or Pisans. For the construction of his sepulcher, "nothing should be done contrary to the letter of the ordinances, except, if possible, placing on his grave his pillow lined with fur [*palandrum foderatum de vaio*] bearing the insignia of his doctorate."[86]

Again, in the plague year of 1374, Pagnus f.q. Maffei, a shopkeeper, ordered in his opening legacy the construction of a chapel in the cathedral of Arezzo, to honor the apostle Saint Mathew.[87] It was to be well endowed (*dotetur bene et congrue*) and to support perpetually "a good and suitable" chaplain at least 31 years of age, "whose only benefice and altar should be the custody of this chapel," where he was to celebrate daily masses. The election rights once again were not bestowed on the custodians of the chapel's host institution, the Augustinians, but were given to the testator's executors, together with his heirs. Again, this merchant expressed ideals contrary to mendicant humility and indulged in the mundane pride of his profession. He ordered his coat of arms and the merchant's insignia used in his shop (*signum mercantie utebatur in sua apoteccha*) to be painted and sculpted in this chapel and on his burial vault (*avella*).[88]

Also in 1374, another merchant, "the discreet man" Matheus Giontarini Bruni, of Arezzo, opened his testament by choosing his burial grounds within his preexisting chapel, again within the confines of the Augustinian church. He used his testament to refurbish and to redecorate the site of his grave by first wishing to have painted, "honorably and decently," the Annunciation of the Virgin Mary with other figures "according to the desires of his heirs." Second, he left to his chapel and for the use of the friars a silver chalice, an alter screen (*unum palium pro altare*), and a vestment for the priest while officiating masses. And on each of these—the chalice, altar screen, and priestly vestment—he demanded the placement of his coat of arms and insignia.[89]

The fourth testator, the citizen Franciscus f.q. domini Johannis Ser Baldi, ordered the construction of a burial chapel which may have resurrected and co-opted the one endowed 45 years earlier in the will of the doctor of laws from the Acceptanti family. At any rate, Franciscus demanded to be interred in the church of the minor friars "next" to where he proposed to build a chapel—a place "now" authorized (*in uno loco iam deputato*) next to a wall in the middle of the church. The chapel was to be named "Saint Francis with the Stigmata," and the feasts (also called "Saint Francis with the Stigmata") and that of Saint

Anthony of Vienna were to be celebrated here yearly. For its construction and for paintings, ornamentation, vestments, the chalice, and other necessities, the testator left 150 florins.[90]

After 1374, new burial monuments and chapels became less pronounced just at the moment when the Aretines (similar to, though later than, their Florentine neighbors) began to rely on the already constructed burial vaults and chapel complexes established by kinsmen and ancestors. For instance, in 1377 the "honorable" widow Margarita f.q. Mani Dietavive donated a strip of land to cover the expenses to be interred and dressed in her widow's gown in her "constructed" chapel called San Bartolommeo in the Dominican church of Arezzo and left further sums for her chapel to buy a missal.[91] Although, as in Florence, testators demanded new burial monuments and chapels less frequently in the Quattrocento than did the previous generation, the new chapels of the early Renaissance were generally on a more grandiose scale.

By far the most spectacular of these Quattrocento burial complexes was stipulated in a testament dated 1410. A merchant from Arezzo, then living in Florence, Lazarus f.q. Johannis de Braccis,[92] whose local fame endured even to the time of Giorgio Vasari,[93] began his testament with stipulations and plans for his burial grounds, which were to lie opposite the major altar of the Franciscan church of Arezzo and to have placed on them a marble tombstone containing "his letters" and coat of arms. Within one year, the friars were to spend 100 florins on an altar banner and various altarcloths and vestments made of special silk fabrics for use at the major altar. All of these holy accouterments were to bear the merchant's arms and insignia. He further offered the friars 300 florins to rebuild and ornament this major chapel, which he had assumed as his own burial grounds. The funds were to be used for painting "on one side" the story of the resurrection of his namesake and on the other the story of Saint Francis "having suffered in his body the stigmata of Christ," and above these narratives were to be placed paintings of the four evangelists.

The merchant's plans did not end with these fresco cycles. He left another 200 florins for building a stained-glass window displaying his insignia and coat of arms. He then added (almost as though in debate with the friars) that his plan to glorify his corpse with the mundane symbols of his lineage at the most sacred place in the Franciscan church was not "due to vainglory [*ob vanam gloriam*]" but instead was to serve "as a good example for posterity." Toward the end of his lengthy testament, the merchant repeated these arguments and further expressed his zeal for earthly memory: "conceding . . . these sums of 500 florins from his inheritance to the Franciscan friars . . . for his memory and the memory of his ancestors and for their example." Out of fear of future encroachments on his soon-to-be privatized holy space, the merchant expressed sentiments and tried to erect safeguards for the preservation of his familial signs of honor similar to the ones stipulated by his contemporary the Florentine Frescobaldi. The Aretine made his grant "on the condition that no one in the future ever be buried in the sepulcher of the said Lazarus." He then returned to matters of the body, desiring his corpse to be draped in the habit of the Franciscans and his coffin (*bara*) covered in the cloth (*veste*) of his confraternity, Saint John the Baptist.[94]

Five years later, another Aretine merchant, "the honorable and excellent man" Baccius f.q. Masii (who happened to be Lazarus's son-in-law and business associate),[95] competed to decorate this same space, which Lazarus had sought to corner as his burial complex and for the display of his personal and familial regalia.[96] In contrast, Baccius's plans for decoration (specified in another testament, redacted in 1408, and in a codicil of 1411) were far less detailed and more open-ended. They placed no time constraints on the friars, made no demands or presumptions about personal insignia (although the chapel would ultimately celebrate Baccius's coat of arms and not those of the more emphatic and visionary Lazarus), and did not place his body at the Franciscan's high altar with grandiloquent schemes that eventually would in fact underwrite the immortal frescoes of Piero della Francesca. Baccius simply left the funds "for painting honorably with figures [*facere honorifice depingi et figurari*]" the major chapel of this church and for constructing there a stained-glass window, if it had not yet been done during his lifetime.[97] Despite Lazarus's claims that he did not seek "vainglory," his zeal for self- and lineage promotion through the placement of his corporeal remains at the base of the high altar and his detailed programs for incorporating its major altar as his private burial chapel and illustrating the walls with the resurrection of his namesake must have proven too much for the Franciscans to allow; they opted for the vaguer, less demanding plans of his competitor, which gave them a stronger hand in determining the decoration of their major chapel according to their taste and iconography. Lazarus died in 1425 and was buried in the *plebis* church of Santa Maria in Arezzo.[98]

New constructions do not appear again until nearly the end of my documentation, when three came in testaments dated 1419. First, a silk manufacturer and citizen of Arezzo, Nicholaus f.q. Bartolommei f.q. Michelis, chose his tomb in the church of San Pietro Piccolo. If both his sons died, his inheritance would support the building of a chapel in that church for his namesake saints, Bartholomew and Nicholas. For the testator's soul and those of his deceased relatives, 300 florins were to be spent on the chapel's construction, endowment, and ornamentation and on the priestly vestments. In the same year, Meus f.q. Fini, a grain dealer and citizen, requested that his body be placed in "his monument," which lay beneath the chapel he had constructed during his lifetime and named for his namesake, Saint Bartholomew. For its endowment, he left numerous strips of land, a house with a courtyard, a well, and a hut in the city. He insisted that the chaplain of his chapel should always be a "secular" priest, never a monk (monacus). Furthermore, the ius patronatus of electing this "secular priest" was more complex than any thus far seen in this documentation: one vote (voce) was to go to the abbot of the abbey of Agnano, one to the operarios of the plebis church of Arezzo, one to the flagellant confraternity (sotiete battentium) of Sant'Angelo in Arezzo, another to the testator's brother, the cobbler Antonio f.q. Fini, another to the swordsmith Gerolinus Baccii, and a final vote to the testator's heirs and, after them, their successors. The elected testator would be required to perform a "respectable and praiseworthy" (laudabilem et condecens) feast on Saint Bartholomew's Day and during the lifetime of his wife, and 11 staii of "baked bread" were to be distributed to the poor of Christ.[99]

In Arezzo, not only the rich and powerful with massive amounts of landed property to finance chapel-burial complexes sought to individuate their graves. Others commissioned more modest works to demarcate and memorialize their bodily remains. These art commissions reach back to 1328, when the citizen Taddeus f.q. Ser Iacopi de Baronanis elected his burial in the parish church of San Biagio, offering eight lire to burn four large candles each year on the anniversary of his death. He then ordered his executors to build his sepulcher (eius sepulturam videlicet unum ulivellum), and above it to paint saints according to the wishes of these executors. They were to spend 25 lire for "beautification and pictures."[100] In the year of the Black Death, a man from the village of Citerna, Cecchus f.q. Raneroli, sought to distinguish his bodily remains by demanding that the figures of the Virgin Mary and Child and, on each side, saints John and Christopher, "be painted above the place of his burial, wherever he happened to be buried." For this commission he left a pittance, the smallest art commission found in these documents, a candle and three lire.[101]

In 1362, Duccinus f.q. Andrea, a wool manufacturer and citizen, left the larger sum of 100 lire to have painted above his sepulcher in the church of San Michele the "ymaginem" of the Virgin Mary with other figures which the testator would specify to his heir and only son, Donatus. After this task had been finished, the residue should be distributed to those persons selected by his heir.[102] In the plague year of 1374, Domina Bona f.q. Pagani, wife of Johannes Vanni Johannis, from the parish of San Michele, left half her dowry of 145 lire to her brother and universal heir. From this sum he was to commission a painting of Saint John and Jesus Christ "to serve at her sepulcher [qui servixit de sepulcro] in the church of Saint Augustine in the city of Arezzo."[103]

PERUGIA   Of the three cities (Florence, Arezzo, and Perugia) that less strenuously embraced the mendicant ideal of rejecting earthly forms of memory, Perugia showed the weakest tendency toward memorialization through tombs. Nonetheless, the percentage of specially demarcated graves in the Umbrian capital more than doubled that of neighboring Assisi, whether measured by the total number of testators or by those who actually chose their burial places (15 and 16 percent, respectively; see table 11).

Here, the number of burial complexes demanding chapel constructions and schemes for their ornamentation, endowments, and ius patronatus were less numerous and less luxuriant than for Florence or Arezzo. None could compete with the vast expenditures of a Tarlati, the decorative program of the merchant Lazarus, or the intricate plans of the Florentine rector of Santa Cecilia for feasts and perpetual masses. In contrast, only three testators from the Perugian samples designed burial chapels in their testaments. The first of these did not even appear until 1385. Finus f.q. Johannis domini Rufini elected his burial in the church of San Francesco, demanding the construction of a chapel and an altar "above" it "at the site of his burial." Its expenses were left to his executors, and its furnishings and the vestments were to be financed through the sale of all his clothes. The friars were responsible for "continually" chanting divine offices in return for an annual 6 emine of grain, 6 barrels of wine, and one castrated lamb (castrone). The testator made no assumptions about the chapel's ius patronatus or the mechanisms for passing these rights on.[104]

In 1390, a notary of the Commune of Perugia (*abreviator reformationum*) but from the Tuscan hill town of Montepulciano, Francescus f.q. Ser Iacobi f.q. Ser Pierdederiis, wished to be buried in the tomb (*tumulum*) of his children and ancestors in the church of the minor friars in his native town. If his son and universal heirs all died, this communal official would leave the *plebis* church of Montepulciano, Santa Maria, as his heir with the obligation of "erecting" a chapel under the name of saints Jacob and Bartholomew to be built "above" the tomb of his relatives. The church would, moreover, have the responsibility of making the necessary furnishings for the altar and of "always" appointing a chaplain to celebrate masses and divine offices for the souls of his "relatives, brothers, wife and neighbors [*propinquorum*]."[105]

Finally, at the end of the century, Bartolommeus, called Boscone f.q. Pietri Magistri Johannis, left the largest legacy found in these Perugian documents to memorialize a corpse. He chose to be interred in the church of San Francesco "in a decent place." His executor was to spend 200 florins solely for construction and another 300 florins for the "rule, sustenance and officialdom" of this chapel. Again, unlike the provisions for burial complexes found in Florence and Arezzo, particularly by the late Trecento, the testator's program remained vague: no stipulations about wall paintings, coats of arms, or inscriptions; no obligations for the feast days of the testator's patron saints; no rules for the election of the chaplain or the devolution of the *ius patronatus*. He only "held that the friars were to celebrate masses at the newly constructed altar in this chapel."[106]

The demarcation and individuation of graves at Perugia instead made use of more modest tools. Deathbed commissions of paintings to identify and hang above graves was more prevalent here than anywhere else, including Florence or Arezzo. The earliest reached back to the year of the Black Death. Nullus f.q. Pepi, from the village of Castro Casalalte, just across the border in the Commune of Todi, elected that his grave be on the Perugian side of the border in the church of Santa Maria in Castelleone. For his burial, the praise of God, and the health of his soul, he commissioned for a mere 10 lire "the making of a *Maiestà*" for this church; "the money was not to be spent for any other endeavor."[107] In the same year, Nutius Cioli desired to be buried in his parish of San Pietro. To this convent and church he left 25 lire for the painting of a *Maiestà* on the wall (*in illo muro et pariete*) above his sepulcher. He further stipulated that "in this *Maiestà* there ought to appear the figure of Our Lord Jesus Christ on the Cross, his Mother, the Glorious Virgin Mary and the figures of Saint John and Saint Constantine." Later in his will, he sought to shed further light and recognition on his grave by granting his brother a house and a mill in the village of Pontignano, with the proviso that his brother supply two *mediolia*[108] of oil a year for the first 10 years following Nutius's death—one to be burned in the church of San Francesco in front of a painting of the blessed Saint Constantine, the other in front of the "figure" he commissioned for his grave.[109]

In 1362, Egidius Martini Crescebene left a larger sum for decorating his burial grounds but was less specific about the iconography. He bequeathed an amount not to exceed 250 lire to be interred in the Chapel of Saint Catherine in the church of Saint Augustine, for the expense of restoring this chapel, and for a "picture" above his sepulcher.[110] In 1367, Martinus Fortis Johannis, from the nearby fortified village of Corciano, wished to be buried in his parish of Santa Maria; he left two florins for his funeral and six "for the reverence and praise of the Most Glorious Mary" and the health of the souls of the testator and his relatives to commission "the making" of a figure of the "Most Blessed Virgin Mary" and Child on the wall above his sepulcher. Concerned with its preservation, he insisted that "this figure" should be covered and "ornamented well."[111]

In 1383, the immigrant Johannes Pietri, from Ruano de Francia (Rouen), elected his grave in the church of San Francesco and ordered his executors to clear a space (*depurgi*) near his grave for a "figura" of the Virgin Mary and one of Saint Catherine, for which they were to spend a meager four florins.[112] In the same year, the married woman Vannutia provided more details about her burial painting, to be placed above her sepulcher in her parish church of Santo Stefano, ordering "the Blessed Mary with her child Our Lord Jesus Christ in her arms," along with the figures of Joseph, Mary Magdalene, and saints Bartholomew, Catherine, and Margaret.[113]

Finally, in 1400, the widow domina Angelina wished to be buried in her ancestral vault (*pilo*), located in the church of San Gregorio, and ordered that the church "renovate [*renoventur*] those figures above her ancestral vault and protect them by making a cover."[114] The most grandiose of these burial frescoes, however, came in 1390 from a woman, domina Johanna, daughter of Ser Stephani (most probably a notary), widow of a druggist, and remarried to a Pauli Pietri Rubei. She wished to be buried in or near the chapel that she planned to construct in the church of the Servites. Naming them as her universal heirs, she obliged them to continue work on this chapel immediately after her death. The friars were to restore a certain wall near the choir, contiguous to the chapel of Saint Julian, where they were held to build a chapel with an altar. On the wall above the altar they were to have a painting of an annunciation, along with the figures of the testatrix and (curiously, since she was at the time remarried) her former husband, Andrea. To complete the project within two years, the friars would receive 200 florins.[115]

PISA   Of the testators who most vehemently shunned the temptations of earthly memory in structuring their pious bequests, Pisans appear to have been the least indifferent to individuating their corporeal remains. In specifying the precise location of graves or memorializing their remains through tomb or chapel construction, they lagged only slightly behind Perugians. Twelve percent of all Pisans, and 13 percent of those who indicated their burial churches, specified precise locations for their tombs. (See table 11.) Part of the reason for this high percentage (at least in relation to Assisi and Siena) was due to the transformation in ideals after the recurrence of pestilence in 1362 — the increase in particular of familial and ancestral tombs. In the early years of the Quattrocento, 44 percent of those selecting their burial grounds did so with precision — a rate surpassed only by the Florentines. As in early fifteenth-century Florence, the vast majority of these (over three-fourths in Pisa) were tombs already established by fathers, husbands, or ancestors. Moreover, exactly half of these ancestral tombs (12) are found in the cathedral's unique mausoleum-cemetery, the Campo Santo, initiated by Archbishop Federigo Visconti under the direction of the *capomaestro,* Giovanni di Simone, at the end of the thirteenth century.[116] This remarkable burial ground, which contained ancient sarcophagi alongside contemporary vaults and frescoes, accounted for less than 16 percent of all burials selected in these testaments but for nearly 40 percent of the precise locations stipulated in the Pisan wills.[117] Testators who chose their burial vaults here were more likely to map out where their bodies should end up. In 1348, a woman from Vico asked to be interred "next to the olive trees in this Campo Santo."[118] In 1411, a furnace maker's widow sought to be buried in the campo "where the tabernacle of the Holy Trinity usually stood."[119] In 1422, a furrier's wife chose a place in this holy field, "in the cloister on the upper side towards the middle."[120]

These communal grounds, moreover, provided ready-made tombs, so that testators, such as the knife maker Domenicus f.q. Bernardi, could be interred there in monumental vaults without incurring huge expenses. He chose to be buried in the "Avello Corporis Domini nostri Yesu Chrispti" for 35 lire — a price that also included his funeral, masses, and handouts to the poor on the seventh and thirtieth days.[121] Nigerius f.q. Bondi, from Casciana, then living in Pisa, selected his grave in the "tomb and monument" of his religious company, the flagellant society of San Gregorio, located in "Campo santo, the cemetery of Pisa's major church."[122] Similarly, the tanner Vivianus f.q. Francesci sought interment there in the *"avello"* of his confraternity, the *disciplinati* of Santo Stefano.[123] Here, testators could simply receive tombs assigned to them by the officials of the cemetery, the *operarii* of the Opera del Duomo, as was the wish of the Pisan canon and priest of the *plebis* of Cascina, who in 1418 requested a vault (*avello*) or a new tomb (*sive tumulo novo*) "conceded and assigned" by the *operarii* "in an honorable and respectable place in the heart of this campo."[124]

Examples of testators buying their burial vaults (found nowhere else for these six towns) suggest further the ready-made character of the sites and monuments in this vast communal cemetery. In 1417, another Pisan canon, dominus Lazzarus, from the neighboring village of Marti, wished to be buried "in that tomb being purchased from my property which lies in the Campo Santo, that is outside the cloister, above the road that runs from one side of the Campo to the other and near the gate over which is painted the Assumption of the Blessed Mary."[125] Similarly, the widow Johanna and daughter of domini Bacciamei Sampantis chose her burial "in that vault [*avello*] existing in the above-mentioned Campo Santo being purchased by me . . . over which my name ought to be inscribed . . . and the coat of arms of my father drawn [*designari*]." For the cost of this vault and her other burial expenses she left 60 lire.[126] As these documents suggest, the special cemetery of the cathedral was not solely the preserve of the wealthy and powerful. For as little as 100 soldi,[127] a testator might hope to have his bones conserved in these Elysian fields. Its vaults were open to a wide spectrum of the work force of Pisa: innkeepers, saddlemakers, carpenters, black-smiths, leather workers, and even servants.[128]

When burial in Pisa is considered more closely, its resemblance to Siena and Assisi and its distance from the other three cities come into sharper focus. Despite the infrastructure provided by the Campo Santo, efforts by Pisan testators to immortalize their earthly remains with monumental burial projects were extraordinarily rare. The one striking exception comes in fact not from a native of Pisa but instead from the cosmopolitan archbishop of Pisa, Giovanni, whose body we have already seen still encased by Nino Pisano's masterpiece.[129] No other chapel-monument project or burial plan involving such an expenditure appears in these Pisan testaments. The archbishop set aside 500 florins for his body's immortalization, a large outlay, to be sure—although, as we have seen, an amount not so unusual for Florence or even the less wealthy and more provincial Arezzo. Moreover, in Pisa, unlike Arezzo, Florence, and, in particular, Perugia, only two burial monuments called for paintings or even ornamentation. In 1381, Andrea of Massa f.q. Pieri, who chose to be buried in his parish of San Martino Chinzica "in front of our altar, that is in our monument," ordered his heirs to purchase for 60 florins "a beautiful panel-painting" now located in the church of San Michele in Veruta. He demanded that it be transported to San Martino and placed above "our altar."[130] In 1390, the furrier Pierus, son of the furrier Iani, elected his burial in the cemetery of his parish church, the monastery of San Giovanni Battista, "in our monument and the monument of our ancestors and descendants," located in the first cloister of this monastery. He ordered the monks to have painted in the *scontipitio* and *arcu* above his ancestral sepulcher "the figure of the Crucifixion of Our Lord Jesus Christ and two saints on each side," its costs left to the discretion of his executors.[131] With the exception of these expenditures for burial monuments and works of art—60 lire here, 60 florins there—Pisans paid closer attention to, and spent more on, the ephemeral charities that composed their funerals than did their contemporaries in Florence, Arezzo, and Perugia. These were matters, however, that literally soon went up in smoke—wax and candles for masses on the day of their burial, "the seventh," and "the thirtieth." As seen earlier, these funeral costs could often climb above 100 lire. In contrast, a burial monument with coat of arms could be purchased in Pisa even in the latter decades of the Trecento for as little as 10 florins, far less than in any of the other cities.[132] But despite these market advantages provided by the commune's unique Camposanto, Pisans, like Assisani and Sienese, rarely invested in the more durable and worldly funerary accouterments—sepulchers and the regalia of their lineages to enhance their earthly fame.

Change over Time

Thus far I have stressed the differences among these six city-states. The efforts to individuate one's bodily remains and to preserve earthly recognition through tombstones, coats of arms, frescoes, and chapel constructions match the differences among these cities seen earlier in their allocation of pious resources—whether to shun earthly memory through the liquidation and fragmentation of pious donations or to stockpile them into gifts that would remind heirs and beneficiaries alike of a testator's life and largess. But as the multiple regression models have indicated, time more than place separated the two broad approaches to the afterlife. In all these places, new constructions of shrines, graves, and chapels began to increase from the Black Death on and reached their pinnacle in the years immediately following the second recurrence of pestilence in 1363. Nowhere did generational graves appear in significant numbers before the Black Death, but by the last decades of the Trecento they flourished, predominating over new constructions and other means of locating graves in all six towns. By the early Quattrocento, new construction projects began to wane, precisely because testators could increasingly rely on the existing monuments erected by their fathers or other ancestors. (See table 12.) The practice of burial to preserve one's name and lineage had become established, moreover, for the long term against the mendicant ideals, which recalled the contempt of early Christian fathers, who had railed against the *selpulchrorum ambitio* of Romans bent on conserving their names through graves and profane art.[133]

With burials, as with the allocation of pious goods, testators in all six cities began to view the afterlife in fundamentally different terms after the plague of 1363, if not immediately during those summer months. From the mendicant ideal of consciously and carefully shunning all forms of earthly hubris—whether it concerned gifts to monasteries in coin with no obligations attached or an indifference toward the precise place of the body's burial—testators sought out new ways to make their lives felt and remembered among the living. A cult of remembrance had already cut socially deep and geographically wide at least a generation before the rise of civic humanism[134] in Quattrocento Florence. This cult of remembrance, however, was neither the antithesis of spiritual indifference nor a loss of fear and passion for what the afterlife might soon bear for the testator, as some art historians in Burckhardtian guise would have us believe.[135] My examples have shown the opposite. As monumental graves and funerary decorations grew in frequency and in expense, and as familial graves and chapels increasingly became the physical embodiments of these artistic schemes, testators devoted large portions of their wills to the election of private chaplains and poured increasingly large sums into the celebration of perpetual masses to ensure the salvation of their ancestors' as well as their own souls. Quantification and further discussion of these masses and matters of the soul will come later, in Chapter 6. But on the basis of evidence assembled in this chapter, I can safely assert: Earthly memory and the salvation of the soul, instead of being in opposition, came to be tied inextricably together in the strategies of the afterlife for men and women of all six cities after the recurrence of plague, 1362–63.

5

Property

Naturally, we all desire to extend the memory of our names through fame;
even more so do those who sense so acutely the brevity of the present life.
—Giovanni Boccaccio, *Epistole,* to Pino de' Rossi (1361)

The quest to live on in human memory often assumes bizarre forms.
—Robert Davidsohn, *Geschichte von Florenz* (1927)

he testaments chart differences among these six societies
and over time in attitudes toward property that match
differences in the patterns of pious bequests and concerns over corporeal remains. As seen earlier, testators
increasingly tended to liquidate their properties, both
landed and mobile, into cash. (See tables 6 and 7.) For
most of these city-states, the extent of liquidation peaked in the last
decades of the thirteenth or the opening years of the fourteenth century,
when testators everywhere converted the bulk of their pious bequests
into coin (from 84 percent in Arezzo to 92 percent in Pisa). Then, from
the early years of the Trecento through the end of this documentation,
testators directed their executors less and less to convert their property
into reified sums for charitable and pietistic ends. In a sense, although
headed for the grave, they held on more tightly to their cherished
possessions.[1] By the early Quattrocento, less than half of all pious be-

quests were in coin in Pisa and Perugia, where pious legacies outnumbered nonpious ones by as much as three to one.

This refusal to relinquish ties to property can be seen in the growing complexity of conditions that the dying heaped on their beneficiaries. Reflecting changes in notions of the afterlife, particularly after the recurrence of pestilence in the 1360s, these tendencies worked against the rational administration of pious patrimonies by hospitals, monasteries, and confraternities. The unwieldy character of dispersed and inalienable estates certainly affected the economies of institutions such as the hospital of the Misericordia, which the Commune of Siena was forced to bail out of its financial straits on several occasions before its bankruptcy in the early Quattrocento,[2] or the Bigallo and the confraternity of Orsanmichele in Florence, which, despite the outpouring of gifts to both these institutions following the Black Death of 1348, would have gone under in the early Quattrocento had the Florentine government not intervened in the administration of their affairs.[3] These difficulties in ecclesiastical and charitable organization and administration may not have resulted solely from the mismanagement of too many fortunes unleashed by the drastic mortalities of 1348, as historians since Matteo Villani have assumed.[4] A change in the character of gift giving—one that did not simply convert properties to the convenience of coin with few conditions or strings attached—certainly contributed a host of new problems for pious beneficiaries.

The most common of these conditions placed on gifts, both pious and nonpious, were restrictions on the alienation of real property, whether urban palaces and large estates (tenimenti, poderi) or strips of land. These clauses prohibited not only the sale of properties but also rights of donation and even leasing, mortgaging, or placing other obligations on the properties. In gifts to friends and relatives and particularly to universal heirs in their minority, these clauses were often not absolute but contingent on the permission of another relative or executor or until an heir reached a certain age. Table 11 charts the frequencies of these alienation clauses across geography and over time.

Again, the differences among cities follow the two-way division seen earlier. More restrictions on property came from testators in the three towns with a mixed character of pious giving before the Black Death—Florence, Arezzo, and Perugia. In Florence and Arezzo, one in four testators placed such restrictions on their bequests; in Perugia, nearly one in five did. The most emphatic of these nonalienation stipulations came from Arezzo when the plague returned in 1374. The "Provident

Table 11.
Nonalienation Clauses

Period	No. Testators	No. Nonalienation Clauses in Pious Bequests	No. Nonalienation Clauses in Nonpious Bequests	No. Nonalienation Clauses Governing Universal Heirs	Total	No. Nonalienation Clauses per Testator	Proportion of Nonalienation Clauses per Total No. Bequests
AREZZO							
< 1276							
1276–1300							
1301–25	56	6	4	0	10	0.18	0.011
1326–47	92	3	21	8	32	0.35	0.022
1348	84	3	8	3	14	0.17	0.013
1349–62	63	2	15	4	21	0.33	0.026
1363	71	2	6	1	9	0.13	0.012
1364–75	88	13	7	5	25	0.28	0.025
1376–1400	94	2	4	4	10	0.11	0.013
1401–25	100	11	11	12	34	0.34	0.039
Total	648	42	76	37	155	0.24	0.020
ASSISI							
< 1276	18	0	0	0	0	0.00	0.000
1276–1300	22	2	0	0	2	0.09	0.005
1301–25	19	0	0	1	1	0.05	0.004
1326–47	27	1	0	1	2	0.07	0.006
1348	27	0	1	0	1	0.04	0.003
1349–62	5	1	0	0	1	0.20	0.009
1363							
1364–75	14	0	0	0	0	0.00	0.000
1376–1400	30	0	4	3	7	0.23	0.018
1401–25	128	0	4	4	8	0.06	0.009
Total	290	4	9	9	22	0.08	0.007
FLORENCE							
< 1276	14	0	0	0	0	0.00	0.000
1276–1300	43	0	3	2	5	0.12	0.007
1301–25	52	8	11	6	25	0.48	0.029
1326–47	57	2	7	6	15	0.26	0.024
1348	63	6	0	3	9	0.14	0.011
1349–62	31	2	4	3	9	0.29	0.027
1363	68	5	4	4	13	0.19	0.014
1364–75	77	15	12	7	34	0.44	0.044
1376–1400	91	11	5	5	21	0.23	0.024
1401–25	85	2	11	7	20	0.24	0.030
Total	581	51	57	43	151	0.26	0.023

Table 11.
Continued

Period	No. Testators	No. Nonalienation Clauses in Pious Bequests	No. Nonalienation Clauses in Nonpious Bequests	No. Nonalienation Clauses Governing Universal Heirs	Total	No. Nonalienation Clauses per Testator	Proportion of Nonalienation Clauses per Total No. Bequests
PERUGIA							
< 1276	2	0	0	0	0	0.00	0.000
1276–1300	4	0	1	0	1	0.25	0.032
1301–25	10	2	1	0	3	0.30	0.017
1326–47	61	3	4	3	10	0.16	0.014
1348	79	0	1	0	1	0.01	0.001
1349–62	20	0	2	1	3	0.15	0.013
1363	28	1	1	1	3	0.11	0.009
1364–75	51	0	4	3	7	0.14	0.015
1376–99	196	22	15	12	49	0.25	0.026
1400–1425	73	10	5	7	22	0.30	0.032
Total	524	38	34	27	99	0.19	0.018
PISA							
< 1276	14	2	0	0	2	0.14	0.010
1276–1300	42	0	0	0	0	0.00	0.000
1301–25	232	6	9	2	17	0.07	0.004
1326–47	100	7	5	1	13	0.13	0.009
1348	15	1	2	1	4	0.27	0.021
1349–61	64	10	1	0	11	0.17	0.013
1362	39	0	0	0	0	0.00	0.000
1363–75	49	1	0	0	1	0.02	0.002
1376–1400	110	5	4	1	10	0.09	0.011
1401–25	72	1	4	1	6	0.08	0.016
Total	737	33	25	6	64	0.09	0.006
SIENA							
< 1276	35	2	2	0	4	0.11	0.008
1276–1300	44	1	2	3	6	0.14	0.008
1301–25	50	3	0	0	3	0.06	0.003
1326–47	67	2	1	0	3	0.04	0.003
1348	55	0	1	0	1	0.02	0.002
1349–62	40	0	1	0	1	0.03	0.002
1363	24	0	0	0	0	0.00	0.000
1364–75	25	0	1	1	2	0.08	0.008
1376–1400	61	0	1	1	2	0.03	0.004
1401–25	45	1	3	0	4	0.09	0.010
Total	446	9	12	5	26	0.06	0.005

Table 11.
Continued

Period	No. Testators	No. Nonalienation Clauses in Pious Bequests	No. Nonalienation Clauses in Nonpious Bequests	No. Nonalienation Clauses Governing Universal Heirs	Total	No. Nonalienation Clauses per Testator	Proportion of Nonalienation Clauses per Total No. Bequests
TOTAL							
< 1276	83	4	2	0	6	0.07	0.004
1276–1300	155	3	6	5	14	0.09	0.005
1301–25	419	25	25	9	59	0.14	0.015
1326–47	404	18	38	19	75	0.19	0.015
1348	323	10	13	7	30	0.09	0.003
1349–62	223	15	23	8	46	0.21	0.024
1363	230	8	11	6	25	0.11	0.011
1364–75	304	29	24	16	69	0.23	0.026
1376–1400	582	40	33	26	99	0.17	0.023
1401–25	503	25	38	31	94	0.19	0.027
Total	3,226	177	213	127	517	0.16	0.018

man" Pierozius f.q. Ser Federigi named the Misericordia as his universal heir, on condition that the rectors place a plaque (*lapidem*) over the door of his house (*super hostio*) "with the letters cut and sculpted in stone" of the year, month, and day he gave it to the fraternity and of the name of the notary redacting his testament. Pierozius then ordered these rectors not to sell, alienate, or trade any of his landed properties, "neither with the advice [*consilium*] of the Commune of Arezzo, nor with the advice of this confraternity, nor through the advice of our Lord the Pope, nor by 'his Cardinals,' nor by the archbishop, nor by the churches, nor with the dispensation of the Emperor, nor through Papal privilege or privileges granted by the Emperor, the Cardinalate, the Bishop or Archbishop, nor by any other person, except out of use and necessity for assisting the poor." One vineyard situated in Villalba might be sold so long as the money was spent for purchasing other landed possessions located there; in that case, the money had to be left on deposit with a designated banker (*apud unum campsorem*) in the interim. If the rectors went against these conditions, the properties would pass to the Olivetan "friars" and the hospital of the Oriente with the same stipulations. If they in turn "contradicted" these clauses, Pierozzus finally called upon a non-Aretine guarantor, the principal hospital of Siena, Santa Maria della Scala, to take over these lands and from their income build within one year a hospital in the city of Arezzo, to be called the hospital of Santa Maria della Scala, after giving notarized public notice to the Olivetani and the hospital rectors of the Oriente.[5]

In contrast, testators from the other three towns—Pisa, Assisi, and Siena—tried far less often to control their real estate once they had passed to the grave. Only 9 percent in Pisa, 8 percent in Assisi, and 6 percent in Siena placed such conditions on their beneficiaries—less than half the frequency found for Perugia and less than one-fourth for Arezzo and Florence. A better measure of these differences, however, would be the number of such conditions per legacy, since a single testator could (and often did) tie up several grants of property, whether to charitable institutions, friends, or universal heirs. For instance, in 1312 the Aretine widow Lucia, from the quarter of Piscaria, gave her house and several strips of land to the Misericordia on condition that they use the revenues from these properties for the sustenance of the poor of this fraternity and "that under no guise or at any time should they attempt to make any alienation or take away any of these lands"; otherwise, the properties would pass to the hospitals of the Ponte and the Episcopatus. She then gave a small patch of vineyard (two *starii*)[6] to the Augustinian friars, a piece of arable land (three *starii*) to the nuns of Santo Sperandio for vigils and Holy Offices, and yet a fourth donation of land to the nuns of Ognissanti, attaching to all of them the same restrictions against alienation.[7] With legacies as the denominator, the differences among these cities become even more accentuated. Florence, Arezzo, and Perugia look more alike with 23, 20, and 18 alienation clauses per thousand legacies (pious and nonpious), respectively, and the gulf widens between these cities and the other three; Assisi, Pisa, and Siena recorded, respectively, only 7, 6, and 5 restrictive clauses per thousand legacies.

Although the frequency of these conditions per testator did not increase steadily and progressively from the earliest documents through the opening of the Quattrocento, the direction of change was unmistakable: it reached its low point in the earliest records (7 percent) and its pinnacle (23 percent) in the years immediately following the recurrence of pestilence (1362–63). By the last period of my investigation, the opening decades of the Quattrocento, the high point was nearly the same (19 percent). If the frequency of such restrictions is expressed as a ratio of all bequests, the change over the long haul becomes stronger: from 4 per thousand bequests in the earliest records, such clauses increased by over six times to 27 per thousand at the beginning of the Quattrocento. Yet, a qualitative and textual examination of these property restrictions, which grow in complexity after the plagues and into the Quattrocento, provides a better guide for assessing the differences over geography and time. Let us begin with testators' attempts to determine the flow of their nonpious properties.

Directions from the Grave

PISA AND ASSISI   In Pisa, Assisi, and Siena, these restrictive conditions on property rarely went beyond the notarial formula forbidding the recipient "to sell, alienate, mortgage, trade or exchange."[8] When applied to nonpious parties, the phrases were often no more than an entitlement to enjoy the *usufructus* during the lifetime of the beneficiary. Such was the nature of the restrictions that Moccia, the widow of the warehouse manager (*fundacarius*), placed on the house that her illegitimate sister was "to use and enjoy" along with the testatrix's servant. She then prohibited her "natural" sister from dividing, apportioning, or in any way assuming the ownership of this residence.[9]

As for the lion's share of a testator's properties (usually the principal residence and landed properties), testators from the three cities that most fully adopted mendicant ideals in allocating their pious bequests rarely specified at what age an heir might alienate an estate, which properties could or could not be alienated, and, if alienated, with whose consent or to whom they might be sold. In these cities, the exceptional cases when testators went beyond simple and direct transfers of property and entered into the future affairs of their friends, relatives, and heirs came predominantly in the latter part of the Trecento and early Quattrocento.

There were a few exceptions. In 1302, the Pisan retailer of woolen cloth (*apothecarius pannorum de lana*) named his four daughters as his universal heirs, with the stipulation that a certain piece of land with a house, a terrace (*solariatio*), and a garden "remain and always be held in common among all his daughters and that they never divide or in any way or at any time sell, alienate, or give [the property] to their daughters as a dowry. Instead, they were to have the property in common and to enjoy and use it communally for all time."[10] In 1309, Gerardescha, the widow of Lord Gionchelli from the noble "house" (*de domo*) of the

Sismundi left her grandsons (the children of her deceased son) as her universal heir but prohibited them from alienating any of the properties during the lifetime of their mother.[11]

After these rare exceptions—perhaps holdovers from a previous more feudal milieu—the next appearance of a restriction that meddled in the future affairs of one's relatives does not occur until 1360, and this appearance hardly mapped out a testator's future beyond the grave through the planned succession of landed estates. Instead, the Pisan citizen Petrus f.q. Celli, from the wealthy and important Gaytani family, divided various articles of clothing equally between his two sisters, provided that neither ever sell or give any of her belongings to their brother, the priest Francescus.[12] (In a previous legacy, Petrus gave his brother a cloak, specifying that he was not entitled to any more of his estate, "since on many occasions" the testator had given him money totaling over one thousand lire.)

After the recurrence of pestilence, these clauses became more frequent and more complex. In 1381, "the merchant and citizen of Pisa" Iustus f.q. Ser Johannis Manninghi made a contingent gift to any daughters who might be born to him. They were to receive as a dowry 500 florins as well as another 500 florins for their inheritance *in parafernum* (that is, the nondotal properties that Roman law allowed daughters to manage outside their future husbands' control).[13] He then "wished" that neither his daughters yet to be born nor anyone else should alienate the sum, which formed that part of the *parafernalia.* However, should no sons be born, these to-be-born daughters might freely "dispense with" the 500 florins that formed the *parafernalia,* once they came of age.[14]

The 1391 testament of Michele f.q. Bindi Malacalse, after he had "elected" his burial, conveyed only one itemized bequest. He left his brother as universal heir on condition that he never sell, alienate, donate, or in any way transfer any of the inheritance so long as their mother, domina Duccia, was alive. If he failed to abide by these conditions, the property would pass to their mother.[15] In 1382, a citizen from Perugia, who had moved to Pisa and was redacting his will there, named his son universal heir, prohibiting him from alienating any of the property unless he was convicted of a crime.[16]

But not until the Quattrocento did Pisan testators evince new attitudes toward property, which conflicted with earlier mendicant ideals of the afterlife: now there was an attachment to earthly goods and a zeal to preserve real estate within the lineage. This new attitude infiltrated beyond the ranks of the old nobility and the merchant elite, and it pertained to more than just the prized pieces of urban real estate or large landed possessions. In 1414, an émigrée from Cremona then living in the *contado* of Pisa, the widow of a gravedigger, gave a friend, the married woman Teccia, her pillow of monk's wool (*pilandram meam monachinam*), only if she would retain it for her own use and not "sell it, alienate it, use it as a pawn, or barter it."[17]

Concerns over the future state of one's property and the destiny of one's beneficiary went beyond cherished monk's-wool pillows. In 1402, the first instance of a testator entailing property down the male line appears in the Pisan samples. Teccia, a widow and native of the Arno village of Navacchio, then living in the Pisan parish of San Paolo in Orte, gave a plot of land with a house and a sun terrace, located in her parish, to a married woman, domina Guiduccia. She then went beyond this simple transaction by insisting that the property be passed *in perpetuum* "to her children of the 'masculine sex' and from them to their descendants."[18] We have already seen the case of the rural notary from Palaja who redacted a will in 1405 during a period of political turmoil and military strife. With his gift, "a large farmhouse, recently burnt down" in the village of Calci, he pried into the future affairs of his beneficiaries. It was given to two brothers (unrelated to the testator) on condition that within six months following the testator's death, they finish roofing it and afterward agree to reside there always with their families and household possessions.[19]

Finally, in 1420, the Pisan citizen Antonius f.q. Francesci, from the Casapieris family, hammered out the details of the entailment of property with redundant clarity. He wrote his testament when he had no living sons or daughters. If he were to father sons, then they would become his universal heirs. If no sons survived him, all his houses in the parish of San Clemente would pass "to my house [*de domo mea*]," that is, to the "consortium" of the Casapieri family. Before returning to the affairs of "his house" and lineage, he gave several gifts in cash to female members of his family. He then ordered his executors to sell for 100 florins his share of a cheese shop, which he held with the cheesemaker Nicholaus, called Canneto. The executors were then asked to buy "a good piece of landed property" in the city, the *contado,* or the district that had been Pisan territory before the Florentine conquest. This property was "to remain always *ad usufructum* and always to be passed down to the single closest male relative of the testator "from our house of the Casapieri" (*uni de domo nostrum de Casapieri mihi propinquinori in gradu parentele*), starting with his "consortio," Marianus f.q. Johannis de Stateriis. Then he amplified the above: "His executors should purchase this legacy of *usufructus* and give it to Marianus, then to his legitimate male children. Those [in turn] born legitimately from them should succeed one at a time . . . and after [the deaths of] Marianus and his male children, it should devolve successively on those of the male line and legitimate offspring of our house of the Casapieri [*ad alios successive maschulos et legiptione procreatos de domo nostrum de Casapieris*]." Its succession, he added, should pass "without controversy" and "always to the nearest surviving kin [*et semper ad propinquiorem in gradu descendenti*]." And at no time or in any way should the property be left as collateral: rather, it was to be "possessed and cultivated simply and in good faith."[20]

In Assisi, testators' efforts to tie up property and to manage its future direction from the grave were even less pronounced than in Pisa. The earliest nonalienation clauses placed on gifts to friends, relatives, and heirs reached back only to the Black Death of 1348[21] and only went beyond notarial formula at the beginning of the Quattrocento. In 1400, Cichus Macthioli Massioli Taddioli left his son as universal heir with restrictions against "selling, mortgaging, and alienating his property" unless "for the necessities incurred through illness or any other evident necessity." In these cases, his son might alienate up to one-half these properties but only with the permission of the testator's two nephews.[22]

In the same year, the "prudent man" and merchant Amatatius Magistri Angeli left the first signs in these documents of entailing a prized piece of property. He gave his wife his house of residence with its courtyard located in the parish of San Francesco, next to the communal piazza, on the condition that she never "sell, mortgage, trade or in any other way alienate" the property. "On the contrary, it is to remain always and in perpetuity in common with the testator's heirs and their successors."[23]

A testament of 1415 spelled out the directions of entail more precisely. Ser Nicholaus Lutii left his only son as universal heir. If this son were to die without heirs, "three portions of four parts" of the inheritance should pass *per fideicommissum* (or through entail) to the sons of the daughters of the testator and the fourth part to the Sacro Convento of San Francesco. Ser Nicholaus further demanded that his son and his heirs never sell any of the landed property "by any manner, right or reason" without the "expressed permission" of his executors.[24] This document, however, was exceptional even for Quattrocento Assisi.

FLORENCE   In contrast to those from the cities above, testators from Florence, Arezzo, and Perugia tried far more often to manipulate from the grave the fate of their property and the future affairs of heirs. From almost the earliest testaments, Florentines were obsessed with the flow of their patrimonies and prized possessions through successive genera- tions in ways that do not appear in the Pisan records until the 1420s or in the Sienese testaments until the beginning of the sixteenth cen- tury.[25] In 1291, dominus Consillius f.q. Ser Olivieri de Cerchis left his patrimony equally to his six sons and stated emphatically that no daughter fathered by him or to be fathered by him or by his sons should inherit any of his houses in Florence; instead, they should pass only through masculine hands. If all six sons should die without male heirs, half his patrimony should be spent on building a hospital on his lands to care for and receive "poor, religious and special persons." This merchant magnate then looked to the future through the ideological prism of the male line. He left the *ius patronatus,* the right to elect the *"hospitalarium et familiarem,"* along with the privileges of overseeing the business affairs of this hospital and its property, to those who were at least 18 years old and of his house (*de domo sua*). He defined those heirs further as "his descendants through the male line [*de descendentibus per lineam masculinam*], originating from his father Ser Oliverio and his mother domine Emel- line." As for the other half of his patrimony (which included all his houses in the city of Florence), Consillius again looked to the future of his properties through his lineage and their flow through the male blood- lines. In the case of the death of all his sons, he left them to the male children of the two brothers Domini Gherardini domini Lapi and Domini Nicchole "and to their male descendants and then afterwards through their male line by family stock [*stirpe*] and not by head [*pro capite*],"[26] thus ensuring the rights of the lineage over possible claims or divisions by individual heirs.

Nor does this early document from a powerful merchant on the rise[27] stand in isolation. In 1301, the nobleman dominus Schiatta f.q. domini Bocche f.q. domini Rayneri Rustici, from the Abbati family, continued an entail of property rights and restrictions, which may have existed in the family for generations. He bequeathed one-eighth part, which was to be indivisible (*pro indiviso*), of 30 parts from all the palaces, houses, lands, and buildings located in the Florentine parishes of Orsanmichele, San Bartolommeo al Corso, and San Martino al Vescovo to his relatives (*consortibus*) and blood kin (*consanguineis*) of the Abbati family (*stirpe*). These properties and their divisions, in turn, "had derived from his paternal bloodline [*ex paterno sanguine derivatus*]."[28] As we saw earlier, this testator did not end his conditions and demands with the continued flow of these properties down the male line but added various charitable tasks to be performed by his *consortes* for the health of his soul.

These strategies and impositions placed early on by Florentine testators on future generations of heirs, as well as the direction of the flow of property through the male line, were not found exclusively among the Florentine *ottimati*. In the same year, Andrea f.q. Manni, after naming his son as universal heir, added the itemized command "that no woman should inherit or be the heir to the household of this testator at any time so long as there was any legitimate male members of his family [*in ipsa domo*]; rather women should have sufficient funds from their fathers for their dowries or for entering a convent, according to the capacities [*secundum facilitates*] of those male heirs down through his lineage [*ex linea masculina*] in perpetuity."[29] While a male orientation defined lineage in almost every instance, entail could travel through both sexes. In a testament drawn up in 1314, Solius f.q. Martini de Tedaldis, "acknowledging the fidelity" of a certain Donatus, of the parish of San Pancrazio, left him "and his descendants male and female" a house with a plot of land in Petriolo.[30]

The next example of entail in the Florentine documents does not occur until the year of the Black Death. Niccholaus f.q. Cini Monaldi, from Poggibonsi, divided his patrimony between his son and his two grandsons born of a deceased son as well as those to be born *ex eis ex recta linea*. If his son and grandsons should die without heirs, Niccholaus "substituted all his property" to build a nunnery "for sisters or recluses" under the rule of Sant'Agostino, "under the protection, regime and discipline" of the Augustinian priors of the province of Pisa and the rule and counsel of the confraternity of Santo Stefano. The testator's generosity did not, however, come without strings attached—conditions which in fact would benefit the well-being of his future offspring and lineage. He demanded that this new convent accept without a dowry any girl wanting to enter who descended from his lineage (*aliqua filia descendens ex recta linea*).[31]

A month later, Gabriellus f.q. Mazze de Ramagliantibus named his two sons as universal heirs. If both died, the inheritance would pass to his three cousins and "their descendants through the male line." Again, a testator strove to ensure the property rights of the lineage's collectivity against the claims of the individual: the patrimony was to pass *in stirpe et non in capite*.[32] In July of that year, Albertus f.q. Lapi, from the powerful Florentine Alberti family, left the revenues from one of his farms (*poderis*) to support a *sacerdos* delegated (*deputatur*) to celebrate daily masses in the Florentine hospital of Sant'Onofrio for the souls of the testator and his ancestors. Albertus specified that this income was to be derived (*possit percipere*) only through renting (*locare et dislocare*) and thus prohibited the sale, alienation, or donation of his property. The lineage-minded testator then assumed the rights of election of this priest and channeled the *ius patronatus* (for the second time in the Florentine testaments) down the male line of his future descendants (*per infrascriptos heredes vel eorum discendentes masculos per lineam masculinam*).[33]

In the interval separating the first two plagues, only one testator entailed his patrimony. In 1355, Michus f.q. Lapi Guidolotti designated his brother as universal heir. If the brother was alive, the estate would pass to this brother's sons and descendants through the male line and by family stock (*stirpe*), not by head.[34] After the recurrence of pestilence, the imposition of entailing property, the granting of special rights, and insistence on the devolution of patrimonies through the male line intensified, infiltrating testaments beneath the ranks of the Florentine oligarchy and merchant elites. In the year of the plague's return, the bulk of Francescus f.q. Masi de Alferriis's will consisted of contingency plans for the division and allocation of his patrimony, if his son, then in his infancy, should die without male heirs. Here for the first time in these documents we encounter the term *agnatus* — well over a century before it surfaces in the Sienese samples. After several pious and nonpious gifts, Francescus divided the remainder of his estate between two cousins and then channeled the properties to his "closest agnates" (*proxiomores agnatos dicti Francesci*), that is, "through the male line of the stock of the Alferi of Florence."[35]

The following year, Alamannus f.q. Tolosini, who bore the family name de Tolosinis[36] but who was identified as the son of an ironmonger from the parish of Santa Maria Novella, appointed his only son as universal heir, along with "all others born through the male line and all their sons and all their legitimate and natural male descendants [*seu omnes filios et descendentes masculos legptimos et naturales*] of this Alamannus through his male line." If his son were to die without heirs, the estate would devolve on his nephew, Tolosinus, and would then pass, once again, through the male line. In a separate itemized act later on in the document, the ironmonger's son further explained this devolution, boosting still more his recently minted family name: the estate would pass to the *consortes*, the legitimate male descendants of the house and stock (*domus et stirpe*) of the Tolosinis and "through its great masculine line [*per lineam masculinam magnam*] and to those kin closest to the testator," but in this case, "divided proportionately by head and not by stock."[37]

On the same day, Alamannus's nephew, Tolosinus, grandson of the ironmonger, made a will directing his estate to ascend through "his male children to be born and their descendants through the male line and through what was commonly called true entail [*substituit pupillaniter vulgariter per fideicommissum verum*]." If it happened that he fathered no sons, his uncle Alamannus and his descendants through the male line were to inherit his patrimony, except for a farm (*podere*) worth 500 florins and another 200 florins in cash to be given, in this case, to his sister and his three aunts. Nor was this property given outright; instead, the nephew and his offspring for successive generations would be forced to channel it through the male members of "his house" and the "stock" of the Tolosini; again, the testator spelled it out: "through the male line."[38]

By 1368, the language of family stock and the distinctions in the passage of family properties through individuals or family groups penetrated even lower down the social scale of the Florentine urban population. Iacobus f.q. Pieri Martelli, a carder in the wool industry (*cardator seu conciator pannorum*), left his estate to any sons to be sired by him and otherwise to his son-in-law and his brother and to their heirs, and despite the absence of a family name, this worker emphasized the rights of his lineage over future claims of the individual, stressing that his property devolve *in stirpe et non in capite*.[39]

The first woman in these documents to practice entailing property down the male line was domina Diana, daughter of Lippus, from the Giambullari family, and widow of Iacobus Strozze, of the powerful Strozzi family. In 1377, she named as universal heir her only son, Alexio, a friar at Santa Maria Novella, later to be celebrated as a *beatus* and to figure in one of the biographies of Giovanni de' Caroli.[40] She left him, however, only the *usufructus* to and the rights of leasing a *podere* with a house and arable lands (the single most important property mentioned in her testament).[41] After this son's death, the farm would devolve to the testatrix's four brothers and then "to their male children and descendants in perpetuity through the legitimate and naturally born members of the male line, by stock and not by head." She further forbade any of these descendants to sell or alienate this farm or to rent it beyond a five-year lease and then envisioned other measures to prevent her brothers "from compelling or coercing her son the friar to loan them anything from the revenues of this property" after her death. These provisions were certainly not formulaic but instead must have been the fruits of this patrician lady's forebodings that these brothers might initiate years of court battles, since earlier they had so vigorously contested the young Alexio's paternal inheritance.[42] In her will, she further forced these four brothers and, after them, their male descendants once in possession of the above-mentioned farm to pay six florins each year to Sister Nastasia, the daughter of one of her brothers and a nun at the Convent of Saint Julian in Monterone.[43]

Ten years later, another woman from the Florentine elite, domina Francesca, the window of a man from the Guidalotti family and the daughter of Nardus Juncte from the Rucellai family, entailed one of her prized landed estates, a *podere* with a house and considerable property, 136 *starii* of arable land, in the village of Castellonchio in the district of Prato. Unlike the lady married into the Strozzi family and her contemporary male testators, Francesca did not fully endorse the male strategy of entail. Instead, she left the estate to her son Francescus, but only during his lifetime. Afterward, it was to pass to his legitimate children, both male and female. If he were to die without heirs, then the estate would go to her other son, Michaelis, who was a friar at Santa Maria Novella, and her daughter, Sister Piera, who was a nun at San Iacobo a Ripoli. They were, however, prohibited from selling, alienating, or mortgaging any property worth more than 300 florins. Then, after they had extracted 300 florins apiece from this estate and after their demise, the remaining property would pass, half to the confraternity of Orsanmichele and half to the hospital of Santa Maria Nuova and its poor.[44]

By the early Quattrocento, entailment of choice pieces of Florentine real estate entered these documents more frequently, as other properties, at least among the aristocracy and the merchant elite, entered the lists of goods never to be alienated and instead to be channeled down successive generations of potential heirs. In 1406, the nobleman Nicholaus f.q. Nobilis Militis domini Luisii f.q. domini Pieri de Guicciardini (an ancestor of the renowned historian) left his estate to his three grandsons born to a deceased daughter, who were 17, 9, and 6 years old. If any died without heirs, the other brothers and their progeny were to be substituted *in stirpe et non in capite* and enjoined to dower their female offspring with 1,000 florins from the patrimony. If all three died, Nicholaus demanded that his estate be "substituted to one or more of his closest relatives by degree, who were legitimately born males of the family and stock of the Guicciardini [*maschulos legpitimos et naturales de familia et stirpe* de Guicciardinis]." The testator then earmarked his domus sive palatium, demanding that "it always remain for the use and habitation of his sons and daughters and his descendants or those most closely related to him by order of succession [proximiorum ordine successivo] and that this palace "by force of the present testament" never be alienated. He further ordered that his shares in the Office of the Monte of the Commune of Florence, the ius patronatus to the church of Saints Nicholas and Biagio in Poppiano, and other property in the parish of Santa Maria alla Torre never be alienated "as long as the last legitimate male of his family and stock should survive."[45]

In 1413, the "nobleman" and "honorable citizen of Florence" Antonius f.q. Africhelli domini Alamanni, of the "house" of the Medici, who was then living in the Castro di Scarperia (Mugello), left his residuary estate to his closest male relatives, Johannes or Nanne f.q. Gucci de Medicis, and Vanne Andree f.q. domini Alamanni de Medici and to their sons and then to any sons fathered by them, divided by stock and not by head. After the deaths of each of these sons born to the "first degree," the inheritance was to devolve on the hospital of Santa Maria Nuova with the stipulation that no "hospitalarius," rector, governor, or administrator sell, alienate, "extract," or rent on a long lease any of the landed properties (bona immobile) of his estate.[46]

Again, women, at least noblewomen, played their part in the transmission of property down male lines. In 1415, domina Pellegrina f.q. domini Basili Teldi de Venetiis, the widow of Antonius Lapacci Rimbertini, from the parish of San Pancrazio, left to her son Iacobus "out of love and charity" 600 florins in coin and in Monte shares. She required Iacobus, however, to spend "this dowry" to repurchase the house and former habitation of her deceased husband along with all its household possessions (cum omnibus masseritiis) and then to continue living there. She further prohibited him from ever alienating the residence or even bequeathing it through a testament "for matters of the soul." Instead, the house was to pass (transire) to his descendants forever (eius descendentes infinites). Lady Pellegrina made further demands regarding her nonlanded properties, insisting that her son "conserve" her linen, rings, and jewelry until he married or reached the age of adulthood.[47] In 1422, "the noble lady" domina Tessa f.q. Francesci, widow of the "nobilis viri Antonio Naldini de Altovitis, bequeathed to her grandsons a farm (predium) with a house and arable lands, "urging them" to leave the property "to one or more of their male descendants and allowing their father to enjoy the usufructus of this property during his lifetime.[48]

Nor were testators' attempts to direct the future flow of their properties limited to the old Florentine families. In 1416, the "good man" (*probus vir*) Johannes f.q. Pasquetti f.q. Mei de Locteriis, a cobbler from Vinci, who had lived for some time (*aliquando*) in the Florentine working-class parishes of Santa Lucia Ognissanti and San Frediano,[49] but who had recently returned to his native village, entailed his "new" house in Vinci, along with its small plot of vineyards and olive trees measuring eight *starii*. Childless at the time of his redaction, Johannes gave the house to a Johannes Mei Tirici for the recipient's lifetime and thereafter to the sons of this Johannes and then to their sons in turn, favoring the rights of the family stock over those of the individual, *in stirpe et non in capite*. This Johannes and his future sons and grandsons were then required to have a mass celebrated for the cobbler's soul once a year at an altar that he had commissioned to be built in his parish church of Sant'Andrea in Vinci; otherwise, half the property would go to supplement the endowment of the chapel and half to assist in the dowries of poor girls marrying for the first time (*de novo maritari*). Finally, the cobbler secured the inalienability of the property in another itemized act "imposing on the said Johannes, his sons, and grandsons" the restriction against selling or alienating the property "in its entirety or in any particular so long as those sons of the said Johannes and any of their descendants should live until the infinite degree [*usque infinitium gradum*]." If they "contradicted" this command, these properties would be divided equally between the Florentine hospitals of San Gallo and Santa Maria Nuova.[50] In 1423, another artisan-shopkeeper, the vintner Johannes f.q. Landi della Malvagia, appointed his wife and two sons as his heirs, along with any male children sired by him. He then entailed the properties for the next generations through his male descendants and, despite the absence of a family name, in family stock and not by head (*filios descendentes masculos in stirpe et non in capite sub vulgariter pupillaniter per fideicommissum*).[51]

Not only did Florentine testators attempt to channel the flow of their properties, on occasion they also tried to block possible transmissions to particular persons at a future date. For the most part, these acts of disinheritance involved in-laws. In 1362, domina Francia, the widow of Mattei and the daughter of a notary, left her son and daughter as her universal heirs, but on condition that "no rights," whether in use or in ownership (*in usufructu vel proprietate*), be converted to Thomassus, her daughter's husband.[52] In 1374, Arnoldus f.q. Petri Sassetti de Sassettis gave his sister 400 florins but debarred her husband from any rights to this property either in *usufructu* or in *proprietate*.[53] On the same day,

the noble lady domina Ceccha f.q. domini Buondalmentis, of the Buon-
dalmenti family and the widow of the noble knight domini Simonis, of
the Bardi family, left her estate to a granddaughter (married into the
Pazzi family), provided that no rights pass on to her husband.[54] In 1393,
Matheus f.q. Pieri Boni left his daughter a quarter of his property, if
his son were to die without heirs, on condition that neither her present
husband, *Magister* Ludovicus, nor any future husband acquire any of the
rights to this inheritance.[55]

On at least three occasions, these circumventions in effect disinherited
blood relatives. In 1348, Filippus f.q. Rosselli de Bacherellis ordered that
his brother not receive any of his patrimony.[56] In 1386, the cloth dealer
(*ritagliator*) Francescus f.q. Vanni named his nephew Vannus Domenici
Vanni as universal heir, provided that "no rights of ownership or possession or usufruct be acquired by his nephew's father," the testator's
brother.[57] And in 1397, the furrier Pierus f.q. Nuti did not make his
son Bernardo a universal heir along with his three sisters and a brother,
but instead gave him 70 florins and demanded that he ask for no more
and not live in the paternal home or go to and from (*vel ire seu redire*)
it or the furrier's shop "or become a partner in any of his father's
businesses or in any way practice or become enmeshed in these affairs,
directly or indirectly."[58]

Stringing the succession of rights to prized properties through future
generations of friends, universal heirs, and relatives or blocking them
were not the only means by which Florentine testators attempted to
pry from the grave into the future affairs of their beneficiaries. As early
as 1313, Florentines, such as the doctor Pierus f.q. Dati, from the parish
of Santa Felicità, tried to rule their roosts after they would no longer
be around. The doctor named his four sons as his heirs but prohibited
them from selling or alienating any of his "immobile properties" (which
he specified as "houses and lands and his other things") without the
"permission and spoken consent" (*absque licentia et parabula*) of their
mother, "since he wanted this property to remain in the family." The
doctor then commanded his sons "to obey, honor and revere" their
mother and "in no way impede or trouble her use of his properties."
Each time they violated this condition, they would lose 100 florins of
their patrimony, which could be collected by those sons who remained
obedient (*applicandum aliis suis fratribus obbedientibus*).[59]

Florentine testators attempted to control the future behavior of their
relatives, friends, business associates, and universal heirs in ways that
went beyond simple obedience to a surrogate father. As early as 1301,

Andrea f.q. Manni Palermine left his blood relative (*suo consanguineo*) Lottus Uberti a clothing allowance of five lire a year for 10 years on condition that Lottus "behave well and live honestly."[60] In 1320, Petrus, the emancipated son of Guido Uguiccionis, from the Florentine parish of San Leo but living in Empoli, left his nephew an income of a florin a year for four years provided he "stay and practice a trade" that the testator's father, Guido, would approve.[61] The international merchant Martinus f.q. Bizzi, stating in his 1351 testament that he possessed 2,000 florins or more in money and merchandise in his business (*fondaco*) in the city of Avignon, required one of his business partners (*sotius*), a certain Ciutius, to make "suitable" yearly accounts of his affairs in that city and "wished" him to administer "these monies, merchandise, and affairs" to the benefit of his heir, Bizzius. If Bizzius's guardians (*tutores*) should judge that Ciutius was not administering these affairs well and for Bizzius's "utility," they were empowered to seize these 2,000 florins from the said Ciutius and to invest them in the city or *contado* of Florence.[62]

The Florentine merchant Iacobus de Iuochis, then working in Paris, confessed in his 1396 testament to have fathered an illegitimate daughter named Thomasseta, whom he had "nourished over the past 10 or 11 years." He gave her a dowry of 400 gold francs if she married by 16; otherwise, the funds would be spent on the poor of Christ and other pious charities.[63] In her brief will of 1406, domina Vanna, the widow of Guidone and afterward the wife of Brogognini, presently living in the Muggello parish of Sant'Agata de Mucciano, named Johanna, a daughter from her first marriage, as her universal heir if within five years of the testatrix's death she returned to live in the village of Sant'Agata; otherwise, the patrimony would be split between the parish church and the sons and daughters born to Johanna.[64]

In considering the character and future behavior of relatives and heirs, Florentine testators did not simply look to controls and the threat of disinheritance; they also wished to ameliorate future conditions to be faced by their kin. Such was the spirit behind the additional comments attached to the end of the 1390 testament of the citizen and merchant Barna f.q. Luce Alberti: "Mindful of the abundance of his patrimony and the needs of his brother, Pazzinus f.q. Luce, who has eleven children, and being attentive to problems that such a large number of children poses, and having affection for this offspring [*prolem*] and his blood relations [*consanquinitatem*], and having deliberated and consulted with others, and moved by a fraternal spirit, the testator gives to these children of the said Pazzini, his nephews, four thousand florins."[65] Similarly, the nobleman Nicholaus, from the Guicciardini family, sought in his 1407 testament to alleviate the possibility that loved ones would slip into dishonor when confronted with unexpected tribulations: "In case any of his daughters should marry and afterwards, on account of the impoverishment of a husband, or because of some other misfortune or unforeseen reason, should wish to become separated from her husband and family to preserve her honor or for necessity . . . she should be free to return, to stay and to inhabit [the testator's] palace and home, to live with his sons and to be fed well from the sumptuous inheritance of this testator."[66]

The most common impositions that testators made on the future actions of their beneficiaries in Florence, or any other city, were the demands husbands placed on their widows-to-be. These will be discussed later. But one arrangement deserves mention at this point, for it reflects the length to which testators might go by the latter decades of the Trecento in attempting to mandate for the future the very movements of their heirs. In 1371, Johannes f.q. Dietisalvi Nigri named his male children still to be born as his universal heirs. If he were to sire no sons, the *usufructus* to all his property would pass to his sister, domina Tessina, although not without qualifications and obligations. She was held to spend 100 florins "to construct and build" within three years a cottage (*domucula*) in the place of the testator's residence in the parish of San Lorenzo "for the utility and convenience" of living there. He then left his wife for as long as she remained a widow the right to remain there as well, but insisted on mapping out the details of her rights of passage in the new edifice. "She might enter by the main passageway [*volte*] and have access to the entire building above the entrance to this passageway using the steps that lead to a newly constructed passageway, except for that part of the building reserved [for his sister] existing above the stairs and under the study [*scriptorium*] and the cloakroom [*guardarobas*]"; that is, as long as she remained a widow, his wife would have "the right of habitation [*habitaturio*] to half of the land and the cottage."[67]

AREZZO   The number of examples of channeling property down a lineage was almost identical for Arezzo and Florence.[68] Although they appear later in the Aretine samples, the first does not come from a testator from one of the old feudal lineages but from a simple *probus vir,* a rural notary and citizen of Arezzo, suggesting that such practices may have already been well entrenched by the early Trecento. In 1334, Ser Andrea f.q. Bettini, from Poppi, chose his son, his two grandsons, and any other grandsons to be born and his descendants through the male line, in this case, by head and not by stock as universal heirs. They were forbidden to sell, alienate, or loan any of these properties unless there was general consensus among those aged 20 or older. Otherwise, the estate would devolve on the Misericordia.[69] As early as 1344, a woman testator— again, not from one of the old families—enforced the devolution of property down the male line, this time in bequeathing not property but the right to control it. Domina Lucia f.q. Donati Aquiste gave her nephews the lands with "perpetual rents" of 26 *starii* of grain and one *mezziolo* of olive oil, provided that they "in no way, for any reason or at any time" sell or alienate these lands without the "express permission" of Friar Bonifazio, the brother of these two nephews. After the friar's death, these rights would pass to the closest blood relative directly down her line of descent (*proximioris consanguinei recta linea descendenti*).[70] In 1358, another rural testator, formerly from the village of Ponzo and then living in Castro Foiano, left his modest residual property to his brother and niece and then funneled it through the descendants of his niece, both male and female.[71]

In addition to sending properties and rights down the tracks of the lineage, Aretine testators enforced the communal restrictions of the consortium over their blood relatives. For instance, in 1362, the friar Martinus f.q. Vati de Testis, a citizen of Arezzo, who was then resident in the monastery of SS. Cosmas and Damian, left a third part of a courtyard and an oven, along with an entire house in the Villa Mori, to his two illegitimate sons, provided that they not alienate the property until one of them, Iacobus, reached the age of 15, and then only with the consent and permission of the testator's brother or his closest blood relative. Moreover, he gave his nephews a third part of the houses in this village, which they held in common, on condition that they alienate these properties only with the consent of his relatives (*consortes*).[72]

The preponderance of such cases from Arezzo, however, comes later, after the return of the plague in 1363. The most remarkable of these appears with the third strike of pestilence in 1374. The merchant-citizen Matheus Giontarini Bruni entailed his "palace" in the street of San Lorenzo to his two brothers and then to their sons; a third portion of his residuary estate would go to his sister if his son should die without heirs, and then to her children, male as well as female, this time in family stock and not by head.[73] More extraordinary were the demands of a citizen, again from a notarial family, Landucius f.q. Ser Andrea Giotti de Acceptantibus. After ordering his arms, plaques (*targia*), and crests (*cimerium*) plastered on his ancestral chapel in Monte San Savino for his memory (*ad memoriam*) and that of his ancestors, Landucius entailed his residence in the *contrada* of Borgo in the city of Arezzo. Here the testator's reasons for prohibiting alienation were made more explicit than for any such entail found even in the lineage-conscious records from Florence: "The testator wishes, demands and insists that the said house of the testator, where he is now living, in no way be sold, alienated or in any way mortgaged by his heirs or any other person; rather it is to stay and must stand in perpetual memory [*ad perpetuam memoriam*] of the testator and his ancestors."

To concretize the survival of his memory, Landucius went a step further, commissioning one of the very few works of art found in these testaments in any city not destined for display on the walls of an ecclesiastical institution. He demanded that his heirs have his coat of arms carved in stone (*intagliata in quodam lapide*), painted, and displayed "so that they could be seen easily and clearly [*ita quod bene et clare videantur*] on the back portion of his house facing the street of Burgi." He then reiterated his demand for entail, that this urban dwelling should be neither sold nor alienated "but always pass through the direct line" to his sons' sons and, if none survived, to their closest male relatives. If it were ever put up for sale, the Misericordia could then intervene and claim the property.[74]

The year afterward, a sister of the Franciscan tertiaries, Francisca f.q. Francisci de Altuciis, divided her estate, giving half to her nephew and subdividing the other half between a Franciscan tertiary, "the honorable sister" Pia, and the testatrix's biological sister Cinella. She prevented both from "diminishing" the property "for reasons of *falcidie* or *trebellianice*[75] or by any other form of alienation or by any donation *inter vivos.*" Instead, after their deaths, this portion of the estate was "to be restituted" to "those male descendants" of her brother and then down the male line. If these male descendants should die before reaching 25 and without fathering male children, the portion of the estate should devolve on her nephew, Augustinus, and then to his sons and their male descendants.

The tertiary then pried further into the biological future and sexual behavior of her lineage, ordering that if any of these male descendants should sire "one or more" legitimate daughters, they should receive dowries of 300 florins apiece. If, instead, an illegitimate daughter (*feminam naturalem vel expuream*) was sired, she would receive 200 florins, whether she married or entered a convent. Furthermore, if Augustinus happened to sire a bastard son, this offspring would receive 400 florins, and if he died without legitimate sons, his portion of the estate would pass to another blood relative, a certain Ser Johannes, to whom she attached the same prohibitions against the alienation of properties, the same devolution of property down the male line, and the same price list for dowering legitimate and illegitimate daughters as well as those of his male descendants. If any of these stipulations were broken, the properties would pass to the Misericordia. The tertiary did not, however, let matters rest even here with this final ecclesiastical guarantor, but instead heaped obligations on this contingent heir several times removed. The fraternity was to pay the Augustinians, the Franciscans, the Dominicans, the Servites, and the monastery of San Marco six florins a year each for annual offices of the dead for her soul and those of her ancestors. Moreover, this last contingent heir was prohibited from alienating this portion of the patrimony, or else this half residuary portion of the estate would pass to yet another contingent heir, the hospital of Arezzo.[76]

Even more complex was the 1416 division and entail of the estate of a spice and clothing merchant, Baccius f.q. Masii, who, you may remember, left funds without details "to paint and make figures" in the main chapel of San Francesco. Unlike Lazarus, his competitor for the chapel ornamentation, Baccius wasted few words on this pious and honorific scheme and instead devoted the bulk of his long testament to determining the precise property rights of his heirs. He dealt first with his son, "the egregious physician and doctor of medicine" *Magister* Thomassus, and Baptista, the doctor's son, by giving them rights in common over the dowry of *Magister* Thomassus's deceased wife, domina Ghita, valued at 475 florins. To the sons and to any sons the doctor might later sire went houses, farm huts, vineyards, olive groves, arable lands, the goods as well as the immovable property that the merchant-father possessed in the Villa and curia of Marcena; half a mill called the "molino dal Raggio," situated on the Arno River, and its equipment; and a *podere* and all its houses, vineyards, etc., in the curia of Corte and Nofri near the Arno. The merchant then went on to enumerate the farm animals, clothing, cloth, ornaments, and books that should ascend to this "stock" of his family. In one of these itemized bequests, two mules were grouped with "all the books pertaining to medicine and its science" and the wine casks found in the merchant's home in Florence.

To equalize the patrimony among his sons, the merchant-father made an accounting of the expenses already incurred by the doctor: 1,000 florins, which the testator maintained he had spent on Thommasus's education, books, and doctorate; 300 florins, which the father loaned to that son while a resident in Florence; 79 florins, which the doctor owed to the cloth business—to its shop (*fondaco*) and for its "traffico," managed by another son, Francescus, and his partners. The father next entered the credit side of the doctor's inheritance: his other two sons were to pay the doctor two parts of their mother's dowry of 450 florins. Finally, the testator declared that his company and cloth shop had earned 2,400 florins in goods, equipment, and credits over the past five years and that his son the doctor was owed half the profits from this capital.

The father assigned his estate in like manner to his other two sons, Francescus and Girolamo. Again, he made these legacies not as simple gifts to each son but as gifts to be passed down from son to son. They involved not only farms and agricultural properties but the shops and the tools of the cloth industry—*purgi, caldarii, domibus tinte*. Moreover, the business divisions between the two sons extended to the fine lines of architectural blueprints for the division of a house containing the testator's shop and warehouse (*apotheca sive fondacis*) with its giant basement and storage bins (*cella magna cum celletta*). Their father imposed on these two brothers, who were also his business partners in the cloth trade, their future rights of passage in this shop and home: Girolamo was to have the ground floor in *"principale parte"* and Francescus in *"secunde parte"* and with the right "to enter and leave the upper bedroom [*superioris camera*] by the upper veranda."[77]

As this last testament suggests, Aretine testators, as in Florence, tried to govern the future affairs of their heirs, weaving their demands and last wishes into the intricacies of daily life and business once they had departed the temporal scene. Again, I reiterate, cases of similar complexity and character are completely absent from the thousands of testaments found for the other three towns. In Siena, where I have read testaments through the eighteenth century, similar wills *do* appear but not until the sixteenth century. In Arezzo, testaments detailing property rights of male heirs and wives to the extent of ascribing the rights of passage in communally owned or occupied homes and palaces outnumbered those for Florence. Moreover, in Arezzo these practices involved properties less imposing than large urban palaces. They slid farther down the social ladder, spreading into the villages of the countryside, and included "houses" that from the descriptions must have represented nothing more grandiose than the cottage of a rich peasant.

The first of these future impositions of rights of passage is found in the testament of a rural notary from Poppi, Ser Andrea. It guaranteed his wife her rights of habitation in the testator's residence down to the details of her future movements. If she lived "honestly" and did not remarry, she could enjoy during her lifetime and together with one of her servants "free habitation" of the first sun terrace off the master bedroom (*sala matrimonialis*), "the room of this Ser Andrea," and a kitchen terrace, along with the rights of passage to "come and go freely" by the stairs leading to the master bedroom. These rights of habitation and *usufructus* were to be acknowledged by his heirs without any molestation or contradiction.[78]

In the plague year of 1374, the villager Masius f.q. Francesci, from Fronzola, determined through his will the future movements within his house of a blood relative (*coniuntus*), Goro Johannis Ser Baldi, and the testator's brother Bettino. To Goro he gave (as a right to be then passed down to his sons) half of a courtyard (*claustrum*) located behind the house. To Bettino and Bettino's family he gave the right to enter the courtyard to fetch water from a well inside it so long as Goro happened not to be entering this courtyard at the same moment. He further ordered his brother to build a wall to divide the courtyard.[79]

In 1415, another villager carefully divided between his heirs their precise property rights and rights of passage. Cristoforus, called Pela f.q. Cecchi, a citizen of Arezzo, living in the village of San Lorenzo, appears to have been even less affluent than the villager Masius from Fronzola. He gave his daughters, Bruna and Donata, the rights of habitation in his urban dwelling located in the Borgo of San Vito of Arezzo, which he then divided. Bruna would receive the anterior part of the house as far as the pantry (*cellarius*) and might debar his son, Menchus, from "its use and habitation." He gave the front part of the house (*parte vero posteriorum*) including the pantry, along with a bedroom and a well located in the back part of the house, to Donata with the right to use these portions "communally" with her sister. The sisters were to hold the vineyards, the arable lands, and the house communally except for properties previously given to his wife, domina Johanna. As for the son, Mencho, we hear no more about him in the will; it appears he was disinherited, Cristoforus having named his two daughters as universal heirs.[80]

Like the villager Masius, who required his brother and a cousin to build a wall to separate their rights of passage, other Aretines imposed posthumous secular construction plans on their heirs. Nor did such concerns over property and its future obsess only the rich and powerful. In 1374, Pierozzius f.q. Ser Federigi, who, as we have seen, was so zealous in ensuring that his house would never be sold or alienated that he forbade it even by permission of the pope or the Holy Roman Emperor, made sure in his will that if a certain Bernardus domini Bettini did not wish to "repair and ornament" a wall in his house, then a certain Johannes, his debtor, was to spend half the debt for these restorations.[81] The woman Johanna f.q. Stefani, from the village of Quarata, wife of Paulus from the same place, made only one itemized act in her testament of 1411. Between her selection of burial and nomination of universal heir, she "confirmed" that she had given her husband 10 florins, which, she "asserted," he was obliged to spend on her home in Quarata for "improvements, works, and beautification [*in meliorationem, opere et aconcimine*]."[82] The merchant Baccius, whose division of property rights we witnessed, was occupied on his deathbed with details for the future remodeling of a house attached to a stable (*stalleta*). He ordered his two sons, Francescus and Girolamo, from their expenses, to have the stable removed and to construct in its place a balcony (*unum veronem*) "extending from the back side to the front" of this house, which he had bequeathed to Francescus and this son's lineage.[83]

Besides channeling property through successive generations, Aretines, like Florentines, tried to control its future by blocking its flow. In 1328, domina Beche, widow of an Aretine notary, left her son, dominus Francescus, a cleric at the church of San Bartolommeo, property from her deceased husband and the *usufructus* of her house, which she forbade him to alienate, except for reasons of illness, unforeseen disasters (*inevitabilibus nec expendiendis*) or the health of her own soul. She further intervened in his future affairs by stipulating that these legacies "were intended only for his person," and no rights were to be assumed by the church or its rector.[84] In 1340, the citizen Guiduccius f.q. Bracci Roberti left a maze of contingencies should his son and universal heir die without heirs: one-third of the patrimony was to be distributed to the poor of Christ; a third to two daughters, the nun Margarita and Paula; one-third to another daughter, Caterina, and, beyond that third, to the sons of his deceased daughter. He then attached a final item to his testament: "namely, that in no way or in any form" might his brother or his children assume any rights to his landed property.[85]

In the year of the plague's recurrence, 1363, Ser Francescus f.q. domini Pagni de Sassolis was even more emphatic in singling out someone never to possess (*percipere*) his property or even to enter his home. He left his two married sisters as universal heirs, then insisted that "these sisters, neither one nor the other, at no time, through any acquisition or division of the inheritance" should allow the husband of his sister, Johanna, the cotton manufacturer, Rossus f.q. Cecchi, "the [right] of intervention to the succession of his estate." Nor was this man "for any reason" ever to "come, occupy, enter, stay or live in the testator's residence."[86]

On occasion, these blockages came closer to home. In at least four instances, Aretine fathers or mothers disinherited their sons. In 1330, domina Adinucia, the widow of Paulus Appulliensis, permitted her son Gellus to ask only for 100 lire and a bed valued at 10 lire from her estate; if he demanded more, he should receive only 25 lire and "would be deprived and excluded from any other utility of her property." She left her residuary estate to complete the endowment and for the *ius patronatus* of a chapel in the Pieve of Arezzo, which her deceased son Iacopus had "ordained."[87] Andrea f.q. Rici, from the village of Forgnone in the Commune of Lippiano, was more straightforward in his will of 1350. Since his son Nanne had been disobedient (*sibi inhobediens*) toward his father "for his entire life," the testator disinherited him (*exheredavit*), mandating that he could take only 10 soldi from his property.[88] The central point of the short will of domina Piera f.q..Ceschi, from Borgo San Sepulcro and the widow of a man from Arezzo, was the disinheritance of her son Pierus. Since, according to the testatrix, he had been "an ingrate and a disobedient son," she gave him 10 lire and then "deprived him of all rights to her inheritance."[89] In the year of the plague's return, 1363, Pietrus f.q. Tegghiarii "disinherited" his son Augustinus, leaving him an honorific five soldi and ordering him not to plead for any more. The father's reasons for disinheritance were the most extraordinary ones found in these testaments. He accused his son of being "always disobedient to his father, treating him with evil magic [or witchcraft] and loiter[ing] about from place to place [*cum malis maleficis moratrahit et conversatur discurrendo per mundum*]."[90]

A testament of 1373 contested the legitimacy and thus the rights of inheritance of a certain Bartolus, who, according to the testator, "asserted himself" to be his son. The testator, named Priore, used his will to refute this man's claims, barring him from any entitlement to any of his patrimony. Bartolus "was not to plead for anything." Nonetheless, for unstated reasons, Priore granted him five florins.[91] Finally, in a testament of 1424, Petrinus f.q. Ceccherani, from Giovo, began by "declaring that fourteen years or so had elapsed" since his son Cecchus left him. At that time, the testator maintained, he had arranged a division of his property assigning his son a share of the movable and landed properties, but had failed to redact a written contract at that time. "Thus, wishing to follow the truth and to have his son approve it and be content," he left this departed son several strips of land, a vineyard, several casks of wine, and a house with a dovecote but "instituted" his other son, Stefanus, as his universal heir.[92]

More common in Arezzo than even in Florence were testators' concerns, often mixed with threats of disinheritance, that sons and daughters treat their mothers "benignly and with charity, devotion and obedience," as in the 1312 testament of Fucius f.q. Cristofori, from Montozzi then living in Arezzo,[93] the 1329 will of the butcher Tosus f.q. Arducii (who added that his sons "should submit themselves to the paternal benediction of his wife, reverently following her counsel, advice and precepts"),[94] the 1344 will of Cecchus f.q. Betti, from Celaria, who lived in Arezzo,[95] and the 1347 will of the notary Ser Cecchus f.q. Neri Bindacchi.[96]

These were not, however, the only familial relationships that testators tried to coax and govern from the grave. In 1318, an innkeeper and citizen of Arezzo, Anzianus f.q. Benedetti, beseeched two of his sons "to advise, correct and treat benignly and with charity" a third son.[97] In 1327, the citizen Gilius left two-thirds of his residuary estate to his granddaughter and the remainder to three cousins, whom he beseeched to treat his granddaughter "benignly, with charity and without molestation," or else their portion of the patrimony would devolve on the Misericordia.[98] The ironmonger and citizen Bertus f.q. Iacopi gave a Neria f.q. Pauli a green cloak and the right to live in his house until she reached the age of 25, provided she treated his children kindly.[99] The citizen Cecchus f.q. Ghini Pucci Grassi in his 1328 will named his four sons as universal heirs, "commending" them to submit to "the power and regimentation, the governance and tutelage" of their uncle, toward whom "they should behave with reverence."[100] A year later, the citizen and grammar teacher (doctor Gramatice) Caroncius f.q. Ser Iacopi, from Vitiano, designated his nephews as his heirs, urging them to pay the same respect and obedience to his brother as they had paid their father.[101] In the year of the plague's return, Duchus f.q. Aghinolfi ordered his two sons to govern his daughter and treat her well; if not, their patrimony would go to the daughter.[102] In 1400, domina Johanna, the wife of Dinus Girelli, left her estate to her grandson, ordering him to obey her husband (his grandfather) like a father (obedire debeat dicti Dini tamquam patrii).[103] In 1412, domina Caterina f.q. Bartolommei Pucci, the widow of Bernardi, a citizen of Arezzo, chose her son's daughter as universal heir, provided that her son "live and be obedient under the benevolence of the rulers of the Commune of Florence and Arezzo [*infra gratiam Magnifici Communis Florentie et Aretii*] and provided that her son live and stay with his children."[104] Finally, in 1418, Niccolaus f.q. domini Mattei Dinufei de Bezolis left his brother as universal heir, "commending" him to revere his mother and treat her benignly in all matters.[105]

Testators' anxiety about possible criminal behavior or even civil disputes increased after Arezzo's submission to the Florentine state in 1384 and particularly in the opening years of the Quattrocento. Curiously, a high proportion of these testators came from country towns and villages. In 1411, Cristofanus f.q. Johannis Godi de Rosellis left his daughter as his universal heir; however, if his daughter should marry and if his cousin, Nofrius, provided her with a dowry of 300 florins and the expenses for her clothing, the inheritance would pass to Nofrius, who then was not to alienate any part of the estate "for any urgency or permission," except to pay off his conviction of a crime should the need arise.[106] In the same year, domina Caterina f.q. Stefani, widow of Mariotti Johannis Ser Astoldi, took the opposite position toward the future possibility of criminal charges against her future heirs. She left her estate to Iacobus and Andrea f.q. Tome Cecchi on condition that they pass the inheritance (*teneantur comunicare dictam hereditatem*) to their cousin (*coniuncto*) Cecchus, provided that "this Cecchus stay and live in the city of Arezzo and not be condemned to exile or declared a rebel [*non esset exbannitus nec rebellis*] of this city."[107]

Again, in 1411, the citizen Nannes f.q. Contucci, called Grancapo, gave a certain Johannes Vive, from Faltone, the *usufructus* to his property on condition that he never become involved in any dispute or court action; otherwise, it would pass to the hospital of the blessed Ann.[108] In 1424, Brunus f.q. Ricci, from the village of Lorenzano, took an even longer view of the behavior of his heirs, declaring that "if any of his children or their descendants should commit any delinquency or crime against the Commune of Arezzo, they would be stripped of their inheritance, and it would pass to the Misericordia."[109] The ultimate obeisance toward the state was paid, however, in a testament redacted several weeks later. The nobleman Johannes f.q. Lazari Niccholai de Barbolanis, from the family enclave of Montaguto Barbolanarum, made his nephews universal heirs. If they were to die in childhood or without heirs, his patrimony would pass to "the Magnificent and Powerful Commune of Florence and to the Magnificent and Powerful Lords in the Great House and Palace of the People of Florence."[110]

PERUGIA   In Perugia, testators' efforts to channel their properties down successive generations did not originate as early as in either Florence or Arezzo. Only three examples, in fact, predate the recurrence of pestilence in 1363. These earliest attempts to control the future flow of property came not from the old urban elites but from a widow in the countryside, from the *castro* of Casalina. She left her sons as universal heirs, and if they were to die without heirs, "she wished her property to remain" with two men who were apparently unrelated to her, Bello and Cangno, and with their sons and the family stock of their house (*domus eius*).[111] Nor did the terms of these stipulations become any more elaborate at the hands of a scion of an important noble lineage, de Oddonibus (Oddi),[112] who named his only son as heir. If the son were to die without heirs, the property would pass to the testator's two brothers and then to his male children by stock (*filios masculos stirpes*).[113]

Even after 1363, when these testamentary entails increased in frequency, they retained their laconic, formulaic character. The Perugian testaments offer no examples as elaborate as the vigorous attempts of Florentines, such as the *nouveau riche* Tolosini, to preserve their "houses" through the eternal flow of properties down the male line, or as explicit as the bid by an Aretine from the Acceptanti family to preserve his prized palace through the flow of his male line for "his perpetual memory." Technical terms such as *stirpe, agnatos, per fidecommissionem, consortes*, and *consanguineos*, and other words such as *semper* and *ad perpetuum*, or the distinction drawn in *in stirpe et non in capite*, scarcely appear here to amplify testators' demands in the flow of properties through the generations. In one of the few instances when the terms *affines* and *consanguineos* did appear, it was not to channel properties down the male line but instead to dismiss claims to a testator's patrimony. In 1383, the knight (*magnificus miles*) dominus Francescus f.q. domini Ugolini "instituted as his heirs all his blood relatives and those related through marriage, both males and females [*eius consanguineos et affines tam mares quam feminas*], up to the fifth degree of relation." The knight gave them five soldi apiece and demanded that they keep quiet.[114] Nor was such wholesale disinheritance the preserve of the nobility. In 1421, a slipper maker with a will consisting of only two items "instituted as heirs" Pellolus Luce and all of his other blood relatives to the fourth degree, giving them five soldi each and demanding that they be content.[115]

Terms such as "lineage" or "through the masculine line" rarely appear in the Perugian testaments. The 1373 will of a noble lady, domina Bianca f.q. Arlocti Arlocti, from the influential Guelph family de Micheloctis,[116] widow of Pandolfi f.q. domini Balionis de Balionibus (one of the ancient bastions of family power in Perugia),[117] was an exception. She left a complex set of contingencies for the future flow of her estate. In the first instance, she named her mother as universal heir, but only during her lifetime and only if her male children remained outside "the benevolence of the Commune of Perugia." If her two sons, Malatesta and Nellus, returned to Perugia, they would become her heirs, and if they should die without sons, she would "substitute" for one-fourth of her estate her cousin Veraginus Symonis Arlocti de Micheloctis and then his male children, and one-fourth would go to another cousin and his male children. If this cousin were to die without heirs, his fourth would pass to Veraginus and his male children by family stock and not by head. As for the other half of her estate, again she emphasized that if her son did not return to the "benevolence" of the state, half of this portion would go to her daughters and the other half would be divided between the above-mentioned cousins (i.e., each would receive one-eighth of the entire estate), and then the legacy would go to their male children and thence down the male line (*et filios masculos et per lineam masculineam*). If both these cousins were to die along with their sons and without surviving male heirs, the noble lady's property would pass to the "male descendants and through the male line" of another male relative on her father's side, "the magnificent man," Biordus Michelocti de Micheloctis (a man not unknown to the chronicles of Perugia, whose "treason" against the Raspanti rule in 1384 enabled the nobility to return to power in Perugia).[118] Another exception was the 1389 will of Paulutius f.q. Nini Pelloli, who left his three sons and his wife as his universal heirs so long as she remained chaste and retained her dowry in the home together with his children. Paulutius then declared that the estate was "always to remain with his descendants through the male line so long as a male survived from that lineage."[119]

Although this careful tracking of the multiple possibilities of the flow of an estate through male descendants was exceptional for the Perugian testaments and found only in the wills of patrician magnates, entailment of property and in particular of the residuary estate was considerably more frequent here (33 testaments) than in Pisa (4), Siena (5), and Assisi (6). Once again, testamentary practice and the ideology of property appear in Perugia to have been more in keeping with sentiments and structures seen in Arezzo and Florence, where the numbers of entails were 38 and 41, respectively. As the frequency of nonalienation clauses (cited earlier in this chapter) suggests, Perugian testators and their notaries may have achieved the same results with less fanfare and a less technical vocabulary. They simply and succinctly demanded that their properties go to "the male children" of their appointed heirs and then to those children's male descendants.

Testators from Perugia, moreover, pried into the future affairs of their heirs, both relatives and friends, in ways other than entailing properties. Not only did they prohibit the sons and descendants from selling their ancestral houses,[120] on occasion they asked their heirs for structural changes and specific improvements in their houses once they had departed the temporal scene. In 1389, domina Angela Peruti Cennini gave a married daughter a house with a garden in her parish of San Savino provided that she spend 20 florins on improvements (cum accomine ad edificationem fiendam) on a cottage given to another, unmarried daughter.[121] The demands of the nobleman Nerus f.q. Nutii Vacrioli in his testament of 1393 reached further into the future affairs of his heirs. He left his cousin (nepos consobrinus) Sagramore as universal heir but required him to build a bridge leading to their ancestral house. The bridge was to be divided equally with a Johannes Mathei and his wife and then to remain "perpetually" the communal property of "all those from his house [debeat comunis dictarum domorum]."[122]

To prevent the sale or division of property, the Perugini, like their contemporaries in Florence and Arezzo, did not always make blanket prohibitions; instead, they interfered in the future affairs of their heirs in finite and concrete ways. In 1363, Tenganius f.q. Angeli Bughi left his four sons as his universal heirs, prohibiting any division of the estate until ten years after his death.[123] In 1371, Stefanus f.q. Nardoli Peri gave the illegitimate son of his nephew a house in the city and landed possessions on condition that he not alienate them for at least 15 years after the testator's death.[124] In 1386, domina Johanna Ciuti de Barsis, the wife of Magi Guidonis Magioli, on the contrary, gave her brother a vineyard, provided that within six years following her death, he sell half the property to pay off her debts.[125] In 1390, Iacobus f.q. Andrutii was even more attentive to the future dealings of his heirs, saddling one of three sons with special conditions: he was not to try to retract his mother's dowry for at least five years, and in that time he was to keep the house communally with his brothers.[126]

In these laconic documents (more so in Perugia than elsewhere), emotional attachment to the future relations of testators' progeny on occasion nonetheless slips into the margins. In 1390, Cristoforus Nigri, from the village of San Cipriano de Boneggio, left his daughter the customary possibility of returning to his home should she become a widow. He then added that he hoped she would be fed and cared for in this home by his son and heir "with fraternal love."[127] In 1417, Francescus f.q. Ser Putii Nelli tried to influence the affairs of his kin down the generations. He left his two nephews a large farmhouse (*casamentum*) with a courtyard and a well, prohibiting any alienation of this property and insisting that his nephews and their descendants maintain it and live in it as a family (*debeant habitare familiariter*).[128]

Concern for the moral and economic well-being of testators' progeny was manifest through other legacies. Like the Aretines and Florentines, the Perugini demanded in their wills the obedience of their children to specially chosen surrogate parents to take their places once in the grave. Pietrus f.q. Angnelelli Maffutii, for instance, demanded that his son and heir stay with and be fully under the governance of his own brothers.[129] In 1362, Egidius Martini Crescebene left his three daughters a dowry of 400 florins each but then added if one of them had difficulty marrying (*non posset commode maritari*), his executors might augment it to 500 florins.[130]

The most extraordinary provision made in these documents, in any city, for the future security of offspring and descendants in fact came from Perugia. In 1383, the knight dominus Francescus f.q. domini Ugolini left his sons as his universal heirs. If they should die without sons, the dowry of his daughter was to be doubled to 2,000 florins. If all his sons and their male children should die without heirs, then his granddaughter's dowry was also to be supplemented by 1,000 florins. In these cases, his residuary estate (which included landed possessions and houses in nine villages) should provide the funds to build (*fiat et edificetur, construatur et fabricetur*) a monastery on the hill (*podio*) called Castellare in the village of Cordigliano. It was to be completed within one year following his death and placed under the rule of the Olivetani. The prior of that order at the abbey of Monte Morcino was to determine the amount to be spent for the construction of "this church and its houses." All the monks were to reside perpetually in this monastery and live well from the property rights and from the fruits and resources of the legacy. If the Olivetani declined his legacy, he would substitute the Sienese hospital of Santa Maria della Scala and ask them to build a hospital on the same hill within one year. In return, the knight Lord Francescus required of the monastery or hospital that if any of the progeny of his house, male or female, legitimate or illegitimate (*spureus*), should prove "deficient in some faculty" and "unable to survive on his own," then the institution was obliged to accept this descendant into its community and to provide food and clothing so long as he remained a member and obedient to the superiors.[131]

The most unusual aspect of testaments in Perugia as compared with the other city-states concerned not so much those who would in the future be provided for by the testators' largess, but instead those blocked and excluded. For instance, domina Iacoba f.q. Andrucciolo Nicole, the widow of Ser Simonis Helemone, called Pellutia, divided her estate between one son, who was a friar, and the son of another deceased son. On the other hand, she gave a second son, Santus, a formulaic 10 lire, instituted him as an heir, and demanded that he plead for no more. She then "deprived him of every right of succession to her inheritance," since "she asserted this Santus had beat her physically on many occasions [plures verberavit eam]."[132]

As we saw above, the same knight, Lord Francescus, who provided perpetual sinecures for his defective kin, at the same time circumvented any claims to his estate by blood kin or kin through marriage by instituting them as heirs, paying them off with the token fee of five soldi and demanding that they be content and ask for nothing more. Notaries and their clients, in fact, employed these tactics for avoiding future claims on estates in all the city-states we have studied. But Perugini entered the future temporal realm of their heirs by these means far more than the rest. More than three-fourths of the testaments in this city that spawned the flagellant movement circumvented the possible future claims of friends and kin by such formulaic devices—double that of runner-up Siena and more than 12 times that of the Pisans, who used these subtle means of disinheritance in only 6 percent of the testaments.[133]

Women and Lineage

The descriptive materials presented above lend texture to the picture earlier sketched from the statistics culled from the charitable legacies. Testators' decisions over property, from the extent to which they monetized their belongings to the rules they attached to the future flow of their patrimonies down lines governed by complex contingencies, carve out precise chronological and geographical patterns. The desire to bind property, direct its devolution, and determine the fate of heirs and their property became more common everywhere after the Black Death and particularly after the second incursion of pestilence in 1363. Increasingly, testaments broke with the earlier practices of mendicant piety, in which properties were simply left unencumbered, and usually in already liquidated sums to be parceled out to beneficiaries, whether pious or nonpious. In a variety of ways, testators failed to accept their total departure from the present world of mundane affairs and attempted to orchestrate from the grave their successors' actions and behavior with the intent (often explicit) of preserving the testators' own earthly memory.

In addition, testators from those three cities where mendicant piety had less influence on the lists and practices of pious giving — Arezzo, Florence, and Perugia — also strove to hold on to their nonpious property beyond the grave by influencing its future devolution and the behavior of their heirs. In Arezzo and Florence, the male-oriented ideal of lineage was the principle by which testators desired to restrict the free flow of their gifts. Here, as against the other towns, testators and their notaries deployed a highly developed vocabulary for directing properties down the male line — *ceppo, agnatio, domus, fidecommissum, consanguineos, affines, stirpes, in ordine successivo, ad gradum, per lineam masculinam* — words and phrases that did not become common in Siena (at least in testaments) until well into the sixteenth century. In Arezzo and Florence, moreover, testators often prescribed the rules of property division for future generations of heirs. Almost invariably, they favored the property rights of the family stock and lineage (*in stirpe*) over those of the individual (*in capite*). While testators from Perugia, similar to those in Assisi, Pisa, and Siena, rarely relied on this technical vocabulary, they were nonetheless as intent on restricting property rights and influencing the ways of their heirs as their contemporaries in Florence and Arezzo.

In line with the conclusions drawn in comparative anthropological studies of societies as diverse as certain American Indian tribes in the nineteenth century and Muslims in medieval Spain, it can be shown that women exercised a weaker control over property in those societies of late medieval central Italy that stressed descent through the male line.[134] However, unlike these anthropological studies, my comparison of complex urban societies in late medieval Italy does not provide the sharp and systemic contrasts between societies structured by patrilineal as opposed to matrilineal systems of descent. In all six cities, the general model of inheritance was roughly the same: fathers as well as mothers named their sons as the universal heirs with equal rights to the estates, while daughters were granted dowries during their parents' lifetimes and at their parents' deaths usually received no more than an "augumentum" to the dowry. Jack Goody and David Herlihy maintain that this arrangement in fact was generally the model throughout Western Europe.[135] For the six city-states, sons and daughters inherited equally as the universal heirs in only 13 percent of the cases in which children of both sexes survived a parent (53 of 409 testaments). Goody further generalizes that, "in stark contrast to most of traditional Africa," women in European societies were "seen as the residual heirs in preference to more distant males."[136] But the inheritance patterns from the city-states of late medieval central Italy do not bear out his claim. Instead, parents chose daughters as their universal heirs before more distant male kin in only 42 percent of the cases (264 testaments out of 631).

Despite the general statutory structure of these patrilineal city-states, they nonetheless show significant differences in male descent over time and space. Before the plague of 1362–63, parents chose their daughters over more distant kinsmen as the first choice to inherit their estates in over half of the cases (135 of 261 testaments); afterward, the figure plummeted significantly to 35 percent (129 of 370).[137] Over space, these patterns of descent roughly reflect the patterns of piety and male lineage ideology found earlier for the six city-states. In Florence, where testators were most conscious of entailing their properties through the male line, parents favored their daughters the least as heirs over more distant kinsmen (36 percent of the cases, or 44 of 123 testaments). Pisa lay at the other extreme of this spectrum; parents in the maritime city entitled their daughters as universal heirs over more distant kinsmen in 55 percent of the cases (59 of 107 testaments).[138] Nor do these differences result simply from the greater numbers of women testators in Pisa. Similar patterns can be found for Siena, where women constituted slightly less than a third of the testators. Contrary to Eleanor Riemer's claims that only mothers named daughters as their heirs, the majority of those naming daughters as universal heirs in the city of the Virgin (at least in the samples studied here) were in fact their fathers (191 as opposed to 137 mothers).[139]

To assess women's control over property in these late medieval communities, the reader of testaments can go beyond patterns of property devolution. First, the very act of women redacting testaments is testimony to a certain degree of discretionary power over property. (See table 12.) In Pisa, where the entailment of property through the male line even among the nobility was extremely rare before the recurrence of plague, women redacted wills almost as often as men (48 percent overall and 49 percent before the Black Death). Florence, where the ideology of lineage and entail down the male line appeared earliest and

Table 12.

Testators and Gender

Town	Women	No. Testators	Percentage of Women	Widows	Married	Unwed	Percentage of Married Women
Assisi	90	292	30.82	32	28	30	31.11
Arezzo	225	660	34.09	134	51	40	22.67
Florence	191	653	29.25	143	19	29	9.95
Perugia	224	564	39.72	83	93	48	41.52
Pisa	355	741	47.91	200	134	21	37.75
Siena	154	476	32.35	63	52	39	33.77
BEFORE 1348							
Assisi	40	115	34.78	11	11	18	27.50
Arezzo	81	237	34.18	55	16	10	19.75
Florence	73	244	29.92	49	8	16	10.96
Perugia	58	161	36.02	17	16	25	27.59
Pisa	198	401	49.38	109	75	14	37.88
Siena	83	274	30.29	36	25	22	30.12
BEFORE 1363							
Assisi	40	120	33.33	10	11	19	27.50
Arezzo	123	375	32.80	77	24	22	19.51
Florence	96	357	26.89	63	12	21	12.50
Perugia	77	211	36.49	22	27	28	35.06
Pisa	242	517	46.81	131	93	18	38.43
Siena	105	339	30.97	44	34	27	32.38

filtered through society most widely, represented the other extreme; less than 30 percent of Florentine testators were women, and before 1363 the proportion was even lower.

These extremes become more patent when the marital status of women testators is considered. Three-fourths of these women in Florence were widows, and under 10 percent allocated their last properties while married. On the other hand, Perugia was the city-state where the highest percentage of married women drew up their own testaments (42 percent), followed closely by Pisa (38 percent, or four times the percentage for Florence). Before the Black Death, however, Pisa was the leader; and while the percentage was roughly constant for Pisans over time, in Perugia its earlier rate was less than one-third (28 percent).

Once the testaments of married women are examined more closely, the distinctions among these towns become even stronger, and the wrinkle in these patterns initially presented by the percentages of women testators in Perugia becomes less problematic. While married women constituted a larger percentage of the women redacting wills in Perugia than in Pisa, the act of writing a will for such women appears not to have been the same in these cities. Over half of Perugian women testators simply used their wills to turn over their dotal as well as nondotal properties to their husbands by naming them as universal heirs.[140] In Florence, nearly 40 percent of married women did the same.[141] But for Pisa the story was entirely different. Of 134 wills from married women in Pisa, not a single one transmitted the bulk of the wife's property to the husband. The closest any testament came to such a property set-tlement was in a codicil redacted by the wife of a nobleman in 1311. Its one itemized gift left Chisluccia's husband, Dominus Chellus, not full rights to all her property but the *usufructus* of all her goods. The testatrix, however, was not a resident of Pisa and instead came from the village of Podio de Lucca.[142] For the maritime city, the customary practice for a married women was instead to leave her husband a mere 15 lire,[143] which after the Black Death certainly did not constitute a sizable gift even for artisans or landed peasants. These women, moreover, would "nominate" as their universal heirs nieces, nephews, or even men and women who bore no apparent relation to them—a practice that the testamentary evidence shows was unthinkable for Perugians and Florentines. In Pisa, some married women wrote wills without even acknowledging their husbands with the customary 15-lire legacy—a far cry from Florence, where a woman had to have the approval of a contracted "protector," her *mundualdus,* who, in the case of married women, was in these documents almost invariably the husband. It is again telling that of these six towns only Florence retained this Lombard custom in its statutory regulations.[144]

As mentioned earlier, the most common dictate from the grave re-garding the future behavior of a beneficiary concerned the property settlements husbands left their wives. A glance at these again reveals the inferior position of women in Florence, Arezzo, and Perugia, vis-à-vis those cities where the mendicant pattern of piety was strong and lineage weak.[145] In all these societies, the individual property settlements that men left their wives show a wide range of possibilities. At one extreme, husbands could name wives as universal heirs over all the husband's property without restrictions, and without barring the wid-ow's freedom to remarry or imposing conditions on her future sexual behavior At the other extreme, they might not even return their wives' dowries or at least might fail to mention the dotal properties in their wills. In all these societies, however, with the exception of Florence, the most usual settlement was one in which the husband left the wife the dowry without restrictions along with the *usufructus* to all of his property so long as she remained chaste ("lived the honest life") and did not remarry.[146] Often itemized within this *usufructus* would appear the wife's *corredo*—her linen and jewelry. In many cases, the husband also granted her an *"ultra" dos* or *augumentum,* a supplement to her dowry, which usually would travel with her regardless of her future behavior or remarriage. In Pisa, unlike Florence, the *corredo* would fall under this latter category. Moreover, of the six cities, only in this maritime town and occasionally in Assisi did fathers and their notaries divide their daughters' inheritances into the two Roman-law categories, distinguishing their dowry from their *parafernalia* or those properties that, under Roman law, the daughter would bring into marriage but could control herself without relinquishing them to her husband's admin-istration. Indeed, Julius Kirshner shows that this Roman law distinction between the *patrimonio dotale* and the *parafernalia* had vanished from the Florentine statutes by the redaction of 1322, and Francesco Ercole has argued that it disappeared in many regions of Italy during the course of the fourteenth century.[147]

Of the six cities, husbands' settlements were the least favorable to their future widows in Florence. The modal arrangement in the city of the lily was distinctly one in which the husband granted his wife the *usufructus* over his property (but often, especially among the merchant class, only a portion of his property—her *camera,* the linen, and her jewelry), provided that she remain chaste, not remarry, and *not* ask for her dowry.[148] This arrangement was unheard of in the numerous wills for Pisa and Siena and put in only a faint appearance in the documents from Assisi (4 out of 115 wills redacted by husbands while their wives were still alive). In these three cities, a woman's rights to her dowry after the death of her husband appear unassailable.

Moreover, in Arezzo and Perugia, where the mendicant patterns of piety competed less forcefully with testamentary designs for earthly memory, women also fared less successfully. Although the most common arrangement for widows was one in which the wife's rights over her dowry remained unimpaired, husbands in these towns commonly left their soon-to-be widows the less advantageous option of taking the usufruct of the husband's property only so long as she relinquished all rights to her dowry. For these cities, it constituted in fact the second most frequent formula found in husbands' settlements for the future widows' welfare.[149]

A General Assessment

This comparative analysis shows Florence, often taken in the recent literature as typifying the condition of women in late medieval and early Renaissance Italy, as the exception.[150] Of the six societies considered here, it appears to have been the worst place to have been born a woman, at least in terms of one's discretionary power over property. Moreover, the situation found in Arezzo and Perugia was roughly congruent with practices in Florence. On this score, the towns divide into the same two triads previously discovered in terms of their patterns of piety and their attitudes toward worldly endeavors and property. With the possible exception of Perugia, whose laconic testaments expressed less about intention than the records in Tuscany, traditions of lineage—the strength of the male line—loomed behind the differences in the patterns of piety among these cities: the strength of mendicant ideals of self- and worldly denial as opposed to the quest for earthly memory. Again, those societies where lineage and the zeal to preserve one's name and the memory of one's ancestors were strongest were also the cities where women played weaker roles in exercising power over property and where the rights over their most basic economic and social resource—the dowry—were in jeopardy. Putting together parts of the testament as diverse as monuments of piety and the property rights of women, a general underlying connection unfolds: those societies where women's power over property was stronger and the ascent of property through the patriliny weaker were the same ones that adopted more vigorously mendicant patterns of piety—the ideal of total humility, the annihilation of self, and the renunciation of the world. More than economy, aristocratic alliance—Guelph or Ghibelline—type of regime, the strength of one order of mendicancy versus another, ancient settlement patterns, or corresponding traditions of law (Lombard vs. Roman),[151] traditions of property ascent help to explain the geographical differences in strategies for the afterlife observed thus far through the wills. We now turn to yet another area of study that can be probed from the testamentary evidence—art commissions and patronage—a subject generally not viewed from the perspective of competing strategies for the afterlife or from the social preserve of artisans and peasants.

III

Art

6

Art and Masses

The idea of seeking perpetual fame through buildings is empty and laughable. If they are thrown down on the ground or are swallowed up by it, along with them, the fame of their author perishes. And many are the traps lurking for them: earthquakes, openings of the earth, thunderbolts, the sun's blistering heat, the rains. . . . And should all these fail and permit these objects to prevail for the longest time, the names of those who build them nonetheless perish, the buildings no longer serving them.

And so dearest friend, in due course all mortal labors perish.

— Giovanni Boccaccio, *Epistole*

he last chapter examined the ways testators attempted to influence from the grave the future devolution of their property and the future behavior of heirs. The secular realm of nonpious legacies was not, however, where testators concentrated their efforts to influence the living. Instead, it was in their bequests to churches and charities that those from all six cities made their most enduring demands on beneficiaries—from new constructions, panel paintings and frescoes, insignia, plaques and coats of arms to be emblazoned on walls and carved in stone to acts of commemoration for their own and their ancestors' souls at designated times in perpetuity.

Perpetual Masses

The simplest of these demands were vague requests for masses to be chanted for oneself and for one's kin, loved ones, and ancestors. Such requests show no clear patterns over time or geography that correspond to those thus far amassed from the other aspects of testamentary giving. In Florence, the percentage of masses peaked after the recurrence of pestilence in the 1364–75 period; in Pisa, during the summer months of the Black Death, 1348; in Siena, once at the end of the Duecento and again in the summer of 1348; in Assisi, after the Black Death; in Perugia, at the beginning of the Quattrocento. Nearly a quarter of Sienese testators requested masses; the Perugini followed with 21 percent, then the Florentines and the Pisans with 20, the Assisani with 12, and last, the Aretines with 9 percent.

Actually, these simple requests for masses (usually unspecified in number) to be performed on a single date (again, usually unspecified) may have been assumed even when the request was not explicit[1] and thus were similar to the one-time gifts doled out to the poor of Christ or to churches and monasteries. Once a request was fulfilled, the testator held no claims on the beneficiary; whatever its recurrent spiritual dividends, the service could be forgotten in the temporal sphere. Testators felt no need to place watchdogs over a church, confraternity, or monastery or to institute "substitute" pious beneficiaries that might wait in the wings to seize the appropriation, should a church fail in its duties.

Requests for perpetual masses to be chanted on certain feast days or on the testator's anniversary or "continuously" or over long temporal expanses from a year to 20 years or the lifetime of a beneficiary or (as was usually the case) forever—were different. With these, the memory of the testator did not end with death, but would be carried on in the earthly as well as in the spiritual sphere. To guarantee these more complex and enduring services, testators placed restrictions on their gifts, often threatening their pious parties with inspection from heirs and executors along with the possible "substitution" of alternative charities.

When these perpetual masses are considered, rather than the simple number of masses, a different pattern emerges. Once again, the rank ordering separates Florence, Arezzo, and Perugia from Siena, Pisa, and Assisi. (See table 13.) Florence led the list, with 43 percent of all testators requesting such masses, followed by Arezzo (26 percent), Perugia (21 percent), Pisa (17 percent), Assisi (14 percent), and lastly, the city that led the list with simple masses, Siena (9 percent). Similarly, over time, these provisions for perpetual masses reaffirm the broad temporal changes charted thus far by the statistics on legacies. In most of these city-states, the percentages of perpetual masses rose after the recurrence of pestilence, 1362–63, through the early Quattrocento. In Florence they hit their highest point immediately after the Black Death, when testators on average demanded more than one perpetual mass per testator; they sank with the recurrence of plague in 1363, then built back steadily over the next half-century to nearly three perpetual masses for every four testators. In Arezzo, on the other hand, the years immediately following the Black Death saw these requests approach their nadir, but, as in Florence, they revived in the second half of the century, reaching their apex of 43 percent in the opening years of the Quattrocento. Pisa's rate reached its high point in the plague months of 1362, then fell, but likewise gradually recovered in the last decades of the Trecento and the early Quattrocento. In Perugia, the years following 1348 marked the low-water mark but then climbed back, reaching their apex of 40 percent at the end of my period of analysis.[2] For Assisi, the apex came at the end of the Trecento.

A better denominator, however, for evaluating variations in time and place is the number of such bequests, since a single testator could oblige more than one institution to chant perpetual masses. For instance, the Aretine surgeon *Magister* Angelus, son of the former doctor *Magister* Benincase, requested the four friaries of Arezzo—the Dominicans, Franciscans, Servites, and Carmelites—to perform masses in perpetuity for his and his ancestors' souls on the feasts of the nativity of the Virgin Mary in September, her assumption in August, her purification in February, her annunciation in March, and her conception in December, and on the feast day of the Madonna della Neve in August. In consideration for what he advertised in his will as his "abundant and gracious charity," which amounted to three *staii* of bread for each mass performed, the surgeon then arranged for the chaplain who was to officiate at his private altar in the church of Santa Maria della Pieve also to celebrate perpetual masses in this church on these same days. He implored his executors and the two rectors of the Pieve to be "vigilant" in seeing that these services were implemented.[3]

The mass programs devised by the Florentine rector of the parish church of Santa Cecilia, Lord Nicholas from the Benucci family, approached the complexity and elaboration later to be found in testaments of a Counter Reform stamp. First, he required daily masses of the priest who was to officiate in his private chapel. In addition, each year on the feast day of the martyred saints, Tiburtius and Valerianus, the chaplain, along with six other priests, was to celebrate a solemn mass and a divine office, followed the next day by an anniversary mass (*unum annuale*) in

Table 13.
Perpetual Masses and Feasts

Period	No. Testators	Yearly Masses	Feast Day Masses	Masses over Extended Periods	Total	Perpetual Masses per Testator	Perpetual Masses per 100 Pious Bequests
AREZZO							
< 1276							
1275–1300							
1301–25	56	12	2	0	14	0.25	2.29
1326–47	92	14	1	12	27	0.29	3.08
1348	84	5	12	4	21	0.25	3.51
1349–62	63	5	4	3	12	0.19	2.49
1363	71	2	3	10	15	0.21	3.85
1364–75	88	6	9	4	19	0.22	3.72
1376–1400	94	3	11	3	17	0.18	4.71
1401–25	100	6	30	7	43	0.43	11.05
Total	648	53	72	43	168	0.26	3.98
ASSISI							
< 1276	18	0	0	0	0	0.00	0.00
1275–1300	22	0	0	0	0	0.00	0.00
1301–25	19	0	0	0	0	0.00	0.00
1326–47	27	1	0	0	1	0.04	0.44
1348	27	2	0	0	2	0.07	1.12
1349–62	5	1	2	0	3	0.60	3.70
1363							
1364–75	14	0	0	0	0	0.00	0.00
1376–1400	30	3	0	8	11	0.37	6.67
1401–25	128	2	3	20	25	0.20	6.70
Total	290	9	5	28	42	0.14	2.42
FLORENCE							
< 1276	14	3	0	0	3	0.21	2.80
1275–1300	43	1	1	0	2	0.05	0.48
1301–25	52	10	5	3	18	0.35	3.49
1326–47	57	8	1	1	10	0.18	2.76
1348	63	8	7	2	17	0.27	3.46
1349–62	31	17	7	12	36	1.16	19.25
1363	68	12	9	0	21	0.31	5.00
1364–75	77	18	19	2	39	0.51	10.99
1376–1400	91	10	25	6	41	0.45	11.45
1401–25	85	39	9	13	61	0.72	22.10
Total	581	126	83	39	248	0.43	7.11
PERUGIA							
< 1276	2	0	0	0	0	0.00	0.00
1275–1300	4	0	0	0	0	0.00	0.00

Table 13.
Continued

Period	No. Testators	Yearly Masses	Feast Day Masses	Masses over Extended Periods	Total	Perpetual Masses per Testator	Perpetual Masses per 100 Pious Bequests
PERUGIA							
Continued							
1301–25	10	3	0	5	8	0.80	7.14
1326–47	61	1	0	0	1	0.02	0.33
1348	79	1	0	4	5	0.06	1.25
1349–62	20	0	0	0	0	0.00	0.00
1363	28	3	2	3	8	0.29	5.93
1364–75	51	6	1	1	8	0.16	4.71
1376–99	196	23	1	28	52	0.27	7.10
1400–1425	73	16	1	12	29	0.40	9.24
Total	524	53	5	53	111	0.21	4.93
PISA							
< 1276	14	0	0	0	0	0.00	0.00
1275–1300	42	4	0	0	4	0.10	0.70
1301–25	232	23	2	1	26	0.11	0.87
1326–47	100	11	2	1	14	0.14	1.55
1348	15	3	0	2	5	0.33	4.31
1349–62	64	20	2	0	22	0.34	4.29
1363	39	4	4	7	15	0.38	3.57
1364–75	49	3	0	0	3	0.06	1.26
1376–1400	110	4	12	2	18	0.16	3.52
1401–25	72	18	2	1	21	0.29	12.57
Total	737	90	24	14	128	0.17	1.95
SIENA							
< 1276	35	0	0	0	0	0.00	0.00
1275–1300	44	4	0	0	4	0.09	1.01
1301–25	50	3	0	2	5	0.10	0.81
1326–47	67	14	0	2	16	0.24	2.55
1348	55	2	0	0	2	0.04	0.55
1349–62	40	2	0	0	2	0.05	0.80
1363	24	0	0	0	0	0.00	0.00
1364–75	25	0	0	0	0	0.00	0.00
1376–1400	61	4	0	2	6	0.10	3.26
1401–25	45	4	0	1	5	0.11	2.55
Total	446	33	0	7	40	0.09	1.30

his chapel with eight other priests, a solemn mass with a vigil, an office for the dead, and seven low masses (*missas planas*). Each priest was to receive five soldi and one candle. Lord Nicholas also left a farm with a cottage (*casolare*) and extensive arable lands (60 *starii*) to the hospital of San Bartolo a Mugnone in the Florentine suburbs effective after the death of his heir. Once they acquired this estate, the director of the hospital (*hospitalarius*) and its rector, the *conversi,* and other servants were obliged each year on the fifth of August "to make a feast and commemoration" for the blessed Virgin, Santa Maria della Neve, at an altar that the testator had previously commissioned in the hospital's church, with four priests singing one mass for the Virgin (*missa de beata* [*Virgine*]) and burning two torches containing a pound of wax apiece. Then the next day they were to celebrate an anniversary mass, along with five plain masses for the dead and one mass sung over the altar of the blessed Mary, with a vigil and an office for his and his ancestors' souls, this time with six priests to officiate, each receiving five soldi and one candle.

Nor did the masses and religious services end here. As long as a certain domina Bilia f.q. Pieri de Macci lived, she was to have masses for his and his ancestors' souls celebrated on the feast day of the Madonna della Neve on August fifth. Lord Nicholas, in addition, gave her the *usufructus* to his residence in the parish of Santa Maria in Campo on condition that from the rent she finance an anniversary mass within the first eight days of each month in the church of Santa Cecilia for his and his ancestors' souls, with 12 priests chanting *sub voce* 11 low masses and singing one solemn mass, a vigil, and an office for the dead. Each priest was to receive 5 soldi and a candle except for the new rector of this parish, who could get "double payment"—10 soldi and two candles; in addition, two other candles were "to illuminate the body of Christ" on the altar.[4] It is important to emphasize that no complex of perpetual masses with anything near this elaboration imposed on future beneficiaries arises in the thousands of testaments examined for Assisi, Pisa, or Siena. In Siena, such programs come only with the Counter Reformation in the last decades of the sixteenth century.

When the number of these perpetual gifts and demands is considered in relation to the number of pious bequests, the differences between these cities are amplified. Once again, Florence led the list, with over 7 such demands on pious beneficiaries for every 100 pious bequests. Next, Perugia, which as a ratio of the number of such masses to testators exceeded Pisa by only four percentage points, now scores two-and-a-half times the Pisan rate (4.93 per 100 pious bequests, as against 1.95);

then, Arezzo (3.98), followed at some distance by Assisi (2.42), Pisa (1.95), and Siena (1.30).

Measured by pious bequests, the trend over time also emerges in much sharper focus. All of these cities reached the high point of demand for such masses in the last quarter of my analysis, except in Siena, where it peaked just before. Moreover, the differences at the beginning of the Quattrocento were striking: in Florence, the rate nearly doubled, from 11 perpetual masses per 100 pious gifts to 22; in Arezzo, it more than doubled, from less than 5 to over 11; and, in Pisa, it jumped by over three-and-a-half times, from 3.5 to 12.5.

Chapels

As the example of the Aretine surgeon shows, a testator need not provide for a private chapel or already possess one to order monks, friars, or priests to say masses over a long periods of time or *in perpetuum*. But, as the example of the Florentine rector of Santa Cecilia illustrates, the private foundation of a chapel was usual in requesting these masses and, more importantly, for ensuring their celebration after a church came to possess the testator's property. We have already examined chapel foundations and constructions in regard to commemorating and enshrining the burial grounds of testators. But burial chapels (at least when described as "next to" or a part of the chapel complex) formed only a fraction of the chapels commissioned in these testaments.

Often testators founded chapels in churches that were not the sites of their burial. For instance, in the year of the plague's return, 1363, an Aretine glassmaker chose to be buried in the Franciscan church. If his sons were to die without heirs, his residuary properties would go to the Olivetani of San Bernardo, where the friars (*sic*) were ordered to build a chapel in their new church.[5] Several wealthy testators, moreover, founded chapels in more than one church or explicitly commissioned chapel constructions where they were not to be buried. The largest number of such multiple foundations comes from Arezzo. For instance, the Lord Symoneus f.q. Ser Benvenuti elected his burial in the Dominican church and ordered perpetual masses on every Monday and Friday for his own soul and all the souls of his blood kin, business associates, servants, and benefactors. He also commissioned the construction of an altar in the cathedral, where his elected priest would perform daily masses with the intercession of the cathedral's canons and clerics.[6] In 1345, Johannes f.q. Cionis Dietavive elected to be buried in the Dominican church and commissioned a chapel to be built next to his grave, but also left extensive landed properties (30 *starii*) to his sister with the obligation of building and endowing a chapel wherever she pleased.[7] In the year of the Black Death, 1348, we have already seen the wealthy Tarlatus, of the Aretine ruling elite, commissioning the most expensive burial tomb found for any of these documents at any time and place, "the middle church" or chapel at the Francescan mountain shrine at La Verna. "The Noble, Wise and Powerful Man" also spent 100 florins to complete the construction of another chapel in the cathedral originated by his deceased wife, the Contessa Johanna of Santa Fiora.[8]

The 1371 will of "the discreet and provident man" and citizen, Verius f.q. Donatini, does not make clear the testator's place of burial. He nonetheless commissioned two chapel constructions, one in the hospital of the Oriente, the other in his parish, the Pieve of Santa Maria.[9] Similarly, Pagnus f.q. Maffei failed to clarify in either version of his testament (redacted in 1374 and 1379) his place of burial. He devoted large portions of both wills, however, to founding two chapels: one to be constructed in the cathedral and to be called Saint Mathew the Apostle, where his elected chaplain was to recite daily masses; and another in the new church of the Franciscans, to be called Saint John the Baptist, which he furnished with books and paintings, desiring his arms and those of his company to be sculpted in its walls, and where his elected chaplain was to sing perpetual masses for his own and his ancestors' souls.[10]

Similarly, the rich of Florence on occasion used their testaments to commission chapels that might not necessarily encase their corpses. In 1367, domina Margherita filia olim Vermigli de Alfanis, the widow of Ugo Altoviti, elected to be buried in the chapel of San Marco in Santa Maria Novella, whose construction was initiated by her father.[11] Later in her will she sought to build another chapel in the Dominican church for the "memory" of her brother and named for his namesake, Sant'Alberto, where a thousand masses a year would be chanted for her own, her father's, and her brother's souls.[12] The Florentine merchant residing in Paris, Iacobus de Iuochis, whom we have already met apportioning his estate between his wife and illegitimate daughter, divided as well his loyalties in his chapel constructions between the Franciscans and the Dominicans. He chose a grave in the church of the minor friars in Paris in a chapel whose construction he had initiated. He then ordered another chapel constructed from cut stone (*lapidis incisis*) in the church of Santa Maria Novella and "completed for his perpetual memory."[13]

The Pisan Johanzeno f.q. domini Iacobi Carionis, from the Lanfranchi family, chose to be buried in the cathedral of Pisa and then founded an altar in the major hospital of Pisa, Santa Chiara, where he "deputed" a priest from the hospital to chant daily masses for his soul and the soul of his wife; in addition, should his children die without heirs, his landed estates in the Collinis (Colline Pisane), held communally in the Lanfranchi family, were to be used for the construction of an altar.[14] Finally the Pisan knight (*miles*) dominus Tighus, of the Upezzinghi family,[15] left 200 florins to ornament his grave in the family vault, situated in the chapel of Santa Maria Maddalena in the Franciscan church of Pisa, and for "a beautifully painted panel painting [*pro tabula una pulcra picta*]" for the altar, whereas his testament concentrated on the construction, decoration, paintings, furnishings, endowment, and election of the chaplain for another chapel, to be named for Saint Francis and to be built in the country church of Santa Maria de Lari.[16]

These demands for chapel constructions were not evenly distributed across the six city-states. The same division between the six found for the other variables thus far examined continues to hold—the number and size of pious bequests, the importance of specific burial sites, the frequency of nonalienation restrictions on property, the frequency of entail, and the number of perpetual masses. This time Arezzo led the list: chapel or altar foundations and construction plans are found in 10 percent of these testaments (65 chapels or altars), followed by 7.7 percent for Florence (45 chapels), 5.5 percent for Perugia (29 chapels), 3.5 percent for Pisa (26 chapels), 2.7 percent for Assisi (8 chapels), and lastly 2.2 percent for Siena (10 chapels).

As we have seen above, testators could make more than one pious bequest for the construction of a chapel, and as the wills of many wealthy testators illustrate, testators of the Duecento and Trecento might pour enormous resources into a great number of pious causes without commissioning a single chapel. When the number of pious bequests is taken as the base (a better denominator), the homogeneity within these two groups of cities solidifies, and the gap between them widens. The Aretines commissioned 15.4 chapels for every thousand pious gifts, while the Florentines and Perugini each commissioned 12.9. Assisani ran a distant fourth (4.6 chapels per thousand pious gifts), followed by Pisans (less than 4.0) and Sienese (3.2 chapels).

Chapel construction was certainly not a poor man's pursuit. Thirty-five percent of those who endowed or built chapels possessed family names, compared to under 11 percent for the population of testament writers as a whole.[17] The average price for a chapel over this long period was 208.90 florins[18]—more than most of the testators' total assets, both pious and nonpious. The most frequent title or profession of the founders was that of nobility (21 cases, or one-fifth of all those identified by a title or a profession). Yet chapel construction and endowment was not the exclusive preserve of the elites. The second most prevalent title or occupation was that of notary (11 cases); and, in several instances, even artisans concentrated their resources to build such a shrine for their perpetual memory and the salvation of their souls.

In the year of the Black Death, the Florentine druggist Stoldus f.q. Berti Upezini made only one pious legacy in his will—to build a "suitable [ydonea] chapel" in his parish church of San Lorenzo in honor of Saint Catherine and "to be called thus." For this construction he left 50 florins, a relatively small sum for such a project. To finance the living of his chaplain (he appointed Francescus Iuncti, from Monte Ugo) and for perpetual masses and divine offices, the druggist left his farm (podere) and all its belongings, located in a place called Allimite (Limite). After the chaplain's death, the druggist left the rights of "assigning" a "suitable" successor to the church and canons (capituli) of San Lorenzo.[19]

In the year of the plague's return, another druggist, Simoneus f.q. Benedetti, from Pisa, devoted the majority of his will for masses to be celebrated in the chapel he had ordered built "within the nave on the side of the bell tower" in the monastic church of San Michele in Borgo. He ordered his sons to have continuous masses celebrated throughout their lives at the altar of this chapel, called San Benedetto, named after the testator's father, with two large candles weighing two-and-a-half pounds apiece and a torch weighing six pounds. Furthermore, they were to prepare a "good and sufficient" commemorative meal (pietanza) every year on the feast day of San Benedetto for all the monks at San Michele "in praise and in reverence" of this patron saint and another yearly feast for these monks and two sacerdotes at a time to be determined by the abbot.[20]

In 1390, domina Johanna, the widow of a druggist from Perugia, ordered her universal heir, the mendicant friars of Santa Maria dei Servi, to "beautify" (reattare) a wall near the choir of this church and contiguous to the chapel of Saint Julian within two years after her death. It was to make way for a chapel with an altar, above which was to be a wall painting of the Annunciation and the testatrix with her late husband, the druggist. For this project she left 200 florins, to cover the costs of divine offices for her soul and that of her deceased husband.[21] In 1361, the ironmonger (ferriolus) and citizen of Arezzo Niccholaus f.q. Ugucci

Orlandi left his residuary estate to build a chapel in the church of the Augustinians "in honor and reverence of the Passion of Jesus Christ," should his brother be negligent in returning the monies, which the testator had gained through usury. This ironmonger was no typical artisan, however, given the considerable sum of 500 florins he left for the project.[22] But, in 1390, the more humble Aretine wife of a beltmaker left her house in the Borgo Rosellorum and its garden to endow a chapel to be constructed in the Abbey of Santa Fiore,[23] and in 1411, the widow of a mere tanner ordered her executors to sell her house for the construction of a chapel in the church of Monte Morcino.[24]

Finally, the cobbler from Vinci, who had lived in the artisan-worker parishes of Santa Lucia Ognissanti and San Frediano in Florence before returning to his native village, left only 50 florins to build a chapel in the church called Santa Croce and Sant'Andrea in Vinci. He ordered it to be called San Michelangelo of Locteriis (his family name); "furnished and ornamented" with a panel painting (de tabula lignea) of the Virgin Mary and "the blessed saints" John the Baptist, Paul the Apostle, Michael the Archangel, and Anthony; and supplied with a missal, a chalice, and all the other necessities. The 50 florins were also to include the living for the priest charged with officiating at the altar and obliged to celebrate masses and a Holy Office at least three days a week—on Mondays, Wednesdays, and Fridays—in perpetuum.[25]

Chapel commissions could even penetrate the ranks of the disenfranchised workers (i.e., those who practiced professions without guild recognition). In 1348, the Aretine domina Giana, the widow of a weaver, stipulated in her short will that "all her property, both movables and immovables, that lay beyond the new city walls of Arezzo" ought to be the property of the chapel and altar that she had had constructed in the church of Santa Maria in Gradibus.[26]

Furthermore, a considerable proportion of chapel founders (26 percent)[27] resided in the countryside or in small towns of the hinterland or were émigrés. To be sure, these were not impoverished rural artisans or peasants; 11 bore noble titles, and others were even of prominent families, such as the Sienese Tolomei,[28] the Salimbeni who resided in the village of Catignano, the Tarlati of Pietramala, the Barbolani of their ancestral village Montaguto Barbolani,[29] the Mainetti of Montelupo, the Pellini of San Gimignano, a noble lady from Castel Focognano married into the noble family of the Ubertini,[30] and the Ubertini of Foiano.[31] Nonetheless, some were certainly rural artisans, and others even peasants. I have already described the chapel plans and endowment of the cobbler from Vinci. In addition, a master carpenter, *Magister* Niccolaus f.q. Magistri Covari, from the small town of Asciano in the *contado* of Siena, in the year of the Black Death bequeathed the modest sum of 20 florins to build a chapel for the salvation of the souls of his mother and father in the *pieve* church of Sant'Agata and "in honor and in reverence" of Saint (sic) Nicholas[32] of Tolentino.[33] In 1358, a *"magister"* Matheus f.q. Venture, who had once lived in the village of San Salvatore a Pilli outside of Siena and now resided in the small town of Castro Foiano in the *contado* of Arezzo, gave several strips of arable land and a garden to construct a chapel in the Dominican church of Foiano. Despite the negligible proportions of his gift, this master artisan, grammarian, or possibly medical doctor expected it to provide for a chaplain, whom his executors would elect to celebrate continually divine offices in his chapel. If the elected priest "did not officiate well and diligently," Matheus authorized his daughters to elect a new one.[34]

Other chapel donors from small villages bore no family names, titles, or occupations, but from the size of their gifts and testamentary holdings may well have been only peasants, even if relatively well-off. Stefanus f.q. Iacobus, from the *plebis* of San Giovanni in the *curia* of Capolona, who had recently moved to Arezzo, left "all of his goods" in his 1374 will to erect an altar in the *plebis* church of San Giovanni.[35] In 1396, a villager from Sant'Anastasio, again in the *contado* of Arezzo, left his residuary estate to found a chapel in the Francescan church of Arezzo under the name of the blessed Anthony.[36] In 1401, Guido f.q. Neri, from Torciana in the Pisan *curia* of Parrano, left several strips of land varying from 4 to 12 *starii* to endow the altar of Santa Caterina in the rural parish of San Martino in Torciana, which he had recently constructed (*nuper pro me constructo*).[37] Finally, the 1325 testament of the countryman Barone, from the village of Santa Maria Castello in the *contado* of Pisa, certainly reveals no impoverished peasant but instead a country gentleman. His will suggests nonetheless that at the lower limits, altar construction, at least in the countryside, may not have been beyond the reach of ordinary peasants. Barone gave a pittance of only 10 lire to roof the church of San Giovanni at Monte Barlani and another 5 lire "for constructing an altar there and purchasing an icon to be placed in front of the figure of Saint Nicholas in this church."[38]

Besides confirming the differences among these city-states, the foundation and construction of chapels and altars corroborates the previous findings on the chronology of piety and property. (See table 14.) Only 22 constructions predate the Black Death — 12 percent of the total as

Table 14.
Chapel Constructions

Period	Arezzo	Assisi	Florence	Perugia	Pisa	Siena	Total
< 1276							
1276–1300		0	1	0	0	0	1
1301–25	1	0	1	1	7	1	11
1326–47	4	0	3	0	4	1	12
1348	7	1	9	0	2	2	21
1349–62	11	2	1	1	3	2	20
1363	5		3	0	0	0	8
1364–75	13	0	19	5	3	0	40
1376–1400	11	2	5	17	2	0	37
1401–25	13	3	3	5	5	4	33
Total	65	8	45	29	26	10	183

Period	No. Testators	No. Pious Bequests	Total No. Chapels	Chapels per Testator	Chapels per 1,000 Pious Bequests
< 1276	83	629	0	0.00	0.00
1276–1300	155	1,728	1	0.01	0.58
1301–25	419	5,044	11	0.03	2.18
1326–47	404	3,298	12	0.03	3.64
1348	323	2,149	21	0.07	9.77
1349–62	223	1,596	20	0.09	12.53
1363	230	1,442	8	0.03	5.55
1364–75	304	1,438	40	0.13	27.82
1376–1400	582	2,312	37	0.06	16.00
1401–25	503	1,715	33	0.07	19.24

against nearly half of all the pious gifts found in this documentation.[39] The Black Death was a spur to chapel building. From 1325–47 to 1348, the rate more than doubled, from 3 to 7 percent of all testators, and almost trebled, from 3.64 to just under 10 per thousand pious bequests. Perhaps again it reflects a desire to immortalize earthly remains in the face of this unprecedented mortality and the threat of ignominious mass burial. 1348, however, was not an aberration but the beginning of a new trend. Between the first two occurrences of pestilence, the rate per pious bequests continued to rise, quadrupling the pre–Black Death rate and peaking in the years following the recurrence of plague in 1362–63, when it nearly trebled the 1348 rate and towered nearly eight times above the pre–Black Death frequencies. In the last 50 years covered by this study, new constructions subsided, but remained almost double the Black Death figure.

Here, the data from burials are instructive. Although not all chapels were to enshrine the testator's burial grounds (such chapels were in fact rare in the sites commissioned before the Black Death), increasingly chapels took on an association with the grave. As we saw in Chapter 5, by the latter years of the Trecento, testators could rely on the previous endowments of their fathers, husbands, and ancestors. Increasingly they chose ancestral burial grounds for their last remains and often in family chapels.

Although we know of chapel foundations and altars that go back to the early Christian period,[40] no such endowments or construction plans emerge for any of these cities in the earliest testaments until the last decade of the thirteenth century. The first chapel endowment in these documents appears in 1291 and not in a church but in a private palace. Dominus Consillius f.q. Ser Olivieri, of the Florentine merchant family the Cerchi, ordered his heirs to maintain a chapel or oratory (*capella sive orratorium*), located in his palace in the piazza (*plano*) Bisastici. In this chapel, a sacerdos with a cleric was "to stay and to live" in perpetuity to celebrate divine offices for the souls of the testator and his relatives. For "the expenses and necessities" of these clerics, Consillius left his farm (*podere*) with all its properties in the village of Terrenzano (near Settignano); "all the *ius patronatus*" and the rights of "electing, protecting and defending the priest and rector and all that they should judge expedient for the honor of God and the Virgin Mary" were to fall to his sons and "their legitimate male descendants and to pass down the male line."[41] This is the only example found at any time or place in these samples of a private chapel constructed for a private palace.

The first chapel construction in an ecclesiastical institution in these samples comes instead from a Pisan of an old family lineage. In 1306, Johannes, called Vannes Zeno f.q. domini Iacobi Carionis, of the Lanfranchi family, left 400 lire to the hospital of Santa Chiara to build an altar in their church "over which" the hospital friars were to celebrate daily divine offices for his soul.[42] He left no instructions regarding the actual construction of the altar or its furnishings and decorations and, more importantly, nothing in regard to the *ius patronatus* or rights of election of its chaplain. We have to assume that these rights must have been left with the religious institution, the *hospitalarius* and the friars of the hospital of Santa Chiara.

This second chapel foundation, with its lack of detail concerning ornamentation and, more particularly, the *ius patronatus,* was more the rule for the laconic endowments found in these documents, especially from before the Black Death. The noble founder from the Lanfranchi family did not even impose a title on the new shrine. Besides Consillius, of the Cerchi family, only four testators before the Black Death even alluded to these rights of "presentment," and only one "privatized" them. The remarkable dominus Symoneus of Arezzo, son of a notary, whom we have encountered at several junctures thus far, went beyond even the merchant from the Cerchi family in privatizing sacred space and channeling its rights down his family line in one of the two chapels he founded. For his chapel to be built in the cathedral of Arezzo, he first appointed the priest (sacerdos) Orlandus, who was to say divine offices "perpetually," unless "impeded by illness." Moreover, the priests of the cathedral, along with their canons and clerics, were to appear in his chapel for the daily celebration of "major masses." If the chaplain or these clerics neglected these duties, the lands that were to provide the chaplain's living (*substentationem*) would pass to an altar in the *plebis* church of Santa Maria. Here, Lord Symoneus established a sinecure for his male descendants. The sacerdos of this altar was to be "good and honest, of respectable reputation," and should descend from either side of the line of his late father. If, at the time of election, more than one of his descendants met these conditions, then the prior of the church would appoint the successor. If none of his qualified descendants wished the appointment, then the prior, in agreement with his canons, should select a priest of "sound morals and honest reputation," who was at least 30 years old.[43]

The chapels founded by the Cerchi and the Aretine son of a notary were not only exceptional in their antiquity; throughout this documentation, references to the rights of presentment or election of the chapel's sacerdos or chaplain or to the *ius patronatus* were rare, especially if they entailed these rights down through the descendants of the male line. Such usages of entail for the privatization of family chapels do not appear in Sienese testaments until the sixteenth century. Of 183 chapel foundations recorded in these samples for the six cities, only 39 give any clue as to who would possess the rights over the sacred space once the chapel or altar had been constructed. Arezzo and Florence predominated in specifying these rights, with 15 and 11 cases respectively, comprising 70 percent of the cases of private presentations. Again, the geography charted by these documents corroborates my earlier findings, as does the chronology: the bulk of these elections (73 percent) came in the year of the plague's return, 1362–63, or afterward. In almost half of the instances when these rights were indicated (18 cases), the *ius patronatus* was given to the resident ecclesiastical body where the chapel was to be constructed—the canons of the cathedral, the abbot and monks of a monastery, the prior and friars of a mendicant house. In two cases, the testator did not assume the chapel's rights or channel them down through his family but granted them to ecclesiastical entities other than the ones whose buildings hosted the new altars.

In 1363, an Aretine lady, domina Odda f.q. domini Oddonis de Servinis, from Cortona, widow of domini Bonigiunte, ordered her nephew and universal heir to build a chapel in the episcopal church of Arezzo. However, she gave her executors, the Misericordia and the hospital of Santa Maria del Oriente, the responsibilities of overseeing its construction and the title of *patrones* of the chapel.[44] In 1419, another Aretine, the citizen Meus f.q. Fini, divided the rights over his burial chapel in the church of Santa Maria de Gradibus among several parties: one *voce* was to be held by the abbot of the abbey of Agnano, another by the *operarii* of Arezzo's *plebis* church, a third by the flagellant confraternity of Sant'Angelo of Arezzo, a fourth by his brother, the cobbler Antonio, a fifth by the swordmaker Gerolinus Baccii, and a final one by his heirs and their successors. The testator intervened further in the future affairs of his chapel by prohibiting the patrons from ever choosing a monk as its chaplain; rather, he "was always to be a secular priest."[45]

Of the remaining 19 cases of chaplain elections where the testator, at least in the first appointment, instituted his or her own man, the Florentines and Aretines dominated to an even greater extent with 16 appointments (9 from Aretines and 7 from Florentines). Those who channeled these rights down family lines were rare indeed, and all except the two already mentioned did so late in the Trecento or thereafter. In 1374, the Aretine doctor of both laws from the Acceptanti family founded a burial chapel in the *plebis* church in which his apparently unrelated heir and sons were to "elect and place" the chaplain. If they failed in this task, then the rights would devolve on "all the males of this house born from legitimate marriages." The testator instructed them to appoint a sacerdos at least 25 years old, "a man of constituted good character, condition and family," who was already ordained and would reside continually in this benefice, celebrating masses and divine offices for the testator's own and his ancestors' souls.[46]

In 1375, the Florentine Bencivennes f.q. Turini left his farm in Poggibonsi to construct a chapel in honor of Saint Catherine in his parish of San Lorenzo. For the election of the chaplain he delegated his executors, his wife, a Servite friar, and an ironmonger, adding, however, that the chapter of the canons of San Lorenzo was to "confirm" the sacerdos and his successors, who "would reside continually" at the altar to recite masses and divine offices.[47] In 1379, the Aretine citizen Pagnus f.q. Maffei ordered the construction of a chapel in the cathedral, to be named Saint Mathew the Apostle. He insisted that the chaplain be at least 30 years old and possess no other benefice. Pagnus extended the rights of election to his executors and universal heirs, his grandson, and, if he died without heirs, the Misericordia.[48] In 1383, Fonsus f.q. Bacionis, from Lilliano in the contado of Legoli, then living in Pisa, ordered a chapel built in his parish, the convent church of San Martino, to be named after the apostles Peter and Nicholas. The chaplain and his successors were to be "good and honest priests" and "among the four chaplains held by the special administration of this convent." They were to be confirmed by "the venerable abbess living at the time," but elected by his sons and brother and afterward by their sons and descendants.[49]

In 1389, "the discreet man" Alessandrus f.q. Iacobi Gini [Benvenuti de Ginoris] ordered a chapel built in his parish of San Lorenzo with the advice of the wool guild. He split the rights of election between the prior of this canonical church and his friend Johannes f.q. Filippi de Rondinelli and, after their deaths, to the prior's successors and "to one of the progeny from the line of this Johannes de Rondinelli in perpetuity." And evidence from the early Quattrocento shows in fact that this commission was executed.[50]

In 1396, the Aretine Francescus f.q. Simonis Ghini left his universal heirs the rights of electing the chaplain to his chapel constructed in the Aretine plebis church. In effect, this grant divided these rights between ecclesiastical and secular parties. Heirs to half his property were the Misericordia and the Olivetani of San Bernardo, and to the other half the Florentine citizen Simoneus Ser Pieri de la Fioraia.[51]

In 1409, the Pisan knight (miles) dominus Tighus de Upessingis, whom we encountered earlier founding a chapel, may have gone further in imposing his will on church administration. He ordered that the church of San Bartolommeo de Rapita "be united" with this altar and that its rector be the altar's first chaplain. Afterward, these rights of presentment were to devolve on his heirs, his grandson, and his successors. This scion of an important noble family then went beyond the walls of his private enclave to determine that his chaplain would become, moreover, the rector of the church of San Bartolommeo. He further insisted that this priest was to be an ordained sacerdos and occupy no other benefice.[52]

Of those testators who "entitled" their chapels (*sub vocabulo*), 68 percent came from Arezzo (26) and Florence (19), and over 70 percent of the testaments were redacted immediately after the recurrence of plague in 1363. Stamping a name on one's chapel construction was no trivial act but reflects a testator's encroachment into the affairs of the church hosting these sacred grounds to be dedicated to the salvation of his and his ancestors' souls. Remember the Florentine testator Francescus f.q. Masi de Alferris, who wished to name his chapel after his namesake, Saint Francis, in the midst of the Dominican stronghold of Florence, the church of Santa Maria Novella.[53] Remember the cobbler from Vinci, who named his chapel in the *plebis* church of Vinci, not with his surname, but after the Archangel Michael and then, to stamp it with his newly concocted dynastic designs, attached his family name to it. The noble lady from the Perugian de Gratinis family similarly referred to her chapel in the cathedral as bearing her family name.[54]

Others sought to extend their memories by naming their chapels after namesake saints. Ser Nicholaus f.q. Ser Laurini de Grassis, from Arezzo, named his chapel Saint Nicholas, which may have ruffled the sensibilities of his hosts, the Franciscans of Arezzo, as much as sticking a chapel named after Saint Francis in a Dominican church, since Nicholas was the patron of the Augustinians, whose church in Arezzo as well as in Pisa and other cities bore this saint's name. Nor did the effect of naming end with its simple entitlement. In this case, the friars and prior would have to recall and revere this patron in the perpetual yearly cycle of their services. The testator further demanded that this saint's day be celebrated yearly in his chapel by distributing four *staii* of baked bread to the poor and by the friars saying daily prayers "in honor of the omnipotent God and the blessed Nicholas."[55]

In at least two instances, Perugini went beyond the Aretines or Florentines in extending their memories when naming their chapels. In 1417, Francescus f.q. Ser Putii Nelli left the Olivetani as his universal heirs with the obligation of building an altar in their monastery "under the name of the said Francescus," that is, the name of the testator and not his namesake, the saint.[56] In the following year, another Perugian, Sapiens Vir Matheus f.q. Vanneli Monti, placed a similar demand on his parish church of Saint Florence: After the death of his daughter, he left

400 florins to his parish either to build or to buy a chapel in this church with an altar to be ordained (*deputare*) "under the name of this testator."[57]

Chapel Decoration

Not only were chapels in and of themselves works of art requiring the craft and vision of architects[58] or master builders, they were often the primary receptacles for sacred artworks in churches, from tombs and sculpted inscriptions to tabernacles, embroidered altarcloths, banners and *palii*, a wide variety of embroidered vestments for the chaplain, wall paintings or frescoes, panel paintings, and, toward the end of this analysis, stained-glass windows. Thus, commissioning a chapel could have a reverberating effect on artistic production beyond the expenses allocated at its inception and beyond the plans of the founder. Throughout these documents, but particularly in the later years, testators added to or refurbished previously founded family chapels by commissioning new sacred works of art for the beautification of their ancestral chambers.

The earliest of these goes back to the Black Death of 1348, when Nicholaus f.q. Cini Minaldi, from Poggibonsi, left funds to be determined by his executors "to replenish" his chapel in the Augustinian church in this town and for "making paintings [*pro picturis fiendis*]."[59] In 1365, domina Iacoba, the widow of two Florentines, the first from the de la Tosa family, was more specific in her plans for redecorating a chapel founded by her second husband, dominus Simoneus, in the Dominican church of San Pietro de Murrone. She left 12 florins for her heirs to have this chapel painted with "the images and figures" of "Our Blessed Lady, the Ever Virginal Mary," the blessed Catherine, San Pietro de Murrone, and underneath "these figures and images," the testatrix herself.[60]

In 1371, the Florentine parish rector of Santa Cecilia, whose elaborate schemes for perpetual masses we have witnessed, refurbished the chapel built by a certain Ser Orlandus, his ancestor, next to the new bell tower of Santa Cecilia, to the point of even renaming it after the ancient martyred saints Valerianus and Tiburtius. He then commissioned the chapel's furnishings: a golden chalice with six enameled figures engraved on its pedestal; altarcloths and vestments with silk drapery decorated with red, yellow, and green compasses and with a golden hem embroidered with the figures of saints, lined with a linen undergarment; and a priestly vestment with cuffs. He also left 25 florins for a missal and 6 florins to purchase an altar screen for use on feast days. In addition to iron railings (*cordellerie de ferro*) to cordon off his sacred enclave, the rector commissioned "an honorable" panel painting of the Virgin Mary "in medio," with the blessed Cecilia and Valerianus on one side and the blessed Bartolommeo and Tiburtius on the other, for the relatively large sum of 20 florins.[61]

In the same year, a domina Lena, from the Aretine family of the Guasconi, ordered further decorations and furnishings (*fulciatur et fiat omnibus ornamentis*) for the chapel previously constructed by her late husband, Ser Bindus, "and others of his *domus*."[62] In 1416, the Aretine merchant Mariottus f.q. Blaxii Grisolini bequeathed more, 200 florins "in pictures and ornamentation," to decorate and increase the endowment for a chapel under the bell tower of the *plebis* church of Arezzo.[63] Finally, the noble lady Gregoria f.q. Ugolini de Gratianis,[64] of Perugia, commissioned wall paintings of the blessed Mary with the cross depicted "in gula" (*in culla*) or the nativity of the Virgin, alongside Saint Christopher, Saint Margaret, the blessed Laurence, and Saint Ann for the family chapel (*capella de Gratinis*) founded by her deceased father and located in the cathedral of Perugia, San Lorenzo, at a cost left to her executors' discretion.[65]

What is in a name? We have already discussed the importance of naming for boosting a testator's honor and memory. Such namesakes did not, however, constitute the majority of the entitlements found in these documents. Nonetheless, a testator's selection of a patron saint, whether or not it was the testator's namesake, could impose his will and shape the chapel in concrete ways. As in the case of the Aretine foundation of a chapel dedicated to the Augustinian patron, Saint Nicholas, but placed in the stronghold of the Franciscans, the chosen name often set the chapel's yearly cycle of events—the feast days, meals, distribution of alms, masses, and divine offices to be celebrated on the birth date of the patron saint. These obligations, moreover, could spill over beyond those tasks placed on the elected chaplain, calling on the host canons, monks, or friars to join in the celebrations to honor the testator's named saint and the souls of the testator and his ancestors.

The naming of a chapel also set its decorative schemes. For instance, "the provident man" Marianus, from the Aretine village of Celaria, in 1372 through his will founded a chapel in the new Augustinian friary of Arezzo, leaving 50 florins for furnishings that included the chalice, vestments, missal, wax, and other necessities, as well as "for pictures." In particular, he named it after the blessed Jacob (*et sub eius tituto intituletur*) and demanded that his heirs have the figure of this patron saint painted in it.[66] In 1374, another Aretine, the doctor of both laws, placed his chapel "under the name" of the blessed Francis and demanded that it be decorated with the narrative cycle of "the blessed Francis when he received the stigmata from Our Lord Jesus Christ" and with the story (*ystoria*) of the blessed Francis.[67]

A Perugian widow, Andrea, founded a chapel "to be covered" (*cappella coperta*) in the Olivetani church of Monte Morcino, where she demanded a preexisting altar, "on the right hand side of the door leading to the choir of this church" to be "honorably" furnished with altarcloths (*tobaliis a dossale*) and other beautiful fabrics, a cross, a chalice, *patena et tur[r]ibulo*[68] of silver, and "honorable" vestments for the priest, the deacons, and the subdeacons, according to the prior's discretion (*iuxta conscientiam*). She used her will to name the chapel after the "Sancta Maria della Annuptiata" and demanded that her heirs consign and place there "a large and beautiful" panel painting (*tabula magna apulcra*) of the Annuciation flanked by the figures of the blessed apostles, Peter and Paul, "one on the right, the other on the left," and at the foot of the "images" the "likeness [*similitudinem*] of the person of this testatrix, along with her arms and other signs for her memory and for the commendation of her soul."[69]

In 1411, the Florentine citizen and merchant Antonius f.q. Lapacci Cini Cettini left the substantial sum of 750 florins to the monks of his parish church to finish his chapel named (*sub titulo et nomine*) Saint Nicholas of Bari. It was to have a stained-glass window (*una finestra vitrea*)[70] and every other necessity for its honor and utility, including most particularly its painting and ornamentation with the narrative cycle of the life of Saint Nicholas of Bari. From this sum, the monks were also to celebrate *in perpetuum* the feast day of this saint in his chapel with four large candles (*cerroti*) weighing a pound apiece, two to be burnt on the altar and two above the altar in the candelabras, while the chaplain celebrated a high mass (*missa magna*) and low masses (*misse parve*), all performed "honorably" according to the discretion of the abbot and monks of San Pancrazio. The monks and abbot, in addition, could demand three-and-a-half florins to be spent for a festive meal (*una pietenza*) for the saint's commemoration.[71] Finally, the cobbler from Vinci named his chapel after his patron saint, Michelangelo, and directed its ornamentation accordingly. As we have seen, he commissioned a large panel painting depicting the Virgin Mary and the saints John the Baptist, Michelangelo, and Anthony.

Several testators, among them Lady Andrea, from Perugia, went beyond commissioning sacred paintings to decorate their chapels and used these sacred spaces to enhance their "memory" and the fame of their families by ordering the walls painted with their coats of arms and other worldly insignia. This mundanity—what Savonarola and other preachers would later condemn as useless vanity[72]—was entirely absent from the decorative schemes for these holy places until after the return of the plague in 1363. Then it began to seep into the chapel plans of testators from the same three cities that stressed earthly memory in the structure of charitable allocations, burials, and property relations— Arezzo, Florence, and Perugia. It does not appear in Sienese testaments until the end of the fifteenth century.

"For her perpetual memory," the Florentine domina Mante, widow of Ser Antonii Ghini, ordered in 1369 that her coat of arms and that of her deceased husband "be sculpted and designed, cut in stone, and placed" in her chapel to be built in the parish of San Lorenzo. (Later evidence from a pastoral visitation in 1422 shows that the commission was executed.)[73] In 1371, the Aretine citizen Verius f.q. Donatini Pietri Orlandi left half his estate to the hospital of the Oriente with instructions to build in it "for the memory of his house a beautiful and an honorable" chapel "designated with the insignia of this hospital [signatam de signo] and the arms of this Verius."[74] In 1379, another citizen of Arezzo, Pagnus f.q. Maffei, extended the use of "the mundanities" beyond family and lineage by ordering, along with his family arms, the insignia of his trade (signum merchantie quem utebatur in sua apotecha) "to be painted and sculpted" in the chapel, which he ordered to be built and endowed in the new church of the Aretine Franciscans.[75] The Florentine merchant from the Juochis family who worked in Paris left his palace (magna domus)[76] to the Jacobin friars and the hospital of Santa Maria Nuova, obliging them "communally" to make the shield of the Juochis family out of stone and to display it "always" at the entrance to this donated home above the walled vault.[77]

Finally, in 1406 Filippus f.q. domini Castellani, from the prominent Frescobaldi family of Florence, founded two chapels—one in the monastery of Santa Maria degli Angeli, for which he left the substantial endowment of 500 florins, and the other to enshrine his burial in the Augustinian church of Santo Spirito, for which he left 1,000 florins, the second largest sum found for a chapel foundation for any city in my samples. Filippus jealously guarded his private rights to this sacred space with a rigor that was unusual for these chapel commissions, "holding" that only the arms of the Frescobaldi could be placed in this space and that only the bodies of "this" Filippus and his descendants could be interred there.[78]

Other Construction Projects

Though quantitatively by far the most important, chapel building was of course not the only type of ecclesiastical construction a testator might initiate in a will. Several construction projects relied on the residuary estates from wealthy and important lineages, such as the Tolomei of Siena, who founded four hospitals in the *contado* of Siena at the end of the Duecento,[79] or the conversion of the *poderi* and houses left in the 1395 will of the Florentine knight dominus Nicholaus Cardinali f.q. Pagnozi de Tornaquincis into a nunnery for noble ladies in the suburban parish of San Piero a Careggi.[80]

On the other hand, construction projects could be as modest as hospitals requiring the upkeep of only two beds, or a hermit's cell such as the one the "noble, wise and powerful" Tarlatus founded for the Camaldoli hermits with the spiritual investment of 100 lire;[81] or, for even less, the cell in the "new dormitory" of the preaching friars of Perugia, for which the Perugian notary Ser Simoneus Helemosine Johannis owed 11 lire of 25 lire that he left to "finish and decorate."[82] In these documents, testators founded, built, or totally refurbished 27 hospitals, 6 convents, 4 monasteries or friaries, and 3 rural churches (two by a Perugian, one in the year of the Black Death,[83] another in 1384,[84] the third by a Florentine in the early fifteenth century).[85] The Florentines led the list of these constructions (11), followed closely, this time, by the Perugini (10), then the Aretines (6), the Pisans (6), the Sienese, and the Assisani (4 each). Although the Pisans and Aretines produced the same number of projects found in these samples, the Aretines nearly doubled the number of such ecclesiastical buildings per pious bequest ordered in Pisan wills. Again, the greatest number of these projects followed the recurrence of plague in 1363.

With these projects testators exercised election and governing rights less often than with chapel foundations; nor did they channel these rights down the male line, but delegated them only to existing ecclesiastical bodies. For instance, Petruccius Cicoli Iacobi del Picciche, of Assisi, in 1340 gave his house and garden in the porta San Francesco to the confraternity of Santa Maria Maggiore, which congregated in the cathedral of San Ruffino to convert the house into a hospice for the "perpetual service of God and for the utility, comfort, and habitation of the poor of Germany [*pauperum Theotonicorum*]" who could not find room in the German hospital already existing in Assisi.[86] In 1351, a Florentine merchant with shops in Avignon, Martinus f.q. Bizzi, founded a hospital for the "poor of Christ" to be called San Martino della Fonte. He placed it under the care and correction (*sub cura et correctione*) of the prior of Florence's major hospital, Santa Maria Nuova, "who ought in perpetuity" to elect the *hospitalarius,* or rector of this hospital.[87] In 1362, the Assisan Iacobus f.q. Vanni, called Zuccha, founded a hospital "for the sustenance of the poor, pilgrims and the infirm," which he named Lo spedale della Pietate and placed under the authority of the confraternity and hospital of the flagellant company of Saint Stephen.[88] In the same year, another Assisan left his house to the same confraternity for the care of the poor of Christ, but went beyond his confrère by insisting that the hospital be named after his family—vocetur hospitale Maragonis.[89] In 1363, a Perugian noble lady left her palace and the houses next to it along with its vineyards and arable lands located near the village of Corciano to "the monks or friars" of Monte Oliveto of the *contado* of Siena, whom she obliged to build in the palace and its houses "a place for religious habitation" (*quendam locum actum ad morandum, standum et habitandum Religiosi*) to accommodate 12 monks.[90]

If his heirs should die, the Perugian Ser Bonfiglus f.q. Mathei Petri ordered in his 1383 will that his houses in the *castro* of Papiano be reconstructed into a church called the ecclesiam Sancti Iacobi, where divine offices and prayers were to be celebrated "continuously" for the souls of his relatives and blood kin (*parentorum et consanguineorum*). Its rule, governance, and administration were given to the Dominicans, who were never to alienate any of its properties and were obliged to send at least eight of their brothers to officiate at this church. If they rejected the offer, the gift and its responsibilities would fall to the Servites of Perugia.[91] In 1390, a citizen of Perugia opted to build a hospital from the proceeds of his landed estates (*tenimentum terre*) in the district of Corciano and left the rights to elect its "patron, governor and rector" and the supervision of its construction and administration to the "care, protection and regime" of the banker's guild of Perugia.[92]

In contrast to endowments of chapels, testators were chary about imposing rules about the administration or the daily to yearly cycles of spiritual events to be performed within these sacred enclaves. The one exception was an Aretine, "the Provident Man" Angelus f.q. Rossi de Catenaccis, whose 1359 will (no doubt prompted and guided along by religious figures) set out in greater detail than any other testament a spiritual vision for a monastic foundation, establishing even the principles of its governance. Angelus left the hermits of Camaldoli his urban "palace," all his houses and his rental properties in the city of Arezzo, and 65 *starii* of land in the Villa Vignale located in the curia of Santa Fiora to construct on this last-named property within one year of his death a hermitage (*heremitorium sive heremium*) for "hermits or friars" of "Sancti Camaldoli." He required a minimum of four of these hermits to inhabit this hermitage at all times except in the case of war, including one sacerdos "in the service of God" who would "continuously" celebrate divine offices and prayers.

The Aretine patrician then specified "the rule" (*sub regula*) under which these "hermits or friars" were to live. Those hermits desiring to take up residence and "to serve" in this hermitage were to keep "customs and observances of the Camaldoli order" (*teneantur et debeant morem et consuetudinem et observantiam heremitarum sive fratrum dicti Sancti Camaldoli*). Under no circumstance might any woman enter. No meat could be served except to a brother suffering from illness or "evident weakness" and then "only to that brother and not the others." The hermits were to join together from the feast of Santa Croce in the month of September until Easter and from the feast of the Pentecost to the feast of the Holy Cross on the fourth and sixth holidays (*feria*). When they joined together, they should not expect to receive money, but might collect clothing and shoes if indigent and according to the discretion of their superior. They were to celebrate divine offices during the nightly hours according to the rituals of Camaldoli hermits. The Prior General of the Camaldoli order was to pay regular visits to this hermitage, and for each visit the friars were to pay him 10 soldi. No friar or hermit should be removed or deprived of residence by the Prior General or the General Inspector of this order without the consent of the local prior and the head of this hermitage (*Prioris et capituli eiusdem loci*). If the position of prior should become vacant, only the resident friars and hermits should have the rights of electing their new prior, but the election results must be "confirmed" by the Prior General according to custom (*iuxta morem*) of the "collegiate monastery." Finally, the testator prohibited the alienation of any of his properties unless "equivalent" properties were purchased, except for eight *starii* of rental land to be sold for 70 florins, of which 25 florins should be used for the conversion of his houses into hermit cells (*hermitorii*).[93]

Only the Florentine patrician Consillius de Cerchiis placed the *ius patronatus* of one of these ecclesiastical foundations into family hands.

His 1291 testament bequeathed half of his property, excluding his houses in the city of Florence, to build a hospital on his lands for the care of "the poor and religious and special persons." The executors of this project were to be the bishop of Florence, the prior of the preaching friars, the guardian of the minor friars, and the ministers of the penitential friars of Florence, "who wore black habits." However, Consillius gave the "ius et patronatus in this hospital" to the "oldest member of his house," that is, "of his descendants through the male line from his father Ser Oliverio and his mother domine Emelline." This male relative, he specified, would have "full power [*plenam potestatem*] in this hospital in electing, placing, putting and extracting" the *hospitalarium* and his servant (*familiarem*) as well as in expediting "every other thing" needed for the utility of the hospital and its properties, "according to the counsel of the discreet men of his house [*consilium discretorum virorum sue domus*], and of his descendants down the male line." If the hospital was not built within two years, the properties would devolve to "the Roman church" to subsidize its crusades to the Holy Land.[94]

Again, unlike those who commissioned chapels, testators rarely imposed their decorative schemes on the architecture or ornamentation of these buildings. In several cases, however, they set out to preserve their secular memories through their foundations by emblazoning their familial insignia and coats of arms on these holy places. All such initiatives came from Florentines. The earliest dates from 1303, when the Florentine Lottus, called Berrettinus f.q. Corsi Berrectonis, left his *podere* with its houses and vineyards in the villa of San Marco to found a hospice for the wandering poor of Christ (*pauperes transeuntes Chrispti*), ordering that "in this hospital" his insignia and his arms (*armorum ad birrectas*) be painted "for his memory [*in eius memoriam*]."[95] In 1396, Anfleus Torini Bencivennis, from the parish of San Lorenzo, left one-third of his estate to the hospital of Santa Maria Nuova to build a hospital with only two beds, where the infirm might rest in peace (*requiesciant*) and where the insignia and the arms of the testators should be displayed.[96]

Sacred Art

To display and preserve one's family coat of arms or leave other concrete vestiges of earthly memory in churches or monasteries, testators did not need to commission a major building project. Nor did they have to resort to the mendicant pattern of leaving small sums to ecclesiastical bodies without determining their specific purposes or holding the recip-

ients to certain restrictions and conditions. Instead, they could commission paintings, engraved chalices, altarcloths, priestly vestments, or
wax figures for parish churches, hospitals, monasteries, nunneries, or
cathedrals where their families possessed no altars and had no intentions
of building one. Indeed, such commissioned objects constituted the bulk
of the sacred art itemized in the testaments for the six city-states.

In addition to commissioning works of art, testators could strive for
lasting memory through an association with a work of art, usually by
offering perpetual supplies of wax or oil for the illumination of a painting,
crucifix, or votive image. The most dramatic of these examples comes
from a Florentine testator, "the discreet man" Ricchuccius, from Santa
Maria Novella, who left sums for the "continuous" illumination of three
paintings—the crucifix painted by Giotto in Santa Maria Novella, the
"great panel painting" (the *Rucellai Madonna*) in the same church, and
another panel painting earlier commissioned by the testator in the Dominican friary of Prato by the "great Florentine painter, named Giotto."[97]

Similarly, the Perugian Nutius Cioli wished to extend his memory
by supplying the wax to be burnt for 10 years in the Francescan church
of Perugia in front of a painting he had commissioned of the "blessed
Saint Constantine" and another in front of the figures he commissioned
to appear above his tomb.[98] Pietrus Salvoli del Giordolo, from the Villa
San Sisto, was one of a number of Perugians who left oil to be burnt
"for illuminating the most exalted figure of the blessed Virgin Mary"
found in the "church or rectory" of the *Maestatis de Volta*.[99]

The Pisans practiced a devotional appreciation of art that was almost
exclusive to themselves, at least among the city-states studied here.
Testators in this seafaring capital made offerings of clothing and jewelry
to sacred images. For instance, in 1348 the country woman domina Mea,
widow of Vannis Cionis from Cisanello in the *contado* of Pisa, offered
"to the Image of Our Lady who is in the Duomo of the city of Pisa"
a roll of cotton cloth, a gold ring, and 60 silver buttons.[100] In 1362, the
year of the plague's return, the widow of a notary from Pontedera who
lived in Pisa offered "her best underwear and a cloak to our lady existing
next to the cross at the altar of San Tommaso de Cintuberio [Thomas
Becket] in the Cathedral of Pisa."[101] The closest approximation from
another city-state came in an Aretine will of 1312 in which domina
Deccha, the wife of Redinus, gave her veil with golden sequins (*capitaneis*)
to the church of San Domenico, designating (*deputandi*) it for the painting
of the blessed Mary in Majesty.[102]

For the purposes of comparing the demand for sacred art among these cities and over time, I have defined testamentary sacred art as requests for the construction of chapels, hospitals, churches, monasteries, hermitages, and nunneries, as well as for figures to be made by an artist or artisan in whatever medium and placed in a sacred building. Such figures might be as complex as the Old Testament cycle "from beginning to end" commissioned in 1348 for Santa Maria Novella by the Florentine merchant Torinus f.q. Baldese, who solicited counsel from the famous Dominican preacher Jacopo Passavanti.[103] Or they might be simple coats of arms, plaques with inscriptions, and other familial regalia or objects, such as the wax images valued at 20 soldi that a Florentine widow offered to the blessed Mary of Orsanmichele in the year of the Black Death.[104]

The media for these figures and the arts and crafts required to finish them spanned a wide range—panel paintings, wall paintings, predellas, icons, pulpits, silver chalices, stained-glass windows, tabernacles, wooden crucifixes, beds painted with images, wax figures, candlestick holders (*aste*), altarcloths, priestly vestments, painted religious banners called *palios,* banners (*gonfaloni*), flags, and finally sculpted figures in wood, marble, and stone. I have excluded items that certainly required the skills of a master artisan, such as chalices, priestly vestments, and altarcloths, but where the testator did not specifically call for "images," "pictures," or "figures." I am concerned here more with the artistic designs of the testator than with the finished product. Contributions to works of art or sums given to subsidize a particular Madonna or Annunciation have been omitted as well. These in fact flourished in Arezzo, which, even without them, was the most remarkable of these city-states in the sheer quantity of demand for tombstones, inscriptions, coats of arms, chapels, and (as we will see) other art forms in the Trecento and early Quattrocento. Here, as early as the 1320s, testators such as the tavernkeeper Paulus Appulliensis contributed a mere 40 lire to the "works" (*operi*) of the panel painting of the blessed Virgin Mary "delegated" (*deputande*) for the *plebis* church of Arezzo, which may well have been the polyptych that Pietro Lorenzetti completed in that decade and which still stands above the major altar of this church.[105] The coffers for such collective enterprises required small contributions from numerous donors and could be left open for years. Instead of evoking a cult of memory, these funds resembled more the mendicant patterns of piety, where the church and not the individual donor determined the charity's use and allocation.

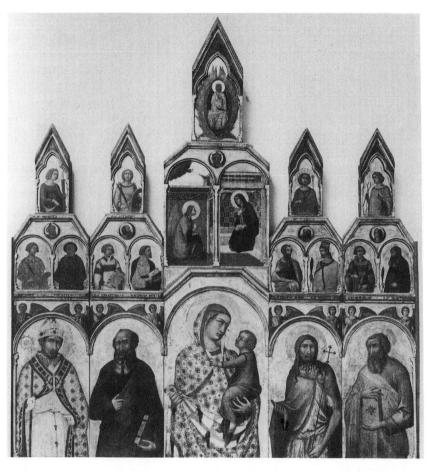

3. Pietro Lorenzetti, *Polyptych*. Santa Maria della Pieve, Arezzo (Courtesy Soprintendenza alle gallerie-Firenze, no. 49797).

Chalices, Vestments, Altarcloths

The number of chalices, altarcloths, and vestments in these samples
containing commissioned figures is small: in only 17 of the numerous

bequests recorded for such altar furnishings did the testator specify engraved or embroidered figures, and these were mostly family coats of arms. In such instances, testators placed their family "mundanities" at the very heart of the most sacred act of the church—the priestly performance of the Eucharist, as when Ser Ridolfus f.q. Ser Ubaldini Bartoli in his testament of 1373 gave a silver chalice with gold trimming and his familial coat of arms to a friar at Santa Croce "for the celebration of divine offices."[106] By the last decades of the Trecento, testators stitched their arms and insignia into the vestments clerics wore while performing mass.[107] In 1382, the Florentine Michele f.q. Braccini Durantis sought to advertise thus his arms simultaneously with the celebration of mass in various churches through the dioceses of Florence and Fiesole. To the church of his burial and to three other specified churches,[108] he gave chasubles worth 10 florins apiece to be made of silk with an *"astola* and *manipolo"* in which his arms were to be inscribed.[109] Of these embroideries and engravings, like the plastering of family regalia in private chapels, none antedated the recurrence of pestilence in 1362–63. Furthermore, none of them derive from Pisa or Siena, and only one comes from Assisi. Again, despite the small numbers, Florence (nine examples), Perugia (four) and Arezzo (four) were distinctive in relation to the other three cities.

Surviving inventories of church possessions corroborate these impressions. In 1391, the Florentine church of the Carmine drew up its first inventory of liturgical possessions held in its old sacristy, dividing them under two headings. The first group— *"calici, patene, terribili et croce"* — comprised 35 items, of which 10 were identified with the engraved coats of arms of Florentine families.[110] Unfortunately, the second group— *"Reliquie, adornamenti dell'altare maggiore d'ariento, di rame, ornati di legno e d'alabastro e veli e altri ornamenti per calici"*—is more difficult to quantify: the possessions were not itemized separately, but were grouped in vague categories such as *"Drapelloni di diverse armi,"* which contained 307 items.[111] The inventory of SS. Annunziata, redacted in 1422, was far more extensive. The prior and sacristan first listed all the priestly vestments, from the ceremonial cape (*piviali*) worn on solemn occasions to their shirts (*camiscie*). Of 97 chasubles (*pianete solenni*) arranged by color—white, red, green, yellow, and the daily red ones (*sanguingne feriali*)—68 were stitched with the personal arms of lay noble or merchant families and 44 of these bore the arms of two families.[112] Of 14 paraments, 11 bore arms, 2 of which had arms from more than one family.[113] Of 19 *piviali*, 5 possessed arms; and of 36 banners (*palii*) for the high altar, 12 bore arms and 6 the arms or shields of two families.[114] The Servites possessed a number of chalices and silver crosses comparable to that of the Carmelites (38), but a larger number had been stamped with family arms (16).[115] This difference over time (even though both points of comparison lie near the end of my analysis) is suggestive. Whether this difference resulted from a change over time, from the late Trecento to the 1420s, or from a difference in these orders' relations with noble and merchant families would require more extensive research into these archival collections.

By contrast, the earliest inventories for the Cathedral of Pisa redacted in the last quarter of the thirteenth and early years of the fourteenth century do not contain a single priestly vestment, chalice, or other liturgical possession stamped with the arms of a Pisan family, even though their lists of properties far exceed the numbers possessed by the Florentine Carmelites or Servites.[116] By the inventory of 1369, however, the picture had changed in Pisa. Of 30 chalices listed, 12 bore the coats of arms of noble Pisan families, such as the Lanfranchi and the Ripafracta, and those of rich merchants, such as the Marci.[117] Yet, arms on altar banners (*palii*) and priestly vestments had not spread as thoroughly as they had in the Carmelite and Servite inventories of Florence. Coats of arms were stamped on only 2 of 39 *palii* in the cathedral inventory of 1369, and only one of 59 chasubles and ceremonial robes had family coats of arms—those of dominus Petrus de Gambacorti, soon to become ruler of Pisa.[118]

Although these cathedral inventories of the last decade of the Trecento and the early Quattrocento listed far fewer liturgical possessions than earlier, the trend over time is unmistakable: of 5 chalices, 4 bore arms, and of 7 *palii*, 6 were stitched with the mundanities of secular and family pride.[119] Still, even by the end of the Trecento, the tradition of stamping private coats of arms on sacred objects appears to have been less common in Pisa than in Florence. While the meticulous inventories compiled in 1396 for Pisa's central hospital of Santa Chiara describe in detail the "figures" engraved on chalices and the colors, hems, and designs embroidered on priestly vestments and banners, the notaries do not bear witness to any familial insignia on the hundreds of such items possessed in the hospital's sacristy and chapels.[120]

Candlestick Holders

Another place for attaching family coats of arms was on candlestick holders placed on or near the altar for "illuminating the body of Christ." Again, stamping these sacred objects with the mundanities of family recognition postdated the plague of 1363 in every case. The earliest example is also the most extraordinary, showing that such forms of family pride reached far down the social ladder, at least in a place like Florence. The biting irony and social scorn of Franco Sacchetti (repeated with bravado 160 years later by Giorgio Vasari) directed against the *"uomo di picciolo affare,"* who was so haughty as to think he could commission Giotto to paint his coat of arms, prove not to have been so far removed from everyday reality, at least in late Trecento Florence.[121] The Florentine wool worker (*cardator seu conciator pannorum*) Iacobus f.q. Pieri Martinelli left a large candle (*torchettus*) to the hospital of Santa Maria Nuova, which the *hospitalarius* was held to "keep burning to illuminate the mass at the altar in the women's section of the hospital." The *torchettus* was to be placed in a "candlestick holder which this worker-testator ordered to be painted and inscribed [*pictis seu signatis*]" with his coat of arms, even though this carder did not even possess a family name.[122]

Unlike a chapel, a monastery, or even a tombstone, these objects for bearing family regalia cost little. The highest payment for a candlestick holder with painted arms was made in 1374 by an Aretine citizen, Masius Neri Mucii Carsidonii de Carsidoniis, from Borgo San Sepolcro,[123] "for the souls of his relatives and blood kin" as well as for the *opera* of the Olivetani church: he left it (his chosen place of burial) 20 lire for two large candles (*cereos*) with iron candlestick holders painted with his arms to illuminate the body of Christ.[124] But such iron holders could cost less, as the 1411 testament of the Aretine ironmonger Nicholaus f.q. Nicholai illustrates; for his painted *ascis* he left only one florin to the parish church of Sant'Andrea.[125]

Painted Beds

Other objects for pious paintings were the beds testators routinely gave to hospitals.[126] The most remarkable of these commissions was again the earliest found in these documents. In 1323 the blacksmith Nutus f.q. Dietiguardi, from Borgo San Lorenzo, then residing in Florence, willed for the honor and reverence of San Lorenzo a bed with all its furnishings (*fulcrimentis*) to the hospital of San Lorenzo in Borgo. No routine donation of a bed, this one was to be painted "with the image in the likeness of the majesty of God [*quodam ymago ad Similitudinem magiestatis dei*]."[127] In other cases, donors of painted beds demanded less dramatic pictorial inscriptions—once again, their familial coats of arms.

But even such commissions could substantially increase the cost of a bed. While beds appearing in these legacies were normally valued between 10 and 15 lire in the second half of the Trecento, the Florentine Silvestrus f.q. Lapi Bini left 60 lire in 1359 for his bed with a litter (*letticha*) to be painted with his arms and given for the use of the poor in the hospital of Santa Maria Nuova.[128] In 1374, the bed of the Aretine émigré citizen of the Carsidoni family cost even more—in fact, as much as an artisan's dowry or a cottage in the city of Arezzo. He left 100 lire to the hospital of Santa Maria della Scala in Siena for a bed with all its furnishings and a new *lectica* painted with his arms.[129] Again, these commissions for beds painted with family coats of arms corroborate the earlier patterns of geography and chronology. All came from Florence or Arezzo, and only one, the remarkable commission for the "likeness of God," antedated the plague's return in 1363.

Coats of Arms, Crests, and Plaques

Other testators simply had their crests (*cimeria*), coats of arms, and other family insignia painted or carved in marble or stone and placed in sacred places or carved directly into the walls of churches, chapels, hospitals, and monasteries.[130] Again, the Florentines and Aretines dominated the production of these symbols for familial pride and memory (11 and 8 respectively of 22 cases), and the vast majority (17) came after the recurrence of plague. In Florence, this trend developed despite the commune's attempts to restrict the plastering of such signs and symbols of family pride on public buildings. As is often the case, repeated legislation bears witness to the endurance of a practice.[131]

While Florence may have quantitatively outstripped the provincial town to the southeast, some of the most noteworthy attempts to extend earthly memory through these works derive from Arezzo. In his will, redacted in 1374, the Aretine citizen Landucius Ser Andree Giotti de Acceptantibus explicitly directed that his arms be plastered in a wide variety of churches and hospitals as well as on public and private buildings. He gave two *panersaria* painted with his arms to the Commune of Monte San Savino and ordered a plaque (*targa*) and a crest (*cimerium*), both bearing his arms, to be placed "for the memory of the testator and his ancestors" in the chapel of Sant'Agata in the *plebis* church of Arezzo. Further, he gave a bed inscribed with his coat of arms to the Misericordia of Arezzo. Finally, "for the perpetual memory of the testator and his ancestors," the "wise and prudent" Landucius required his heirs to have the family arms painted and carved in stone on the back of his palace in the Contrada di Borgo, where they could be "always seen easily and clearly."[132] Another Aretine, the merchant Lazarus f.q. Johannis Bracci, whose decorative program for the major altar of San Francesco we have already considered, ordered his arms and insignia displayed in at least five sacred places: in the stained-glass windows of the major chapel of San Francesco; on the altar's banner or screen (*palio*); and on the priest's vestments, the chasuble (*planeta*), the *cotta*,[133] and the *piviale,* a sumptuous liturgical cope worn only on the most solemn occasions.[134]

But the Florentine Augustinus f.q. Francesci Ser Johannis perhaps went farthest in his zeal for emblazoning the symbols of family pride in sacred places. In 1417, "to conserve and maintain for ever his memory," he ordered perpetual masses and divine offices to be celebrated and his arms displayed in the chapel of Santa Lucia, located near the door to the sacristy of the Augustinian church of Santo Spirito. He further demanded that "no other flags, plaques or other insignia" be placed next to this chapel or in the space leading from it to the church's organ. He further paid 100 florins to commission a stained-glass window for his chapel and ordered his arms placed in two other places in the chapel "so that they could readily be seen by all." Finally, he bequeathed yet another 100 florins to finish construction on the sacristy in the friary church of Santa Maria della Campora and to build a wardrobe (*armarium*) in it. "For the perpetual memory of the testator and his predecessors," he demanded that the friars use these funds to place the arms of the testator carved (*intagliata*) in marble of sacred stone (*in marmo sacre pietre*) at the principal door to the sacristy and "to conserve [them] for ever," in order, he repeated, "to be present and apparent in perpetuity."[135]

Sculpture

Testamentary commissions for coats of arms stimulated demand for the services of sculptors. Combined with the demand for tombstone designs and inscriptions (see Chapter 4), they must have provided a major source of employment for these late medieval and Renaissance craftsmen. Among the most remarkable testamentary commissions found in these documents was one by Archbishop Johannes for his reclining effigy to be sculpted above his sarcophagus with bracketed arches and angels in gold and marble, which was executed shortly after his death by the sculptor-goldsmith Nino Pisano. Less famous or intricate projects for memorializing corpses and preserving emblems of family fame must have been the stock in trade of a great number of sculptors' workshops, just as Ugo Procacci has shown flags and banners to have been standard productions even in important artists' workshops in early Quattrocento Florence.[136]

Marble and stone, moreover, were not the only media in which testators desired sculpted figures. I have already referred to sculpted figures or "images" made of wax, which constituted perhaps the cheapest and most ephemeral art commissioned in these testaments—20 soldi for figures of women to be presented to the Virgin of Orsanmichele,[137] or one florin for a wax "ymagine" to be placed in the Assisan church of Santa Maria degli Angeli.[138] But, as Aby Warburg has shown for the High Renaissance, wax figures constituted a major art form that could draw considerable funds. As Franco Sacchetti's story of the man who promised the Virgin of Orsanmichele a wax image of his lost cat suggests,[139] these traditions certainly antedated the evidence Warburg culled for the famous collection once housed in the Florentine Servite church of Santissima Annunziata.[140] In 1374, a daughter of a cobbler and the widow of a citizen of Arezzo, domina Ysabetta, had her heirs sell a four-*starii* strip of land to finance sculpting a child (presumably the infant Jesus, *in figuram cuisdam pueri*) out of 15 pounds of wax, to be offered to the blessed Annunciation; a similar sculpture from 12 pounds of wax, to be offered to the church of San Bartolomeo; and yet another of the same weight, for the church of San Iacopo.[141] More extraordinary and costly was the wax sculpture ordered by a Pisan merchant, who in 1286 paid 160 lire for a votive figure of himself in wax (*unam imaginem hominis de cera quam ex voto a me facto*), to be placed in a rural church near Marseilles: this constituted one of the earliest and most expensive commissions found in these documents, outstripping even that which the greatest artisans (Cimabue and Duccio) could demand at the end of the Duecento.[142]

Sculpted figures in other media make only a scant appearance in the wills, despite such renowned traditions as the marble figures, bas-reliefs, and elegant painted wooden devotional figures from Duecento and Trecento Pisa and Siena.[143] Except for the reclining effigy of Archbishop Johannes, only three references to statues appear, and two of them come from the same testator. The Aretine wool manufacturer (*lanifex*) Sinus f.q. Pamei gave 10 florins to be converted into clothing (*vestibus*) for the sculpted figure of the Virgin Mary existing in the oratory of his confraternity, the *disciplinati* of Santa Croce. In the absence of surviving sons, he left the altar of Santa Maria in the church of Santa Maria in Gradibus as his universal heir on condition that the clerics have a ciborium built for it. The *lanifex* then made one of the most remarkable and egoistic commissions found in these testaments: he requested that not the Virgin Mary nor any saint but instead "the figure of this testator be made and sculpted" for the altar and chapel (i.e., the one of the flagellants at Santa Maria in Gradibus).[144]

Less egocentric but just as remarkable was an earlier commission for a sculpted roadside shrine. In 1343, the Florentine Andrea f.q. Ugolini, who doubled as a tavernkeeper and gravedigger, bequeathed two pieces of landed property measuring 30 *starii* in the suburban parish of Santa Maria at Novoli "for the poor and abandoned [*pauperibus et piectis seu gittatis*]" of the Florentine hospital Santa Maria della Scala on condition that it never alienate the bequest. The hospital's rector, moreover, was to distribute once a year to the friars at Santa Maria Novella 2 *starii* of "well-baked" bread and one barrel of "good and pure" wine from the "fruits" of this property. Finally, the gravedigger-tavernkeeper ordered the rector to have built within one year, not in any ecclesiastical building but on the field he had bequeathed to the hospital "[*in dicto et super dicto Campo seu terra*], next to the road, a walled column [*unum pilastrum muratum*] with stones, bricks, and limestone" that would stand "at least six *bracchii* above the ground" (about 15 feet high) and would contain a plaque with "the image of the blessed and Ever Virgin Mary with her child in her arms" and the insignia of the hospital of Santa Maria della Scala.[145]

Restoration and Repair

Testators did not necessarily initiate new creations to preserve their earthly memories; they occasionally used their pious sums to restore and repair existing ecclesiastical structures and works of art. These efforts at restoration, though few in number (16), corroborate once again the same patterns of geography and change over time plotted by the other testamentary commissions. Over 70 percent (11) of the restorations came with the second strike of pestilence or afterward, and less than 20 percent (3) originated in the three cities where the mendicant ideals of humility were most pronounced—Assisi, Pisa, and Siena. This time, the Perugini led the list (6 restorations), followed by the Aretini (5) and the Florentines (2).

The earliest of these concerns with conserving existing structures came from Perugia. In 1315, Paulutius f.q. Boncagni gave the Augustinian friars up to 200 lire to remove a wall that separated the chapel of Saints Catherine and Simeon from the choir of the friary.[146] Indeed, the majority of these restoration projects involved architectural renovations. With the return of pestilence in 1363, a Florentine gave the country church of Sant'Andrea de Doccia 50 lire to repair (*pro reattando*) "that part of the church which is destroyed and which lies in front of the altar."[147] In 1387, the Perugian Nicholaus f.q. Marini Bartholi spelled out his architectural improvements more precisely. He gave a portion of his residual estate to the Augustinians on condition that they make improvements (*convertatur in acconcimine*) "by raising the roof of [their] church in its entirety through the section that lies above the vault [*infra in partem de super voltam*], and that it be repositioned above the columns [*super pilastres*] . . . by five feet." If the friars failed to carry out these improvements, the funds would go to the hospital delle Voltole.[148] We have already learned of the desired actions of the widow of the Perugian druggist who in 1390 left 200 florins to restore (*reattare*) a wall near the choir and next to the chapel of Saint Julian in the church of the Servites to make way for the construction of her own chapel. In 1393, the Aretine silk manufacturer Marcus f.q. Angeli gave his confraternity, the *disciplinati* of Saint John the Baptist, 100 lire "to build and to repair" the walls of its hospital.[149]

The largest of these projects came from a Florentine citizen, the "dignetus vir" Bartolus f.q. Bartoli ser Johannis, who left landed properties to rebuild (*reficiatur et reconstruatur*) the church of San Martino de Colle in the *contado* of Pistoia.[150] To raise additional funds for this project he used his will as the instrument for initiating the campaign fund to solicit contributions (*in auxilium construtionis*) from the "men of this parish . . . in whatever amount they pleased and found fitting."[151] Many others, such as Feus f.q. Quaglie, from Santa Maria de Pupigliano in the district of Florence, who in the plague year of 1363 bequeathed a mere florin to repair the roof of his parish church (*in subsidium reparationem tecti*), sought to provide funds communally for repair and preservation of their local churches.[152]

Architectural renovations were not, however, the only restoration projects found in these documents. In 1372 the Aretine citizen and nobleman Michelucius f.q. Pucci domini Michaelis left whatever expenses would be necessary to repair (*reparatur*) in his parish church of Sant'Andrea the crucifix, "which was broken and separated from the body." The expenses were to cover the costs of "attaching it to the body [*applicatur corpori*], painting it seemly [*ut decet*], and placing it on the wood where it ought to remain."[153] At the beginning of 1400, domina Angelina, widow of a Perugian citizen from the village of Ascagnano, left the church of San Gregorio funds to renovate (*renoveatur*) "the figures" (presumably painted) that lay above the tomb of her relatives and to protect them by making a cover.[154]

As the last example suggests, renovations might as easily as commissions for new art be intended to beautify and conserve objects for personal and familial remembrance. In 1409 the Pisan knight Tighus f.q. domini Nini de Upessingis gave the considerable sum of 200 lire for the ornamentation and repair (*pro ornando et reperando*) of "my altar" of Santa Maria Maddalena in the church of San Francesco.[155] But an Aretine, Pierozius, son of the notary Federigi, went the farthest in attaching a repair job to his earthly memory. In his 1374 will, he gave 10 florins to repair the roof of the church of Saints Cosmas and Damian. For this charity, he demanded, however, that his name be inscribed in one of the beams (*et ponatur inscribatur in ligno tetti nominem dicti testatoris*).[156]

In this chapter, I have traced the connections between the demand for perpetual masses and works of art, from 20-soldi wax figures to the reclining tomb effigy of the Pisan archbishop Johannes sculpted by the renowned goldsmith and sculptor Nino Pisano. Such spiritual services to commemorate the souls of testators and their ancestors were best ensured through the construction of chapels, where increasingly, after the second occurrence of pestilence (at least in three of these cities), testators imposed their wills on their host institutions by determining the rights of election of chaplains as well as their age, conduct, and status. The chapels, in turn, became major receptacles for paintings and various other forms of art and familial regalia commissioned to boost and preserve the earthly memories of testators and their lineages. A wide variety of art—painted beds, wax figures, engraved chalices, stone crests, marble plaques, carved candlestick holders—spilled in and out of these sacred niches of family pride, providing employment for minor craftsmen as well as becoming the stock in trade of more important artists' workshops. To a greater or lesser degree, each of these initiatives, from founding monasteries to emblazoning family insignia in sacred places, embodied the antithesis of the mendicant ideals of humility and self-abnegation in the midst of the eternal glory of God—Catherine of Siena's deep, calm sea of self-annihilation or Domenico Cavalca of Pisa's patience, which defined Christianity in opposition to mundanity.[157] Taken individually or collectively, these testamentary commissions of art and counterpoises to mendicant piety bear out the implications drawn earlier from the statistics on pious giving. The six cities taken as a whole show a shift in the frequency of commissions around the time of the second occurrence of plague in the early 1360s, even as two geographically distinct clusters of cities and their territories arose. While Assisi, Pisa, and Siena were embedded in the habits of mendicant humility, Arezzo, Florence, and Perugia early on sought ways of preserving earthly memory not only for the testators themselves as "Burckhardtian" individuals but for their relatives and ancestors as well. Nor did these means of self- and lineage promotion turn away from matters of the soul by drawing a radical dichotomy between earthly remembrance and preoccupations with the afterlife (as Burckhardt and later Panofsky and Herklotz have surmised). On the contrary, perpetual masses, feast-day celebrations, and commemorative meals for monks and friars increased in frequency after the recurrence of plague, just as did testators' efforts to incorporate sacred space for the founding of private family chapels. All served as instruments for the simultaneous perpetuation of an earthly self and the glorification of one's ancestors and lineage—roads to salvation that the mendicant preachers from the early Spiritualists to Savonarola had attacked and would continue to attack as useless mundanities. To complete my survey of commissions for art *in extremis,* I turn now to a form testators commonly embraced in my samples—paintings.

7

Paintings

When the parish priest Arlotto had patched up the church walls, he wanted
to whitewash them; and to make it all white he first needed to plaster over all
the ugly paintings and to leave some of the others. And going around with
the master mason, examining which figures to leave and which to destroy, the
priest spotted a Saint Anthony and said:
— "Save this one."
Then he found a figure of Saint Sano and said:
— "This one is to be gotten rid of, since as long as I have been the Priest
here I have never seen anyone light a candle in front of it, nor has it ever
seemed to me useful; and therefore, mason, get rid of it."
—*Motti e facezie del Piovano Arlotto*

fter chapels and altars, testamentary commissions for
sacred paintings, both panel paintings (*tabulae*) and wall
paintings (or frescoes), were next in numerical importance. The range covered by sacred paintings includes
altarpieces, tabernacles, panels, and column paintings
that were not altarpieces but were placed elsewhere in
churches and convents.[1] The categories and subcategories of sacred
paintings and their relation to altars, recently emphasized by art historians, were not uppermost in the minds of those commissioning paintings in these documents. The basic distinction instead was one of medium—
wall painting (*pictura*) or panel painting (*tabula*). This was still the essential
distinction drawn by Leon Battista Alberti in *Della pittura*. He makes no
mention of altarpieces as such.[2]

As we have already seen, commissions for paintings often accompanied
the foundation of chapels. Moreover, these sacred enclaves formed the

repositories for which later family members could request new artwork, of which sacred paintings were a major component. Testators, however, did not need to found a chapel or to possess one in the family to order a painting for a local church or monastery. In fact, the vast majority of such commissions were not additions to the decorative schemes of one's own chapel.

Commissions for paintings could originate lower down the social ladder than chapel constructions. Despite the minuscule survival rate of such works, these samples show the intentions and activities of butchers,[3] cobblers,[4] bakers,[5] blacksmiths,[6] and even a gardener or green-grocer (*ortolanus*) as patrons of sacred paintings. In 1371, the Aretine Cione f.q. Cinghii, of the parish of San Matteo, who was not identified by profession, left only four lire to his flagellant confraternity of Santo Spirito to paint the narrative of the company (*convertendos in picture cuiusdam ystorie*), to be placed above the altar in the church of this religious company.[7] Although not specified, this commission was probably for a predella under an existing altarpiece. Nonetheless, it illustrates just how little a testamentary commission for a painting might amount to. In discussing the introduction of panel paintings in thirteenth-century Italy, Hans Belting claimed, "In a small size, produced at a low cost, the intimate panel made paintings accessible to a new public, and did so to a degree that would be surpassed only later by mass-produced prints."[8] The possibility of locating surviving paintings from such commissions is extraordinarily slim. As Wackernagel has shown in his efforts to re-construct the Quattrocento appearance of Santa Maria Novella, even works by masters as prominent as Fra Angelico had low rates of survival. Of this church's Quattrocento paintings, only one survives—the much-hallowed fresco of the Trinity by Masaccio—and even this one was only rediscovered in 1860 behind an altarpiece painted by Giorgio Vasari.[9]

With three exceptions (at least when paintings were priced), com-missions for paintings (whether frescoes or panel paintings) found in these samples did not call for vast contributions. While chapel con-structions cost on average over 208 florins, commissions for sacred paint-ings ran a little over one-seventh that sum (27.11 florins). By far the largest, in fact, was not for the decoration of a private chapel. The citizen and merchant of Florence Torinus f.q. Baldese left 1,000 lire for the painting of the "entire" Old Testament story "from beginning to end" in the church of Santa Maria Novella and named Jacopo Passavanti to determine its program and place in the church.[10] But the other two sizable commissions were decorative programs for private chapels: in

1410, the Aretine merchant Lazarus left 300 florins to the Franciscans for the narrative cycles of the Resurrection of Lazarus and the "story" of Saint Francis receiving the stigmata; and in 1362 Egidius Martini Crescebene, from Perugia, left a total of 250 lire for pictures, his grave, and the beautification of his chapel of Saint Catherine in the church of the Augustinians.[11]

The Geography of Painting

The data on demand for paintings reconfirm the geographical patterns found earlier for pious giving, burials, and attitudes toward property and its descent. Testamentary commissions in Arezzo, Florence, and Perugia were considerably more numerous than in the other three city-states. (See table 15.) As with commissions for all forms of art production, little-studied Arezzo, considered "of dubious artistic renown between the two hotbeds of culture, Florence and Siena,"[12] instead led the list in the sheer number of commissions for paintings, both absolutely and relative to the number of testaments and pious bequests, comprising more than 10 painting commissions for every 1,000 pious bequests. Nor does this extraordinary level of patronage result from a simple bias in the documentation, such as a reliance on the rich archive of the Laici. For Arezzo, unlike any of the other city-states, the preponderance of commissions for paintings as well as for artworks in general derives from the public protocols preserved in notarial archives.[13] Perugia closely followed Arezzo with just under 10 per 1,000, then Florence with almost 7. In terms of the number of pious bequests, the list clearly separates these cities from the other triad: testators in Assisi commissioned paintings only half as often as the Florentines and a little over a third as often as those in neighboring Perugia. While the same percentage of Pisan and Perugian testators commissioned paintings, Pisans commissioned less than a third as many in terms of the number of pious bequests. Finally, Siena was at the bottom of the list: before 1425, only one percent of its testators requested paintings in their testaments, which accounted for under 2 per 1,000 pious gifts.

This paucity of testamentary commissions is remarkable for Siena even within the context of the three cities, where mendicant values of humility and pious giving were the more entrenched. Were there factors at work in this center of late medieval art that go beyond testators' efforts to shun the sins of earthly hubris? One cause may have been Siena's stronger tradition of communal commissions on the part of

Table 15.
Testamentary Commissions for Paintings

Town	No. Commissions	No. Testators	Commissions per Testator	No. Pious Bequests	Commissions per 1,000 Pious Bequests
Arezzo	45	648	0.07	4,219	10.67
Assisi	6	290	0.02	1,737	3.45
Florence	24	581	0.04	3,489	6.88
Perugia	22	524	0.04	2,253	9.76
Pisa	18	737	0.02	6,601	2.73
Siena	6	446	0.01	3,088	1.94
Total	121	3,226	0.04	21,387	5.66

churches, convents, monasteries, friaries, confraternities, and the commune itself. Another reason may have been the Sienese predilection not
to cram numerous frescoes onto a single wall as was the case in Florence
and Arezzo, and, because of its "strong bias for lifelike views," to allot
no more than a single picture to a wall. "Tiered schemes among the
Sienese are exceptional rather than the rule. Among these exceptions
it is significant that those by Simone Martini, Barna, and Bartolo di Fredi
were painted for churches outside Siena—at Assisi and San Gimignano."[14] But, as noted before, accidents of documentary survival and
selection do not account for these differences. Roughly the same patterns
of artistic commissions emerge for these cities when only commissions
found in the public protocols are considered.

Of course, situations other than lying on one's deathbed or contemplating the final distribution of one's property occasioned the commissioning of religious art. The differences in the frequency of these testamentary commissions among the city-states may well have hinged,
moreover, on differences in the traditions of corporate as opposed to
individual patronage. Finally, the act of commissioning a painting certainly involved sentiments that went beyond any Burckhardtian notion
of the individual's desire to leave a lasting mark for posterity. Throughout
this period, paintings, from single figures on small planks of wood to
monumental fresco cycles, possessed iconic values,[15] as illustrated in
stories such as that cited above from the second half of the Quattrocento
(Piovano Arlotto's decision not to whitewash the figure of a saint after

it showed the power still to perform miracles).[16] Yet, art historians Boskovits and Belting have recently argued that a transition was occurring in the intrinsic value of paintings from iconic to aesthetic precisely during the last decades of the Trecento when, as we shall soon observe, a groundswell of testators surged to commission religious paintings.[17] Notwithstanding the psychological variability and complexity involved in the commissioning of any work of religious art, my statistics corroborate geographical patterns similar to those already found for other aspects of pious behavior. As with chapel construction, the plastering of family coats of arms, or the funding of perpetual masses, testamentary commissions of religious paintings divide the six city-states into two triads. But, once again, these obsessions with earthly remembrance were not in conflict with other religious urges or the zeal to influence the hereafter. Let us now look more closely at the patterns cast by time.

Before the Black Death

The demand for painting closely followed the trajectory traced by chapel constructions, whether or not the paintings might be destined for such quasi-private chambers. Just as with chapels, no commissions for paintings appear in the earliest documents. The first commission for a painting found in the wills was for neither a panel painting nor a fresco; moreover, it was stipulated for a Sicilian church by a Sicilian who happened to be residing in Pisa. In 1284, Angelus Spina f.q. Ruggeri Spine, from Scala Burgensis Messane (Messine), ordered an icon (*unam choniam*) for the church of Saint Nicholaus de Monimento in Sicily, made from gold to be bought and painted in Pisa with "the image" of Saint Nicholas.[18] The earliest commission for a panel painting or fresco came from Assisi at the beginning of the Trecento. In 1300, Puccius Venture Ascarani left 60 lire to have an image of Saint Mary painted "next to" the altar of Saint John[19] in the church of San Francesco, "similar to that image next to the altar of Saint Anthony in this church [*ad similitudinem illius ymaginis*]," which bore a cross and an image of Saint Peter.[20]

Again, like testators' demands for chapels and altars, commissions remained at a low ebb through the early Trecento until the outbreak of pestilence in 1348. Fewer than 3 percent commissioned paintings, and only slightly over 2 per 1,000 pious legacies were for paintings. (See table 16.) While fewer than one-fifth of these paintings were commissioned before the Black Death, a third of the testators and half of all pious bequests preceded 1348.

Table 16.
Chronology of Paintings

Period	No. Paintings	No. Testators	No. Pious Bequests	Paintings per Testator	Paintings per 1,000 Pious Bequests
< 1276	0	83	629	0.00	0.00
1276–1300	3	155	1,728	0.02	1.74
1301–25	11	419	5,044	0.03	2.18
1326–47	10	404	3,298	0.02	3.03
1348	18	323	2,149	0.06	8.38
1349–62	10	223	1,596	0.04	6.27
1363	13	230	1,442	0.06	9.02
1364–75	20	304	1,438	0.07	13.91
1376–1400	16	582	2,312	0.03	6.92
1401–25	20	503	1,715	0.04	11.66
Total	121	3,226	21,351	0.04	5.67

The pre–Black Death commissions, moreover, were less detailed and precise than the demands testators would later impose on their holy beneficiaries. Not a single narrative painting was demanded,[21] and only two commissions called for the painting of the donor or one's relatives. Little attention has been paid to the portraiture of these donor figures in the Trecento. In his famous essay on portraiture, Aby Warburg jumps in one paragraph from Giotto's depiction of the kneeling donors in the Bardi chapel frescoes to Francesco Sassetti's commission to Ghirlandaio in Santa Trinità, circa 160 years later.[22] More recently, Enrico Castelnuovo has added only the work of Simone Martini in Avignon to the description of Giotto's donor portraits before more fully discussing examples of the second half of the Quattrocento.[23] Other recent works similarly concentrate on the fifteenth and sixteenth centuries.[24]

The earliest example in my samples came in 1315 once again from a Pisan; yet again, that Pisan was a recent émigré, this time from the north. The German (*theotonicus*) Guarnerius f.q. Borlandi, from the city of Liège (*Leggi*), a mercenary of the Pisan commune (*ad servitium et soldatum Pisis comunis*), ordered a painting of "a beautiful and good image and figure of Our Lord Jesus Christ, the glorious and ever Virgin Mary his Mother and other Saints of God" for the church of the hospital of Saint Clare, to be chosen by his executor, the prior of the hospital. He then required that the painting show him genuflecting (*et mei ipsius existentis*

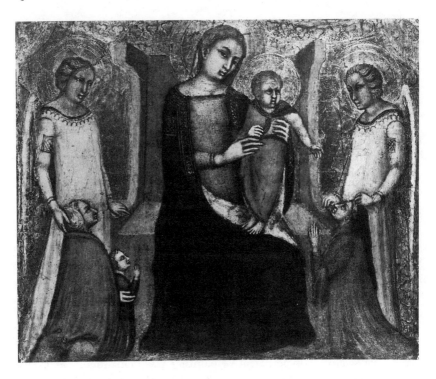

4. Guiduccio Palmerucci, *Madonna and Child between Two Angels Adored by a Donor, His Wife, and Child* (Courtesy Samuel H. Kress Collection, k 1742, University of Kansas, Lawrence, Kansas).

genuflexi in ea).[25] The other example similarly came from the district of Pisa, but once again not from a Pisan native. Gadduccius f.q. Beneciveni, from the commune of San Piero ad Maccadium (Macadio) in the Valdiserchi, north of Pisa, was less precise than the German mercenary. In his testament of 1334, he left 12 lire "for making" a panel painting including "his figure" that would be placed at the altar of the church of San Piero ad Maccadium.[26]

As far as I know, art historians have not observed changes in the language of contracts before the Quattrocento.[27] Nevertheless, earlier shifts can be detected in the testaments I studied. For the most part, testamentary patrons before 1348 were less precise and less demanding than those after the plague, although the German mercenary stationed in Pisa was an exception. Five of the 24 pre–Black Death commissions for painting failed to specify their subject matter altogether. For example,

in 1334 a Sienese woman asked only "to have a panel [*una tabola*]
honorably painted,"[28] and the Aretine Taddeus f.q. Ser Iacopi de Baronani
requested that the space above his sepulcher (*ulivellum*) be beautified and
painted (*reattetur et depingantur*). Taddeus left 25 lire for this purpose.[29]

When testators before the Black Death did specify a subject, their
instructions were less detailed than afterward. Ten of these 24 commissions simply called for the depiction of the Virgin Mary, mentioning
no saints or other figures. Such was the request of domina Bonina, widow
of a Florentine cabinet maker (*capsectarii*), who left a mere 3 lire in 1300
for a panel painting of the blessed Virgin Mary to be put on permanent
display (*ponendam et permansuram*) in the cathedral of Florence.[30] In 1331,
the Perugian villager Martinus Bernardi, from Villa Plancarpinis, left 10
lire to have a *"magesta"* painted in the parish church of San Giovanni.[31]
Of course, this vague designation might have included more figures than
simply the Virgin enthroned, as another Perugian commission in 1345
makes clear. The *Magister* Cinus Bernardi Sinibaldi, from the parish of
San Cristoforo, left the same modest sum of 10 lire for a *"maiesta"* in
the country parish of San Biagio in Monte Pacini for a painting to include
"Our Lord Jesus Christ, the Virgin Mary and the blessed John."[32]

Orders to depict saints or blessed ones further evince the simplicity
and lack of specificity of pre-plague requests for paintings. Of the eight
pre-plague commissions that asked for saints, four called for only one
saint—San Giovanni in a 1327 testament from Florence,[33] Santa Zita in
a panel painting commissioned by another Florentine in 1347,[34] the Pisan
icon of San Niccolò of 1285, and an Aretine commission in 1321 for
Santa Barbara.[35] In no pre-plague request did a testator specify more
than two saints. In terms of the number of figures desired, the 40-soldi
icon (*una ycona*) commissioned by the Pisan villager Martinus f.q. Gual-
fredi, from Vecchiano Maioris—one of the cheapest works of art to be
found in these documents—may have been the most complex of the
pre-plague commissions. Martinus asked that his sons have the icon
made for the altar of San Martino in the church of Sant'Alessandro in
the village of Vecchiano and that it include the images of Saints Mary,
Peter, and John.[36] Of course, the actual paintings once executed may
have been much different, filled with other figures desired by the ecclesiastical hosts or the testator's executors, and vague requests such as
that of the Perugian villager domina Druda f.q. Gili Peruti, from Villa
Planicarpinis, allowed such choices. In 1332, before embarking on a
pilgrimage to the city of Rome, Druda left a testament that ordered the
figure of the Virgin Mary painted with an indeterminate number of figures.

Mary was to be accompanied "with Angels" and the painting placed in her parish church.[37]

The point nonetheless remains: testators in their commissions, as in their other legacies, were less specific and less demanding before the Black Death; they left more to the discretion and freedom of their heirs, executors, and spiritual beneficiaries. Before 1348, not a single commission specified the positions of the figures to be painted. With two exceptions, testators' instructions to executors did not even reach beyond the occasional nearly formulaic adjectives and the adverbial phrase—to make or paint the images with *pulcritudinem et honorabiliter.* The exceptions were Puccius Venture Ascarani, from Assisi, who asked that his Mary be executed "in the likeness" of "that image" above the altar of Sant'Antonio in the Sacro Convento of Assisi,[38] and the Aretine widow domina Iacopa, who desired only that her paintings—one of the Virgin Mary with John the Evangelist and Michael, the other of Saint Barbara—be beautiful and painted with lively faces (*sint pulcre et vive facce*).[39]

1348

Again, like chapel constructions, commissions for paintings during the year of the plague's first strike more than doubled what they had been in the previous quarter-century, from 3 for every 1,000 pious bequests to over 8, and the percentage of testators commissioning paintings jumped from 2 to 6. (See table 16.) The change in mentality suggested by this abrupt change in the statistics did not, however, strike the six cities equally. Of the 18 commissions for paintings found in these Black Death testaments, the bulk came from Florence and Arezzo as against only one each for Pisa, Assisi, and Siena. For these three towns, moreover, the content of the commissions showed no fundamental changes from the earliest commissions through the period of the Black Death. While the 1348 documents from Siena and Pisa listed more saints than did any previous requests for paintings, no testator there attempted to guide the artist's hand by directing where these figures should be placed in the composition. The Sienese lady Francesca f.q. Andrecci left 9 lire for the rector of her parish of San Donato simply to have painted for the church the figures of the Saints John, Christopher, Francis, and Catherine, along with the Virgin.[40] In the Pisan documents, again, not a resident of the city proper but an outsider, Maglata f.q. Lamberti Magliate, from the village of Vico, commissioned a panel painting "to be ornamented" with the Virgin Mary with child, John the Baptist, Peter, Andrew, and Francis to adorn his newly built altar in the *plebis* church of this Pisan market town.[41] The 1348 bequest of the Assisan Putius Lelli did not even specify the subject matter for his paintings but simply left the confraternity of Sant'Antonio between one florin and 10 lire "for pictures or wax."[42]

In contrast, the first narrative painting in these samples came from Florence in the year of the Black Death: the 1,000-lire Old Testament cycle "from beginning to end." And Aretine testators were the first to position their requested figures themselves. Cecchus f.q. Raneroli, from the village of Citerna, ordered a painting to be placed above his sepulcher showing the blessed Virgin Mary with her child on the right and Saints John and Christopher on the left.[43] The citizen of Arezzo residing in Bibbiena, Pasquinus f.q. Montagne, son of a blacksmith or stable master, was more demanding: he devoted the major part of his testament to describing the painting he projected for the friars of the blessed Virgin Mary in this mountain market town. He left landed property for "the major church" of this monastery to have the Virgin painted "with her child in her arms" with Saint John the Evangelist on one side and "Saint" Mary Magdalene and Saint Anthony on the other. He ordered, moreover, that these figures be so labeled (*cum litteris continentibus sic*) and that "an image of the person, Pasquinus f.q. Montagne, its donor [*eius donementum*]" be painted on one side of the Virgin and, "on the other side," his deceased father, Montagne, kneeling. Finally, he directed the future painter to label these two figures *a capite:* "Hic est Montagne Mareschalchus; hic est Pasquinus Montagne."[44]

The blacksmith's son was not the only Aretine testator in 1348 to order himself painted in saintly company. The village notary Ser Donato f.q. Mucii Ser Fei, from Boschetta, ordered a painting of the "blessed Virgin Mary with her child" to be placed above the grave of his ancestors in the Dominican church of Arezzo. At the foot (*ad pedem*) of the Virgin he further ordered "the images of the above-mentioned testator and his brother" the deceased Cione in the act of praying.[45] More remarkable was the commission of the mercenary residing in Arezzo, who appears straight from the pages of Jacob Burckhardt. After leaving all his armor to the Misericordia except his helmet, which was to serve as his memorial "signature" for his tomb in the Servite church, Raynierus from Monte Feyche in the diocese of Liège gave 25 florins to his native parish of Sant'Antonio not for an altarpiece of the Madonna or a patron saint but simply "to have painted in this church the person of this testator [*de persone dictis testatoris et occasione picture sue persone*]."[46]

With the onslaught of pestilence in 1348, testators from Perugia,

Arezzo, and Florence began to fill their frescoes and panel paintings with greater numbers of designated figures. While only one-fourth of the commissions before the Black Death (18 of 24) called for more than a single figure to be painted and none for more than three, in 1348 more than half specified more than a single figure, and most were for more than three figures. As we have seen, the Sienese Francesca demanded four figures; Maglata from Vico, six figures; Pasquino the Blacksmith's son, seven. Similarly, the Perugian Nutius Cioli specified more fully than previous testators the figures to appear in his *maestate* that he ordered painted on the wall (*in illo muro et pariete*) above his sepulcher in the Benedictine church of San Pietro. It was to include "the figure of Our Lord Jesus Christ crucified, his mother, the Glorious Virgin Mary, and the figures of Saint John and Saint Constance."[47] The Aretine Filippus f.q. Gori Ronami contributed six florins to have five figures painted in the Opera of the *plebis* church of Santa Maria: "Our Lord Jesus Christ, the blessed Virgin Mary," and the figures of John the Baptist, John the Evangelist, and Saint Catherine the Virgin.[48] Others asked for fewer figures: for example, the Aretine domina Vanna, the widow of Martinozzi, specified only two figures in a commission for a painting to appear in the church of Santa Maria in Gradibus, but asserted herself as forcefully as those who demanded that more saints appear in specific positions. Instead of the standard fare of the Virgin Mary with her child or the Saints John and Peter, she stipulated that the less common blessed Smiraldus and San Marcellus be depicted.[49]

After the Black Death

In the interval separating the first strikes of pestilence, 1349 to 1362, the number of commissions fell slightly to around 6 paintings per 1,000 pious bequests and to 4 percent of all testators. Along with this fall in commissions came a decline in the specificity of the testators' requests for subjects and figures. Half of the commissions found in the interval between the plagues did not indicate subjects for their paintings. These testators made loose and open-ended demands *pro picturis et aliis ornamentis fiendis,* similar to the 1360 request of Vangnutius f.q. Francesci, of Assisi.[50] Of those who named figures, none named more than a single one, let alone ventured to arrange the placement of figures.[51]

The recurrence of pestilence in 1362–63 led to an abrupt change, in which the trend initiated by the Black Death continued with renewed vigor: the second time around, the number of commissions jumped

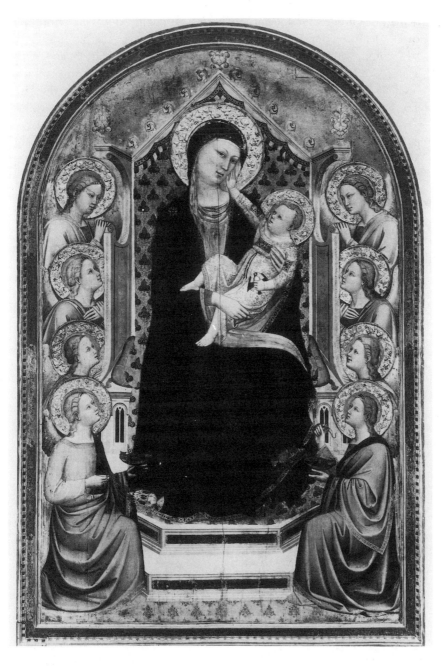

5. Bernardo Daddi, *Madonna and Eight Angels* (Courtesy Soprintendenza alle galerie-Firenze, no. 26997).

beyond the 1348 mark to 9 per 1,000, and testators concretized their demands with greater specificity, detail, and complexity than before the Black Death or during the intervening years between the plagues. Only two commissions failed to specify figures or subject matter; and once again, a narrative scene appears. It pertained, however, only to the predella, which commonly expressed the stories of saints by the late Trecento.[52] The Florentine Francescus f.q. Pieri Noldi de Gherardinis gave funds to the church of San Lorenzo at Cortina to buy a panel painting containing the "images or pictures" of the Glorious Virgin Mary, San Lorenzo, and Santo Stefano, with the "storia" of Saint Francis "in the predella under this panel."[53]

In the years of social and economic dislocation, 1364 to 1375, when several art historians have assumed that demand for art after the plague plummeted,[54] retreated to retrograde workshops in the provinces,[55] or even disappeared completely,[56] demand as revealed by this testamentary documentation runs in the opposite direction. Parallel to demand for new chapel constructions, testamentary requests for paintings reached their apogee in these years. Over 7 percent of the testators ordered paintings to adorn the walls above their tombs, their chapels, or other ecclesiastical buildings on which they wished to leave their mark; they commissioned 14 paintings per 1,000 pious legacies, over five times the rate before the Black Death. This increase, however, was not uniform for the six cities under investigation. The bulk of it came from Arezzo and Florence.

More than ever before, testators concretized their demands with specific figures to fill their surfaces. Instead of naming a single figure and leaving his or her heirs, executors, or the artist to select the background saints, testators of the 1360s and 70s often crowded their frescoes and panels with numbers of figures. This demand by patrons for numerous and specific figures of devotion may have led to the problems of "compressed" space in paintings of the third quarter of the Trecento and to what Meiss has called "the most inflexible and schematic assembly of figures in the history of Tuscan art."[57] In 1374, the Sienese Sinus f.q. Lenzi Compagni ordered his heirs "to construct, build and make" in the Augustinian church of Asciano, above the altar on the side of the campanile, "a predella sufficiently and honorably ornamented and depicted" with the figures of the blessed apostles Peter and Paul and Jacob and the patron saint of Siena, Ansanus.[58] To fulfill this demand, he left the modest sum of 10 lire.[59] In 1368, the Perugian Nicholaus Martini Lelli ordered for his parish church of San Severio a painting of "Our

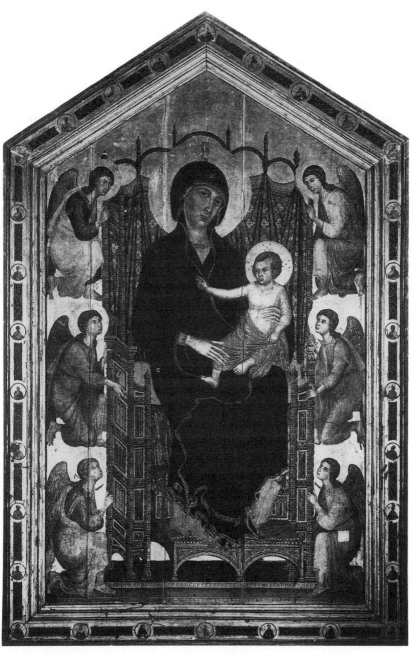

6. *Madonna col Bambino e gli angeli Gabriele e Raffaele.* Florentine school, 15th century. San Lorenzo a Cortine (Barberino Valdelsa).

Lady, the Virgin Mary with her child" and the blessed Antonio, Santa
Lucia, and even the early Irish martyred virgin, Santa Cannera.[60]

The commission of the Florentine patrician-rector and "intimate
friend of Petrarca," Dominus Niccholaus de Benucciis, was more complex. Like those in the year of the Black Death, he entered the frame
of his commission, directing where his chosen figures should appear. He
left 20 florins in 1371 for "an honorable panel" for the altar founded
through his will "named the chapel of the blessed martyrs Valerianus
and Tibertius" in the church of Santa Cecilia. The central figure to be
"depicted" was the Virgin Mary "in the middle," to be flanked by figures
of the blessed Cecilia and Valerianus on one side and the blessed Bartolommeo and Tiburtius on the other.[61]

Even when testators did not specify a number of figures to crowd the
frame of their commissions, they made other demands which went
beyond the laconic testamentary requests preceding the Black Death.
For instance, the Perugian from the neighboring village of Castro Corciano, Martinus Fortis Johannis, "for the reverence and praise of the
most glorious blessed Virgin Mary and for his own and his ancestors'
souls," left 6 florins "for the making of the figure of the most blessed
Virgin Mary with her child," to be "covered and well ornamented,"
above his sepulcher in the wall of this church in Corciano.[62] In 1372
the Aretine citizen Marianus olim Cole, from Celaria (Cegliuolo), left
50 florins to complete a chapel he had founded in the new Augustinian
friary of Arezzo. The monies were for furnishings—a chalice, a chasuble,
a missal, wax, and other necessities, including a wall painting in which
only one figure was specified, that of his patron, Saint Jacob; the testator,
however, insisted that the figure bear its title under the painting.[63]

We know, moreover, from Vasari's description of the now lost fresco
cycle in the Aretine house of Sant'Agostino,[64] that the actual painting
was in fact rich in detail relating to the personal sins, fears, and obsessions
of the testator, who was faced with the realities of his commercial and
contractual milieu. According to Vasari, "Berna" painted "with great
vivacity the affects of the soul" and particularly those in the face of
Marianus, whom Vasari describes as a swindler or moneychanger (barattiere) by trade. Driven by "his lust for money," the testator was,
according to Vasari, depicted giving to a devil "ugly beyond belief" a
contract written out in the testator's own hand, which the devil held
on to and showed to the "throngs of the world." The testator, Vasari
tells us, beseeches his patron, Saint Jacob, to "liberate him" from this

PAINTINGS

promissory note, which the saint succeeds in doing only after Marianus has been led to repent for his sins at this, his final moment of life.[65]

Despite the rhetorical character of Vasari's descriptions (*ekphrasis*)[66] and depictions of usury as a topos in late medieval fresco cycles, the scene described by Vasari was not the standard iconography for usury, which usually portrayed money and moneybags in the company of the other sins and vices and not as here with the devil taunting the sinner with a written contract.[67] In addition, the specificity of Marianus's sin and the guilt aroused by the quotidian acts of his business find traces in his will. While Marianus's profession may not have been stated in his testament, it is clear that he loaned money at usurious rates and felt the pains of guilt from this activity while drafting his will. In the third of only three pious legacies, he left 200 lire to be distributed by his executors to those persons whom he had swindled "through illicit and evil extortion." If the injured persons could not be found, then "for the health of his soul" the monies were to provide dowries for marrying girls or placing them in nunneries.[68] While phrases such as *pro male ablatis* and *pro illicitis et male extortis* had commonly appeared in pious legacies in the late Duecento and the early years of the Trecento, such phraseology (and its underlying motivations) had become rare by the time this will was redacted.[69]

These testators of the 1360s and 1370s, moreover, did not opt for the stock figures current in pre-plague commissions—the Virgin Mary, John the Evangelist, John the Baptist, and Peter. In addition to the above-mentioned blessed Anthony, Jacob, Lucy, the Irish Virgin Saint Cannera, Bartholomew, and the ancient martyred saints Valerianus and Tibertus, the Aretine Masius f.q. Francisci, from the village of Frongola, in his testament of 1374 commissioned a painting of Sant'Urbano for his chapel of the blessed Fumaxio (Sonnazio?) to be built in the Aretine church of San Francesco.[70] In that same year another Aretine citizen, Francescus Pieri Francesci, ordered a painting of the figure of San Leonardo for the Aretine parish church of San Michele,[71] and Cicchus Petrutii Marchuti left 10 lire to have the figure of Sanctus Blaxius Benedictus painted in the church of San Matteo at the Franciscan hermitage of Monte Subàsio.[72]

But the testators of the 1360s and 1370s left their mark and memory even more indelibly by demanding that images of themselves be placed within the frames structured by their chosen sacred figures. The Florentine domina Gemma, daughter of the deceased Fei domini Taddei, of the della Tosa family, and widow of domini Simoni de Soli, ordered a painting of "the images and figures" of the Our Lady, the blessed Ever Virginal Mary, the blessed Catherine, and San Pietro Murrone for the chapel founded by her late husband in the Dominican church of San Pietro Murrone. She demanded that a painting of her own figure appear underneath and left 12 florins for the lot.[73] In 1374, the Aretine doctor of both laws, Dominus Francescus Johannis de Acceptantibus, ordered a *Maiestà* of the Virgin with the figure of the blessed Urban "at the foot of the garden, that is, next to the Aretine church of Santa Trinità." In addition, an image of the doctor's very "likeness" (*cum ymagine sua*) was to be painted "at their feet."[74] In the same year of the plague's third return, another Aretine citizen, Pierozius f.q. Ser Federigi, commissioned for the Aretine church of the Murello the Annunciation of the blessed Mary with his coat of arms and the figure of himself at her feet.[75]

Finally, testators of the 1360s and early 1370s went beyond the simple portrayal of individual figures, commissioning two narrative programs. Again, the Aretine doctor of both laws emerges. For his burial chapel with sculpted coat of arms, which he founded next to the baptismal font in the *plebis* church of Santa Maria and which he named San Francesco, the doctor-lawyer commissioned the painting of "the image of the blessed Francis when he received the Stigmata from Our Lord Jesus Christ," along with the "Storia" of the blessed Francis.[76] In September of the following year, the lawyer's executor and heir, the Misericordia of Arezzo, commissioned the Aretine painter Spinello to carry out the testator's last wishes, further specifying that the figure of Saint Francis receiving the stigmata appear in the rear of the chapel (*in facie anteriori*); the "majestic" figure of Santa Maria de Misericordia, on the side toward the door; and, on the other side, the blessed Anthony. On the upper portion of the chapel (*in parte superiori*) Spinello was to paint four stories of the blessed Francis "as he wished to conceive it." He was to paint the Passion of Christ "well and respectfully," "with good colors," and the crowns of the saints were to be ornamented with gold. On the lower portions he was to paint the four evangelists "with good and fine colors"; on the wall near the baptismal font, Saint John baptizing Christ. Finally, Spinello was to paint yet another story of his own choosing (*pro ut volet concipere*). For these paintings the Misericordia offered him 55 florins. By 1401, these paintings had not yet been executed; the Misericordia repeated its desires, this time offering Spinello 30 florins. Whether these fresco cycles were executed is difficult to know; no traces survive after the 1401 repeat commission.[77] In 1371, another Aretine, though not of such exalted status, the gardener or greengrocer (*ortolanus*) Cione f.q. Cinghi, from the parish of San Maffeo, gave his confraternity, the *disciplinati* of Santo Spirito, four lire to paint (*convertendos in picturis*) the narrative (*ystorie*) of the Holy Ghost, to be placed above the altar of the confraternity.[78] Given its price—one of the lowest found for any painting, for any surface, and at any time in this documentation—this commission was most likely one for an altarpiece's predella. These two commissions for narrative cycles were the exceptions. Until the last years of the period of my analysis (the early Quattrocento), narrative cycles remained rare in all these city-states.[79]

Painting in the Late Trecento and Early Quattrocento

In the last decades of the Trecento, the number of testamentary commissions for sacred paintings declined by half, whether measured as a ratio of pious bequests (fewer than 7 paintings per 1,000) or as that of testators (3 percent). By the latter measure, the rate of commissioning fell to levels comparable to those before the Black Death. Although the share of commissions for paintings in pious bequests rebounded in the early Quattrocento (11.66 per 1,000 pious bequests, the second highest figure found for these data), the last 25 years of my analysis show no substantial change in per capita demand from the last years of the Trecento: only 4 percent of testators commissioned paintings. In Arezzo and Florence—quantitatively the vanguard of artistic demand in the 1360s and 1370s—the decline was even more accentuated. In the years following the second onslaught of pestilence, 1364–75, 9 percent of testators both in Florence and in Arezzo commissioned paintings. In the years 1376 to 1425, demand in Arezzo slipped to 5 percent, while in Florence demand fell even further, to 2 percent of all testators on the eve of the emergence of "the three crowns" of early Renaissance art—Donatello, Masaccio, and Brunelleschi.[80]

In the meantime, Pisa and Perugia appear to have had delayed responses to the societal impulses that touched Arezzo and Florence in the previous generation following the recurrence of pestilence in 1363. In the last 50 years of this analysis, more testamentary commissions (12) derive from the records of Perugia than anywhere else. In Pisa the increase from the period after the second strike of pestilence through the early Quattrocento was even more dramatic. From a complete absence of testamentary commissions in the years 1363–75, Pisans demanded in absolute terms the third highest number of paintings for any city in any time frame, and relative to the number of pious legacies, only Arezzo surpassed Pisa (13.33 paintings per 1,000 pious legacies, as opposed to 11.78—an insignificant difference). These numbers, moreover, fail to reveal another change in the Pisan demand for sacred art. Of the nine commissions found before 1375, only three projected paintings for churches within the city walls and only two patrons were native Pisans, the others coming from neighboring villages of the Pisan *contado* or from as far away as Messina to the south and Liège to the north. In contrast, of the eight testamentary commissions made after 1375, only two were by outsiders to Pisa—one came from the nearby Arno village of Navacchio, the other from Massa—and only two of the paintings were destined for churches beyond the city walls of Pisa: one for San Iacopo in Navacchio, the other for Santa Maria in the village of Lari.

With the overall decline in testators' demands for sacred paintings to levels reminiscent of the period preceding the Black Death, did these commissions likewise resume the more open-ended and loose character of their predecessors? In several respects, this seems to have been the case. More than one-fifth of the commissions after 1375 (8 of 36) failed to specify the subject matter, and few listed more than two figures. The exceptions derive almost exclusively from Perugia. In her testament of 1383, the lady Vannutia f.q. Andrutii, wife of Venture Pietri Tiberti, required her executors to have painted "the figure of the blessed Virgin Mary with her child, Our Lord Jesus Christ, in her arms and the figures of Joseph" along with saints Mary Magdalene, Bartholomew, Catherine, and Margaret.[81] In 1425, another Perugian lady, this time from the nobility, domina Gregoria f.q. Ugolini de Gratinis, left "that quantity of money which her *fideicommissari* would find fitting" to have five figures painted in the burial chapel constructed by her father, namely the Nativity of the blessed Virgin Mary with a crucifix, Saint Christopher, Saint Margaret, the blessed Lawrence, and Saint Ann.[82]

Unlike these two ladies and testators more generally from the 1360s and 70s, by the last decades of the Trecento, those desiring more figures often left more discretion to their heirs and executors or to the artist. The Florentine Bartolommeo f.q. Bati Gregori left 20 florins to have a panel painting made within one year of his death for the major altar of the rural parish of Santa Maria de la Mole in Gangalandi "in which," he vaguely stipulated, "many saints should be painted et cetera." Obviously, this commission was uppermost in Bartolommeo's mind. He ended his testament by repeating it, adding that if his heirs failed to carry it out, their inheritance, along with its obligations, would pass to

the Florentine hospital of Santa Maria della Scala.[83] In 1392, the Pisan
domina Tana, widow of the lord and knight Grinnzelli Buzacchinacci,
of the patrician Sismundi family, and the daughter of the former Guidonis
de Braccis, left 40 florins for "a beautiful and well ornamented panel"
for the altar of San Biagio, which she had endowed in the Pisan church
of Santa Cecilia. The painting was to include the patron of the chapel,
San Biagio, and "other saints," which she failed to name.[84]

Another Pisan, the furrier and son of a furrier Pierus f.q. Iani del
Magrino, ordered his heirs to have his sarcophagus painted; it was to
stand above his ancestors' sepulcher, located in the first cloister of the
monastery of San Michele in Borgo. The artist was instructed to depict
"Our Lord, Jesus Christ, crucified with two saints, that is, one on each
side of this figure of the crucifixion." The furrier did not, however, say
which saints.[85] At that, he was one of the few in these records after
1375 to direct the arrangement of figures in a painting.

Yet, testators of these last 50 years of my analysis did not simply
revert to the traditions and tastes of the pre-plague period. While their
commissions may indeed have been less cluttered with figures than the
testamentary commissions of the 1360s and 1370s, the figures they chose
were not the common fare of the pre-plague period. In addition to the
plague saints, Anthony Abbot, and San Biagio, mentioned above, testamentary patrons demanded the presence of Saint Lazarus, Saint Urban,
Saint (sic) Nicholas of Tolentino, Saint William, and Saint Nicholas of
Bari. The last may have reflected the new charitable impulse to dower
poor girls, which had swept through central Italy in the latter decades
of the Trecento and the early Quattrocento. This Saint Nicholas had
saved three girls from prostitution by providing dowry funds to their
impoverished father, a fallen nobleman.[86] Moreover, patrons from these
sources finally looked to local Tuscan saints of the Trecento to appear
in their burial frescoes and table paintings. In 1392, the Aretine Francescus f.q. Lippi de Chatenacciis ordered his coat of arms posted, along
with a painting of Sant'Urbano and Sant'Agnese de Montepulciano, in
the Aretine church of Sant'Agnese's namesake.[87]

More important, in the last decades of the Trecento more than in
any other period (5 of 15 commissions), testators sought lasting memory
by insisting that their figures and, on occasion, those of deceased relatives
be included within the compositions they commissioned. In 1382 the
Aretine citizen Ceccus f.q. Vive Angeli Pieri commissioned for the
plebis church of Arezzo the painting of the yet-to-be canonized Saint
(sic) Nicholas of Tolentino, "and at his feet the image of his own

person."[88] In 1390, the Perugian Johanna f.q. Ser Stefani, from Artimino, widow of the spice trader Andrea and at present the wife of Pauli Petri Rubei, ordered a chapel to be built in the Servite church of the city and to have the Annunciation painted "in the wall" above its altar with "the person of the testatrix and the said late Andrea her husband." She ordered the chapel and paintings to be completed within two years of her death and left 200 florins for the project.[89] In 1393, a Florentine parishioner of San Lorenzo ordered his executors to have "the image and figure" of the blessed Anthony Abbot, along with "the image of the testator genuflecting," painted "honorably and well" in the church of this Anthony.[90]

At the turn of the century, Tomas Guglielmi, from the village of Certina, then residing in the city of Perugia, exceeded the simple call for the patron's portrayal or the inclusion of the figure of a relative by ordering a more complex composition for "the recently constructed" church of Santa Maria delle Valle called Sant'Egidio. His commission was to depict "the figure of the Virgin Mary with the child in her arms and with the testator's father kneeling and holding a trumpet [tuba] in one hand while flying a flag [pennone] bearing the arms of the Orlandi family in the other and with the figure of Saint George with [his name] written above his head."[91] The commission most obsessed with preserving a testator's earthly memory came, moreover, from another Perugian, Andrea Cioli Gectarelli, widow of Angeli Ser Celloli. After leaving all her landed possessions "large and small" for the building and endowment of a "covered" chapel called Santa Maria della Annuptiata" in the Olivetani church of Monte Morcino, she commissioned "a large and beautiful" panel painting for her chapel. It was "to depict the figure or image of the blessed Maria della Annuptiata with the blessed apostles, Peter and Paul, one on the right, the other on the left," and somewhere else a figure "in the likeness [ad similitudinem] of the testatrix's person" with her coat of arms, which the testatrix demanded was "for her true memory [sue memorie in veritate] and for the commemoration of her soul."[92]

After 1400, testators' requests for figures of themselves, their husbands, or their fathers to appear kneeling at the feet of their commissioned Madonnas and saints suddenly disappear from these records. Even so, the early Quattrocento commissions did not become less complex in terms of the images testators demanded. To the contrary, while narrative programs entered these records with the Black Death, they remained rare until the early Quattrocento.[93] From the onslaught of plague to

the Quattrocento, testators requested only three such programs requiring
various scenes and figures (out of 77 commissions for paintings). Only
one of these, however, was a project with impressive dimensions similar
to those found in the Quattrocento testamentary commissions; the other
two were for inexpensive and most likely tiny predella scenes, which,
according to Sixten Ringbom, had become common for *tavole* of the
second half of the fourteenth century. In the last years of my analysis,
the narrative fresco cycle became the genre most often sought after in
these documents, eclipsing even paintings of the Madonna, which curiously slipped in popularity. Only one testator after 1400 desired the
Madonna's image, and perhaps he reflected the backward tastes of the
countryside. The rural cobbler from Vinci ordered his 50-florin burial
chapel to be adorned with a panel painting depicting the Virgin with
"the blessed saints John the Baptist, the Apostle Paul, Michael the
Archangel and Anthony."

I have already had occasion to describe most of these narrative cycles
in connection with the elaborate and costly construction of burial chapel
complexes, coats of arms, and stained-glass windows. Again, they came
exclusively from Florence and Arezzo. In 1411, the Aretine citizen and
cloth manufacturer (*retagliator pannorum*) from the prominent de Mar-
supinis family, Conte f.q. Dominici Minucci, demanded that the Franciscans of Arezzo build him a chapel in their city church and decorate
it "with pictures from the "Istorie" of Saint Francis.[94] In 1410, the
indefatigable Aretine merchant Lazzaro Bracci, who quixotically desired
to convert the principal chapel of San Francesco into his own burial
chapel complex, left 300 florins to commission two fresco cycles on the
very walls eventually painted by Piero della Francesca. On one side of
the chapel the merchant demanded the "istoria" of the resurrection of
his namesake, Saint Lazarus, and on the other, "when Saint Francis
suffered the Stigmata in his body from Jesus Christ." In addition, the
four evangelists were to be placed on the ceiling, which in fact the
Florentine late Gothic painter Bicci di Lorenzo executed just before his
death in 1452 and which remains today as testimony to the merchant's
largess and schemes for immortal fame.[95] Finally, the Florentine citizen
and merchant Antonius f.q. Lapacci Cini Cetini left one of the largest
single bequests to be found in this documentation, 750 florins to build a
burial chapel with stained-glass windows in his parish of San Pancrazio
"under the title of San Niccolò of Bari" and "to have it painted and
adorned" with this saint's "storia."[96]

The Price of Art

As examination of these patrons and their projects suggests, testamentary commissioning of painting in sacred places had changed social class by the beginning of the Quattrocento.[97] Unlike the patronage of individual panel paintings, tabernacles, and altarpieces for which earlier testators had spent as little as three lire to several florins, all but three paintings ordered in these testaments after 1400 were part of the ensemble in the decorative schemes of testators' private chapels. In addition to the wealthy merchants from Arezzo and Florence whose narrative fresco series I mentioned above, these early Quattrocento patrons included the Pisan knight (miles) from the Upezzinghi family[98] and the noble lady from the Perugian patrician de Gratinis family.[99]

Despite the numerous problems of convertibility of currencies, standardization for real prices, missing data, and the fact that the "asking price" may not have always reflected the final costs (as in any contract, past or present), testamentary prices for commissions are suggestive of the trends in demand over the course of the Trecento and early Quattrocento. (See table 17.) The average sum that testators left for paintings in 1348, the year of the plague, increased nearly sevenfold in nominal terms (from 4.85 to 32.27 florins) and over fivefold in real values from the earlier part of the century (4.01 to 22.89 florins). With such small numbers of priced commissions, the single 1,000-lire commission of the Old Testament cycle for Santa Maria Novella is responsible for a considerable part of this increase.[100] But this spectacular commission does not entirely account for the differences in values; measured by the medians, commissions in 1348 doubled the earlier values (from 3.1 to 6.0 florins). Besides, as Millard Meiss, Marvin Becker, and others have noted, the Black Death gave rise to an unprecedented outpouring of wealth from testaments to church coffers, which may well have led to new works and spectacular prices for commissions, as the fabulous figure for the Orcagna tabernacle in Orsanmichele gives testimony.[101]

Afterward, the sums left for paintings came tumbling down: first, in the interval between the plagues it fell by half (to 16.28 florins). Then, in the year of the plague's second strike, 1362–63, instead of rebounding along with demand, the values for paintings declined even more sharply to 6.82 florins, about one-fifth of their Black Death values. From 1364 to 1375, when testamentary demand for paintings doubled the levels of the period immediately following the onslaught of pestilence in 1348 (see table 16), prices did not rise accordingly, but instead dropped again,

Table 17.
The Price of Art

Period	No. Works	Average Price of Work	Average Price (Constant Florins)
ALL ART (WITH PRICES)			
< 1348	48	63.17	52.21
1348	33	194.36	137.84
1349–63	28	131.82	86.72
1363	15	73.61	48.43
1363–75	37	56.77	26.65
1376–1400	39	69.38	32.73
1401–25	42	173.19	105.60
Total	242	108.90	70.03
PAINTINGS			
< 1348	19	4.85	4.01
1348	12	32.27	22.89
1349–63	7	16.28	10.71
1363	5	6.82	4.49
1363–75	8	8.16	3.83
1376–1400	7	22.71	10.71
1401–25	2	162.50	99.09
Total	60	36.23	22.25
CHAPELS			
< 1348	15	141.81	117.20
1348	13	458.00	324.82
1349–63	10	196.37	129.19
1363	4	235.75	155.10
1363–75	15	105.26	49.42
1376–1400	15	117.83	55.58
1401–25	20	245.50	149.70
Total	92	214.36	140.14

resting at only one-fourth the Black Death level.[102] This drop is all the more remarkable when we remember that testators of this period asked for more figures in their altarpieces than at any other time reflected by this series of documents. In the mid-Quattrocento account books of Neri di Bicci, the best source for prices in the early Renaissance, the number of figures was the principal determinant of price.[103]

In the last decades of the Trecento, prices reversed direction as the values for paintings rose by three times in terms of bread prices. The most dramatic jump, however, awaited the beginnings of the Quattrocento, when, as we have seen, the character of commissions changed qualitatively. In real terms, testators were willing to pay 9 times more for sacred paintings than their relatives had in the previous generation and a fantastic 26 times more than those in the 1360s and early 1370s. The account books of Neri di Bicci corroborate these trends. Although "a prolific mediocrity" often engaged in turning out subjects that were "utterly stereotyped" and produced artworks for a wide class of clients,[104] Neri di Bicci could fetch prices for altarpieces by the mid-Quattrocento that soared exponentially above the prices of the late Trecento; they ranged from a minimum of 60 to 560 lire.[105]

Of course, these numbers can only suggest possible trends and substantial changes in magnitude. For the Quattrocento samples, only two commissions came with price tags. The reason for this paucity of quantitative evidence, however, is indicative of qualitative changes in testamentary commissions, in terms of both the art and the social class of patrons. So few testamentary commissions for *tabulae* and wall paintings are found in these early fifteenth-century documents with individually calculated price tags precisely because the small panel painting had all but disappeared from these records; instead, requests for painted figures (now frescoes) had become part of chapel and burial complexes, financed by large portions of a testator's landed patrimony or monetary gifts as high as 1,000 florins. Not only were all four of the narrative commissions from the years 1401–25 a part of testamentary chapel constructions and endowments, all except three of the commissions for paintings in this quarter-century were itemized together with the numerous furnishings and endowments that constituted the greater whole of chapel foundations. Only one of these separated and itemized the monies to go for the paintings as distinct from the other costs required for founding a chapel—its construction; the sepulcher; the altar furnishings, from priestly vestments to the silver chalices; and finally the support of the chaplain's dowry or living expenses.

Unlike previous commissions for altarpieces, which might cost only a few lire, or less than the price of a chalice, and constituted a small portion of a chapel's total outlay, the elaborate commission of paintings for the major chapel of San Francesco by the Aretine merchant Lazarus constituted the single largest expense in his burial chapel complex, accounting for 300 of the 500 florins his will provided. If testators or their notaries had itemized the values for the narrative cycles and frescoes found in the testaments of patrons, as the Florentine merchant Antonius f.q. Lapacci, who left even more than Lazarus for his chapel construction in his parish of San Pancrazio (750 florins) did not, then the increase in values from the last years of the Trecento to the early Quattrocento certainly would have been even more dramatic than the prices suggest.

To circumvent the problem of missing prices for paintings in the last years of analysis, I turn to a larger body of statistics—the prices for all works of art commissioned in these records, from painted candle-holders to burial chapels. This much larger body of prices (242 as opposed to 60 priced pieces of art) traces a trajectory similar to the one for commissions of paintings alone. In the year of the Black Death, art prices increased nearly fourfold. Afterward they declined again, reaching their low point in constant florins in the years when the demand for art production in fact reached its height, 1364–75. In the last decades of the Trecento, prices began to climb; then, in the first years of the Quattrocento they trebled, and this time my tables offer for this last quarter of analysis 42 individually priced commissions.

Of course, "art" so defined could range from the elaborate construc-tions of sacred buildings to wax images, and thus a shift in the com-position of commissions to a preponderance of chapel constructions would tilt prices significantly upward. But, as we have seen, the tendency after 1364–75 was just the opposite. The number of new chapel con-structions declined by nearly half, from one for every 8 testators at its height in the years 1364–75 to one for every 14 testators in the first years of the Quattrocento. (See table 14.) Moreover, if we look only at priced chapel constructions, the rate of increase was about the same as for art in general; commissions for chapels increased in value three times, from 49.42 in the 1364–75 period to 149.70 florins. The jump in the prices for art from the late Trecento to the early Quattrocento was in fact most remarkable for that city most distinguished by the quality of its art and architecture in the early years of the fifteenth century— Florence. Here, prices for art in general, instead of increasing by three times, soared by nearly four, from 72.20 to 268.30 florins.

How, then, do we explain these price series, particularly for the years immediately after the second wave of pestilence, 1364–75? According to market economics, we should generally expect increases in demand to drive prices upward unless there are countervailing changes in tech-nology or in the organization of production. First, in this case, the collapse in prices might in part be explained by a new demand for smaller works of art. In fact, Offner, Meiss, Boskovits,[106] and others[107] have commented on the smaller devotional works that survive from this period and have assumed that these were tabernacles for private devotion commissioned by a new class of bourgeois patrons. But given the rarity of such small devotional tabernacles in household inventories in the Trecento except for popes, cardinals, princes, and ruling patricians and their total absence in contemporary testaments, these works may instead have been the fruits of artisan, shopkeeper, and even peasant commissions like the ones found in these testaments in the years following the recurrence of pestilence.

But size alone cannot explain this decisive shift in the demand curve (especially when we remember that patrons in these years began to demand more figures within their frames). Little has been written on the organization and the business arrangement of artists' workshops in the late Trecento or early Quattrocento.[108] Work now under way by the Norwegian restorer and art historian Erling Skaug suggests that the year 1363 was in fact of pivotal importance in the organization of painters' workshops in Tuscany. Through a quantitative and meticulous investigation of punch marks in panel paintings—the imprints artists made in halos and other areas where they inlaid gold leaf—Skaug shows that workshop organization became more complex after this date.[109] Previously, it was possible to identify a workshop with a set of punch marks and their tools. After 1363, this became increasingly more difficult as studios began to collaborate and as artists began to move more freely from one workshop to another. Without the assistance of any statistics on demand for art, Skaug has speculated that this change occurred to meet increased demands made on those workshops and artists who survived the second wave of pestilence.

My statistics corroborate his speculations, not only from the supply side (the number of surviving artists),[110] as Skaug has emphasized, but, more importantly, from the demand side, at least from what can be glimpsed through the testaments of those contemplating the fears and rewards of the afterlife. Similarly, van Os argues that the large workshops of the first half of the Trecento—those of Duccio, Simone Martini, and the Lorenzetti brothers—depended on steady commissioning for "huge altarpieces provided by powerful institutions." With the rise of a "completely new patronage," these broke up into smaller workshops in the second half of the Trecento and moved largely into the small towns in the countryside. When van Os's picture of workshop practice is merged with Skaug's tools, it appears that a process analogous to cottage industry or proto-industry characteristic of the manufacture of other commodities during the early modern period began to alter the organization of artists' workshops in late Trecento Tuscany.[111]

Painting after the Black Death: A Reassessment

Through examining the form and content of paintings in Trecento
Florence and Siena, Meiss found a fundamental shift not only in painting
but in culture and mentality, provoked by bankruptcies, famine, war,
and ultimately the Black Death in the 1340s. Painters and their patrons
turned their backs on the achievements of early Trecento masters such
as Duccio, Giotto, the Lorenzetti brothers, and Simone Martini, who,
according to Meiss and others, displayed naturalism and a "modern"
sensibility toward "individual consciousness." The third quarter of the
Trecento "seemed to challenge all at once, in the name of medieval
society and medieval Christianity, the new individualism, the new sec-
ularity, and the new economic order."[112] Through a didactic ecclesiology,
which resulted, for example, in the transformation of the Virgin "as
simple housewife" into a "frontal, elevated, and almost motionless" figure
of authority, the Virgin Queen, painting was "pervaded by a profound
pessimism and sometimes a renunciation of life."[113] Works of art revived
the ideals of asceticism, penance, and guilt, "recovering" the forms and
attitudes of the Duecento.[114]

The evidence from wills, not only on commissions for painting but
also on a wide range of charitable activity and attitudes toward property,
directly contravenes Millard Meiss's interpretation of the impulses underlying Florentine and Sienese culture and society after the Black Death.
With this evidence, I cannot pretend to resolve stylistic debates between
Meiss and others, most notably Miklós Boskovits. The commissions from
wills constituted only one of several forms and moments within the life
cycle of patronage, although an important one, especially before the
Quattrocento. From these data, we can say nothing about the corporate
patronage of lay confraternities, hospitals, monasteries, and the commune; nor can the data shed light on other moments of commissioning
in a patron's life such as at the time of marriage. Meiss suggests, for
instance, that paintings of the early Trecento represent a variety of holy
marriages, "many of them novel," which reflect "burgher values . . .
commissioned by a married couple for their own private devotion." By
the third quarter of the Trecento, according to Meiss, these represen-
tations fell by the wayside. Perhaps the growing obsession after the
Black Death with earthly memory after death stimulated a shift in the
moment of patronage that concentrated demand at the end of one's
life. To date, however, art historians have not been especially interested
in such questions.[115]

Despite these qualifications, the data from thousands of last wills and testaments place the pictorial interpretations of Meiss, Boskovits, and others in an altogether different social and cultural context from the one these art historians have imputed from the visual remains. Testators in the six cities examined here, perhaps in response to fears of abandonment by friends, relatives, and churchmen (as one chronicler after another repeated), turned decisively against the phenomena of mounting corpses and mass burials by specifying more precisely than ever before the places of their final resting grounds. As a result, numbers of ordinary citizens and villagers (as opposed to what had earlier included only prominent churchmen and those from ruling families) began to devise ways to ensure burials that would individuate and preserve for successive generations the place of their corporeal remains. The number of burial chapels started to increase for these cities in 1348 but with renewed vigor when the pestilence returned in 1362–63. Those with fewer resources significantly increased their demand for concrete remembrance by sponsoring paintings to be placed above their tombs or in sacred niches of other churches, hospitals, and monasteries. These testamentary patrons, especially after the return of plague, pursued more earnestly than ever before their own schemes, entering the frame of the painting both by directing its composition and more literally by demanding that the artist place the testator *ad similitudinem* at the feet of the desired saint or the Virgin Mary.

The period after the second occurrence of pestilence, 1364–75, marked a more significant turning point than 1348, not only for Florence and Arezzo but for the other cities in Umbria and Tuscany as well. Demand for all types of art production, from coats of arms on candlestick holders to burial chapels, increased sharply in number. Moreover, the character of the demand for paintings also changed: not only did more testators specify more figures to crowd their commissioned surfaces, but more than at any time before or afterward these patrons insisted that their own "figures" painted in their very likeness be included in their sacred art. As we have noted, this cult of remembrance is paralleled implicitly and explicitly in other changes in testamentary practice, such as the demands testators imposed on their heirs and on their property in attempts to control the future behavior of their beneficiaries and the future preservation, use, and flow of their houses and real estate.

How, then, does this information on the esprit of the period after the Black Death, particularly in the 1360s and 1370s, square with the stylistic and iconographical interpretations of Millard Meiss and other art historians drawn from in-depth searches through actual surviving works of art? After nearly 40 years, *Painting in Florence and Siena After the Black Death* still stimulates lively debate. Several have questioned Meiss's dating of individual paintings, most importantly, the *Triumph of Death* in the Camposanto in Pisa, claiming that its execution predated the Black Death.[116] Others, such as John Paoletti, have questioned Meiss's interpretation of individual paintings, most importantly, the Strozzi altarpiece in Santa Maria Novella, which, Paoletti argues, shows "varieties of spatial presentation . . . far more complex than Meiss suggested."[117] Nancy Rash Fabbri and Nina Rutenburg also have argued forcefully that certain works of art, such as the Orcagna Tabernacle of Orsanmichele, cannot be so easily categorized as "Giottoesque" or "a return to dugento forms." Rather a "duality dominates" this magnificent work, reflecting its sacred functions in the secular setting of what had been Florence's central grain market. From this interpretation of this single cluster of artistic creation the authors maintain that Orcagna's post–Black Death style "provides evidence of continuity" rather than rupture.[118] Still others, such as Bruce Cole, while agreeing that the 1340s inaugurated a new "disturbing art"[119] and that "the mortality of the plague" may have "inspired" the imagery of the Strozzi chapel,[120] have questioned Meiss's bold interpretations, suggesting, "Might not style have its own rhythm and history that has little to do with the events swirling around it?"[121] Yet, in interpreting changes in style in Orcagna and his circle, Cole has replaced Meiss only with a nominalist tautology: "Some of this shift might be a result of patrons' and artists' desire to revive the ancient, and therefore sacred, visual and iconographical vocabulary of the period before Giotto."[122] But the point of cultural history (of which art history is a part) is to understand why artists or patrons changed their minds and desires.

Few have questioned the essence of Meiss's argument—his interpretation of the spiritual, social, and ideological contexts that lay behind these paintings (as well as behind contemporary works of literature). Did the crowded, more simple and rudimentary painting techniques—stark profiles instead of more complex and difficult quarter faces—and the hieratic and didactic arrangement of figures[123] reflect a society that had rejected the naturalism of Giotto and had "recovered" the Duecento, the ideals of self-denial preached by Passavanti and zealously invoked by Saint Catherine of Siena?

Miklós Boskovits's monumental *Pittura fiorentina* is the most thoroughgoing revision of Meiss's interpretation of painting after the Black Death.[124] At the outset, Boskovits claims to shun the politico-social analysis of art found in the seminal works of Frederick Antal[125] and Meiss, arguing that "relations so direct between the conditions of economic, political and social life, on the one hand, and art on the other" cannot be established.[126] Boskovits, instead, finds his inspiration in the master of the generation preceding Antal and Meiss, Richard Offner and his stylistic analysis.

Ironically, Boskovits's complex analysis of changes in artistic style over the course of the Trecento strives to follow the eddies of cultural, political, and economic change much more minutely and directly than that ever proposed by either Antal or Meiss. Instead of the one vague and general transformation in cultural values and artistic style that Meiss chronicles sometime between the bankruptcies of the 1340s and the Black Death of 1348, Boskovits finds four "revolutions" in painting over the course of the later Trecento. The first is almost identical to Meiss's interpretation: "And in opposition to the taste and aesthetic norms of the 'classical' period of Giotto, a true and real rebellion in painting began at the end of the third and at the start of the fourth decade [of the fourteenth century]."

While this break—the rejection of naturalism and "quotidian" values— crossed the great divide of the Black Death of 1348, it was not to dominate for as long as Meiss's dark period. According to Boskovits, Orcagna "inaugurated a new phase in Florentine painting by reconciling the formal traditions of the early Trecento with the latest developments of the style of courtly Gothic," and other artists of the 1360s such as Giovanni da Milano, who momentarily appeared on the Florentine scene, the invented "Giottino," and Niccolò di Tommaso suddenly revived "the vivacity and humor, achieved either through the acute observation of daily life or by pure and simple devotion, the world of Franco Sacchetti's stories."[127] Nor does this turn of the '60s appear to have been confined to Florence. More recently, Christie Knapp Fengler has found a similar "joie de vivre" and "a new appreciation of everyday pleasures" in the fresco cycle of the Sienese painter Bartolo di Fredi in the Collegiata of San Gimignano, signed and dated 1367.[128]

But this "revolution" of the 1360s was not, at least in Boskovits's scheme, to last for long. With the plague of 1374, the war with the Milanese Visconti, the financial burdens incurred through payments to the English soldier of fortune John Hawkwood, the papal interdict, and finally the revolt of the Ciompi, Florence entered an economic depression. As a result, Boskovits argues, "religious fervor increased,"[129] and art, responding directly and immediately to these new social, economic, and religious realities, rejected "the loquacious humor of anecdotes and fables" characteristic of the previous decade. With the emergence of artists such as Jacopo di Cione, "the lively amusements of this world, light-hearted and often even sentimental," disappear in "the glacial immobility of figures, the uniform roundedness of bodies . . . almost mechanical in its form and rigidity."[130] In its "conservative" and "obsequious" attention to the "art of past times," the 1370s' "re-editions of popular images from the first half of the Trecento" lost all "immediacy, spontaneity and freshness, that air of intimate domesticity characteristic of their models."[131]

This downturn, however, was again short-lived. Based entirely on anecdotal evidence—the fact that a man as sensitive to finances as Francesco Datini should decide to return to Tuscany from Avignon— Boskovits argues that the Florence of the 1380s experienced economic revival, carrying in its tow changes in religious sentiment and culture. Here, Boskovits, unfortunately, misreads Hans Baron's thesis on civic humanism, pushing political changes of the early fifteenth century back to the 1380s. He apparently has forgotten that (according to Baron) it was the political and military crisis of the summer of 1402 that triggered the sharp break in culture—the fusion of mercantile patriotism with humanist learning, which created the "civic humanism" of Leonardo Bruni and subsequent generations of political ideology. Boskovits (unlike for the period of the 1370s) does not recall for the 1390s the economic consequences incurred by siege warfare and the Visconti military expansion vividly described by Baron,[132] which, according to Ottavio Banti, brought with it economic depression, famine, and demographic decline.[133] Boskovits's sketchy economic and social analysis, nonetheless, sets the stage for the largest section of his stylistic interpretations, where once again style directly and immediately parallels changes in the social, economic, and cultural spheres: Giovanni da Milano returns to Florence; Giotto's art is revived; and with the painting of Lorenzo Monaco and the Maestro della Madonna Straus, "the measure and dignity of Florentine art of the early Trecento is reaffirmed."[134]

To be sure, the laconic descriptions of testamentary commissions do not allow me to challenge or reinterpret the stylistic trends charted by Meiss, Boskovits, and others who have viewed hundreds of surviving works of art through the Trecento. Nonetheless, the trends followed by the demand for artworks and their prices can be intertwined with the visual evidence and might assist in sorting out certain contradictions in stylistic interpretation. First, those who have challenged Meiss by arguing that the turn from Giottoesque naturalism predated the Black Death and stretched back as far as the 1330s or 1320s have done so primarily from the perspective of Pisan and Sienese art—in other words, from those societies where the testaments evince the strongest penetration of the mendicant patterns of piety. Second, the "revolution in painting" that Boskovits finds in the 1360s and early 1370s—the appearance of Giovanni da Milano and Giottino and the revival of the quotidian values of Giotto—corroborates the shift in piety from mendicant self-abnegation to the cult of re-membrance charted by thousands of last wills and testaments from societies across Tuscany and Umbria.

But how, then, does this testamentary evidence square with Boskov-its's image of art rejecting once again the naturalism and quotidian values, "the spontaneity and freshness" of the *primo Trecento,* or for that matter the longer duration of Meiss's gloomy pessimism and "recovery" of earlier religious sentiments across the later Trecento? From the per-spective of spirituality, instead of being diametrically opposed, both practices could have been present in the same society, and indeed were different sides of the same coin. A new mentality that rejected Augus-tinian self-denial and in its place sought earthly signs of remembrance inspired a rush of new donors, some from artisan and rural backgrounds, to leave concrete memorials for their earthly memory and family fame. One way of doing so (in fact, one of the cheapest) was the patronage of works of art, particularly paintings, while contemplating the afterlife. Demand for art intensified after the Black Death and more so by the 1360s and 70s with its relived trauma that rippled through city and countryside alike across central Italy.

At the level of broad changes in spirituality, the testaments do not record the minute shifts that Boskovits tries to demonstrate through stylistic interpretations of paintings, few of which bear any dates at all. Nor do the testaments bear out his assertion for the 1370s "that those disposed to decorate their family chapels or to make donations to churches for similar reasons, preferred to wait for better times."[135] Instead, the testaments plot a sea change—the rejection of mendicant patterns of self-abnegation and the spread of a cult of earthly memory. This change, moreover, did not turn on facts particular to the political and financial history of Florence—the campaigns of the *condottiere* John Hawkwood, the War of Eight Saints, war indebtedness, papal interdict,[136] and the revolt of the Ciompi—as Boskovits's noncomparative approach assumes. As thousands of last wills and testaments make clear, the transformations in mentalities were not peculiar to Florence but ran through large swaths of central Italy.

The pressure of this new demand, along with a collapse in the supply of artists (perhaps even relative to the general decline in population), led workshops to economize and rationalize in order to fill the orders of this myriad of new patrons, as Erling Skaug and others are now discovering. As a result, paintings became smaller, cheaper,[137] and less sophisticated as more sophisticated organizations of labor and business practices began to expand. Art operated in fact as any other commodity might, given similar market and organizational realities. Like the manufacture of cotton cloth during the Industrial Revolution (or closer to the period, the proto-industry of linens),[138] these paintings cheapened, and the value that their commissions fetched stands as direct quantitative testimony to what the art historians have judged qualitatively. While demand in the 1360s and 1370s increased fivefold over the pre-plague period, prices in terms of constant florins fell from the Black Death mark to one-fifth of their previous levels. This picture of changes in production coincides with descriptions of paintings executed in the decades after the Black Death found in both Meiss's and Boskovits's analyses. Meiss emphasized the "strict uniformity and regimentation of the figures" and commented on the rapidity of production,[139] while Boskovits characterized the works of "these less gifted artists" in the 1370s as "mechanical in form and rigid in expression."[140] But from these signs of increasing productivity in art, both drew conclusions on the societal and cultural level that run directly counter to the evidence provided in last wills. For Meiss, these changes in art production involved "a denial of individuality . . . opposed to the art of the earlier fourteenth century," and for Boskovits (like Meiss), a sudden return to "a more fervent religiosity."[141] Instead, the wills bear witness to the rise of new views of the self, lineage, remembrance, and earthly fame that cut deeply through the social fabric, not only of Florence, but across central Italy in the decades following the return of pestilence.

By the end of the Trecento, and much more profoundly during the first quarter of the Quattrocento, testamentary demand for various forms of sacred art, and more particularly for painting, reversed, and the social character of patronage changed, especially for painting. Prices took a quantum leap, and sacred art changed qualitatively from 10-lire panel paintings, which even peasants could afford, to complex narrative fresco cycles that testators bearing prestigious names and titles demanded from their heirs and beneficiaries to grace the walls of their burial chapel complexes. An increase in the demand for art did not necessarily lead to improvements in quality and the production of great masterpieces, as is often postulated.[142] This evidence for the Trecento and early Quattrocento suggests indeed the opposite: the early Quattrocento, both visually and verbally (i.e., the testamentary commissions), shows a change in taste away from small panel paintings cluttered with individually specified saints and their donors at their feet to the much more costly and elaborate fresco cycles commissioned for private chapels. These changes in taste, moreover, may have been militated by more than aesthetics and the revival of antique notions of space—the "delight in what was rational, symmetrical, and open to mathematical calculation."[143]

As we have seen, testators from early Quattrocento Florence not only feared the encroachment of others' works of art and coats of arms in their privatized sacred spaces, they also demanded that their ecclesiastical hosts keep the passages leading to their enclaves of private devotion and memory clean from the clutter of others' commissioned works. The propagation and reception of new classical notions of ecclesiastical design and space associated with Brunelleschi and later Alberti—"the fashion of whitewashing muralled church interiors in order to give them a neat, clean look"[144]—appear at the very moment when patrician families became intent on dominating these temples for their own political and social purposes. They began the long but steady process, culminating in the renovation plans of Vasari and Cosimo I, of transforming and erasing what Eve Borsook has called "the busy fullness" of fourteenth-century church interiors; and thus this aesthetic, with its sphere of commissions that formerly had allowed artisans and even peasants to leave lasting mementos of their earthly fame and the perpetuation of their lineages for as little as a few florins, came abruptly to an end.[145] As the story of one of Arlotto's sayings suggests, the practice of periodically "erasing" paintings which no longer paid in terms of miracles (as Richard Trexler has emphasized)[146] or in terms of attracting candles and other contributions (as Piovano Arlotto in fact reasons) may have become widespread by the mid-Quattrocento. Years before Vasari whitewashed church walls to clean up a jumbled mosaic of figures and frames,[147] patrician donors reshaped church interiors for their own private devotion, tearing down the more democratic vision of family and self-remembrance supported by a wide array of small commissions.[148]

The rise of patrician cultural hegemony in the Renaissance paralleled changes in political control, in which aristocratic regimes ousted more popular and more broadly based governments. From the 1360s through the 1370s, each of these towns had become ever more open in social, economic, and political terms to new men of the artisan classes and from the countryside (the *gente nuova*) as Black Death demographics opened doors to new men and women of talent and broke down old guild matriculation restrictions.[149] The 1380s, on the other hand, marked the reversal of such developments — the defeat of the Ciompi in Florence in 1382, the return of the aristocratic *fuorusciti,* and the forced migration of thousands of workers; the defeat of the Raspanti and the return of the nobility in Perugia in 1384; the loss of Aretine independence to the Florentines in the same year; and the fall of the government of the "Riformatori" in Siena, the year after, which opened the city gates for the return of magnate political exiles — "i Salimbeni, i Malavolti, i Piccolomini, una parte de' Tolommei, i Cerretani, gli Vgurgieri, e gli altri Gentiluomini" — and caused thousands of artisans to flee the city and territory never to return. According to the sixteenth-century historian Orlando Malavolti, their flight injured Sienese industry for years to come.[150]

The striking exception to this trend comes from the political history of Pisa, where in 1392 Iacopo D'Appiano,[151] a notary and son of a notary, wrenched the reigns of government from the Signoria of Pietro Gambacorta. Supported by a groundswell of popular opposition to the old regime, this proponent of the "Seven Guilds" of Pisa opened the council of elders (the *Anziani*) to members of the artisan classes — *artefices* — and led the anti-Gambacortiana faction comprised of guildsmen from the *"popolo medio"* allied with landowners-cattle herders from the Maremma.[152] Yet, parallel to these political changes, native Pisan testamentary commissions increased, finally rivaling, in these years, those from Perugia, Arezzo, and Florence.

But it was in Florence, where the changes in aesthetics, taste, the class character of artistic commissions, and the testamentary prices for art were the most accentuated from the 1360s to the early Quattrocento, that we also find the most radical reversal in politics and society. From the wide participation in government and society of the *arti minori* and the *popolo minuto,* which expanded their power through the sixties, reaching their apex with the revolt of the Ciompi in 1378, a bureaucratic patriciate trained in law began to shape a new, more autocratic Renaissance territorial state in the 1380s and 1390s.[153]

While the early Quattrocento may have constituted a historic turning point for art, it did not at the same time mark a major shift in values across society, at least in terms of testaments and the structure of giving.

That shift had come earlier and was indeed the stimulus for the increased production of a panoply of smaller panel paintings later to be labeled "the primitives."[154] Nor did the Quattrocento mark a reversal in values for those who could no longer afford to patronize sacred art. Instead, they found other, more domestic ways of leaving their earthly memory. Though largely pushed out of the art market for sacred paintings by soaring prices and patrician consolidation of ecclesiastical space, more than ever before testators imposed their wills on the behavior of their heirs and, through increasingly complex mazes of contingency clauses, guided the flow of their worldly possessions for the preservation of their earthly memories, the glorification of their lineages, and the salvation of their souls.

8

Conclusion

In its most characteristic form, this idol of the tribe of historians has a name: it is the obsession with origins.

—Marc Bloch, *Apologie pour l'histoire*

We cannot assume, as some holistic approaches to comparative sociology have tended to do, that all variations in social action interlock one with another; nor yet can we accept an atomistic view that dogmatically asserts the opposite.

—Jack Goody, *Death, Property, and the Ancestors*

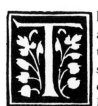he comparative approach to attitudes about property and piety found in 40,043 itemized bequests[1] from 3,389 testators in six city-states of central Italy has neither singled out Florence as the hub of a new Renaissance cult of remembrance nor underscored a deeper structural Mediterranean culture without sharp distinctions over space and time. Instead, this study has unearthed other findings. First, testators' choices of pious beneficiaries do not bear out the conclusions of recent historiography—a change from institutions such as monasteries and nunneries, which expressed the values of penance and asceticism, to those such as hospitals and confraternities, which worked to resolve social ills within the present temporal sphere. In all six cities, contributions to monasteries, friaries, and parishes remained strong over the course of this study, from the earliest records through the early Quattrocento. Of the pious beneficiaries of the old order, only nunneries

suffered a major decline in bequests. Gifts to confraternities and hospitals, on the other hand, did not rise in tandem; the two more often competed for the same social services. Only in Florence did they both tighten their grip on the charitable desires of the pious. The most fundamental shift registered by these pious choices came in poor relief. In all six cities, at least by the last decades of the fourteenth and the opening years of the fifteenth century, indiscriminate handouts to the poor of Christ declined and were supplanted by the foundation of dowry funds for a selected few virgins of *buon costume*.

As I found earlier for Siena, a change in the structure of testamentary giving provides the key for understanding change in mentalities over time. From liquidating estates into small monetary sums scattered among numerous pious entities, testators in all these city-states began to focus their patrimonies on a few select charities. This happened at the same time that testators broke with the mendicant patterns that formerly left legacies unencumbered with impositions, conditions, and constraints governing future use. Instead, testators tried to hold on to their earthly possessions, especially land, controlling them from the grave through the legal channels of the will. In preparing their passage to what Petrarch called "that other side of life," testators of the later Trecento also devised mechanisms for earthly immortality, from perpetual masses and feasts in which their largess and their names would be recalled to the faithful to plaques plastered in sacred places to stand *in perpetuum* for their everlasting memory and that of their lineages. Again, as in Siena, nowhere did the first onslaught of pestilence in 1348 set in motion this transformation in piety. Instead, the decline began earlier, but the decisive break occurred with the recurrence of pestilence in 1362–63 or immediately thereafter. Only at that point did the long itemized lists of pious bequests with few strings attached disappear from these records.

The other five cities, however, were not simply mirror images of Siena, especially before the recurrence of pestilence. While Assisi and Pisa replicated and even exaggerated those patterns seen in Siena, the testamentary mechanisms for earthly memory in Arezzo, Florence, and Perugia delineated another world of sentiment. Not until the Cinquecento do testators such as the Aretine son of a notary, who dedicated a large portion of his will to dividing and then guaranteeing the perpetual survival of his library, even enter the Sienese records. Complex cycles of perpetual masses, which the humanist rector of Florence's Santa Cecilia imposed on the chaplains of his refurbished burial chapel, came even later to the city of the Virgin. Similarly, testators early on in the records from Florence show an obsession with coats of arms and other familial insignia to preserve earthly memories that even reached the wills of wool workers without family names. While the testaments in Perugia were generally more laconic than elsewhere, testators here more than in any of the other towns controlled the future behavior of their heirs and directed the flow of property by blocking the future transmission of property.

Testators from these three cities used their wills far more often than in the others to commission works of art, from 20-soldi wax images to the 4,000-florin construction of "the middle church" of the Franciscan shrine at La Verna. Along with this interest in leaving behind concrete creations for earthly memory, the testators from Arezzo, Florence, and Perugia were more preoccupied with demarcating and memorializing the precise places for their corporeal remains.

How can this geography of piety be explained? Should we look for long-term and distant origins as historians often do and speculate that perhaps deeply embedded character traits from Roman versus Etruscan traditions or even farther back to the tribal configurations of prehistoric Italy underlay the patterns found for the late Duecento and early Trecento? Or, can events and settlement patterns closer in time to my findings clarify the riddle of these regional differences? Did the invasions and three-century-long dominance of the Lombards, which, according to Giovanni Tabacco, finally toppled the Roman social system dominated by the old senatorial families,[2] create a social fabric that enables us to understand these long-term structures of mentality? Certainly, women's property rights were stronger in those provinces where Roman law prevailed over Lombard law and customs.[3]

But these differences cannot be pushed back to the settlement patterns and politics of the fifth through the seventh centuries; otherwise, the island of Byzantine rule and Roman law—the Duchy of Perugia, which included Assisi[4]—would have appeared as the distinctive region in this analysis. The Lombards had conquered all of Tuscany and had transformed its laws and customs, some of which, such as the husband's *mundio* over his wife, survived in the Florentine statutes through the fifteenth century. Instead, Marc Bloch's criticisms of "the idol of origins" appear well-advised.[5] First, the differences among the cities do not appear to have been of such ancient origins. From the earliest testaments until 1275, the differences in the choices and patterns of bequests were minimal. Second, the geographical groupings of cities and their territories do not correspond with any of these earlier settlement patterns; they do not conveniently divide along a north-south, an east-west, a Tuscan-Umbrian, or a Lombard-Byzantine line. It was not even a matter of propinquity; the two city-states in closest proximity, Perugia and Assisi, show as radical a difference in the pre-plague patterns of piety as any two towns in this analysis.

Nor can population size or wealth take us very far. The richest of these cities, Florence, gave the fewest number of pious gifts per capita at its height, while the poorest, Assisi, gave the most; and the obverse of this correlation between poverty and piety does not take us any further. The political histories of these places also fail to lend much help. True, Florence and Perugia were traditional Guelph strongholds, but Arezzo and Pisa (where testamentary giving represented opposite ends of the spectrum) were the bastions of Ghibelline power in central Italy. We also cannot point to the form of government; Pisa and Arezzo, the two city-states that handed the reins of control under the *signoria* to a single noble family were again at opposite ends. Moreover, the importance of antimagnate laws and the extent to which nobles were able to share in the political power of the mercantile elites during the Trecento explain little. Two of the city-states where testators most forcefully attempted to preserve earthly memory and to manipulate future events from the grave were also once again on opposite ends of the spectrum. While the Florentine Ordinances of Justice of 1293 became emblematic of the antimagnate legislation sweeping through northern and central Italy in the late Duecento and early Trecento, the feudal lords from the rural Casentino (Pietramala) took control of Arezzo at the beginning of the Trecento. Moreover, because of its late arrival, Perugia's antimagnate legislation, *Libro Rosso,* never succeeded in ridding its governmental councils of strong aristocratic influence. Nor can we point to the relative severity of pestilence in these places. As best as can be determined from the sources, the plague of 1348 swept through and equally devastated all these towns and their territories and then returned for a second blow in 1362 in Pisa and 1363 in the others.

Should we speculate that the geographical differences resulted from the relative degrees of economic, political, and cultural decline in the late Duecento and early Trecento? Certainly, Pisa and Siena lost ground to Florence and possibly Perugia as well before the Black Death. But what about Arezzo? While evidence from the testaments shows that the city may not have sunk as low as some historians have assumed, the current historiographical picture of culture and politics for this middle-sized city-state by the early Trecento is as bleak as that for Siena, if not more so.[6] And certainly, Arezzo did not become a regional center as did Perugia and Florence. At best, after submitting to Florentine rule in 1384, it became a link in the restructured international economy of Florence.

In addition, these patterns over space do not correspond with religious characteristics, such as Dominican versus Franciscan popularity. While it is suggestive to compare Dominican Florence[7] with Franciscan Assisi, the correspondence ceases to hold when the other cities come into the analysis. In Arezzo, the Franciscan influence looms large in the literary and artistic evidence as well as in the statistics for pious bequests. In this early city of humanist learning, the Dominicans did not even rank second among the mendicant orders. Nor does the presence of universities help us along. Four of these cities—Perugia,[8] Siena,[9] Arezzo,[10] and, to a lesser extent, Pisa[11]—possessed venerable universities before the Black Death, but they do not correspond to those cities that championed remembrance early on. Most notably, Florence's *studium* was lackluster until the Medici began to patronize it in the second half of the fifteenth century, just before Lorenzo moved it to Pisa.[12] The link between early centers of humanist learning and the cult of remembrance might be offered as the key to the patterns of piety in Florence and Arezzo,[13] but then how is Pisa, a center of learning equal to or even more important than these cities in the late Duecento, but on the other end of the spectrum in testamentary giving, to be explained?[14] Finally, despite Paul Grendler's recent and excellent overview of schooling in the Renaissance, we still know little about differences in the systems, curricula, and organization of educations from city-state to city-state, especially before the Quattrocento.[15] The one systematic comparative study with which I am familiar draws a distinction between the emphasis on mercantile or abacus learning in Florence and the more literary or grammatical emphasis found for Arezzo.[16] But these two cities, as we have seen, were similar in their early patterns of piety and in the emphasis placed on self and lineage.

No doubt, more city-states and analyses of other economic, social, and cultural facts not so easily gleaned from testaments alone would shed further light on these geographical patterns; and if the field of examination were extended to France, England, and Germany, other typologies would be discovered. At this point, however, the one structural characteristic that does correlate closely with these differences over space is the importance of the male line in property ascent and its corollary, the disadvantageous property status of women. Where concern with the souls and memory of ancestors and the devolution of property through the patriliny were strong, mendicant values proved less hegemonic. Here, at the heart of Burckhardt's classic formulation of Renaissance individualism, lies a crucial contradiction. Those societies where testators were most obsessed with earthly glory and the preservation of memory, whether achieved through clauses blocking the alienation of property or through the construction of burial complexes advertising the profane symbols of family pride, were also the ones where testators were most governed by the constraints of their ancestors. These testators' attempts to govern from the grave the future behavior of religious beneficiaries and heirs might well be interpreted as evidence for the assertion of "individualism"—what Stephen Greenblatt calls "the attempt to fashion other selves."[17] At the same time, however, these testators succeeded in creating at the societal level new restrictions and barriers to the free and individual disposition of property. As we have seen with the choice of burials and chapel foundations, so too with the channels of property descent, the hand of the ancestors increasingly restricted the limits of individual testamentary choice. Moreover, the "individualism" and cult of memory that intensified during the late Trecento—far from being opposed to those ideals that Burckhardt identified as feudal and antithetical to Renaissance individuality—were instead the very channels through which the most egoistic testators expressed their desires for earthly remembrance, ultimately forming a new ideal of salvation based on this-worldly foundations.

Furthermore, women, in those societies where the ideals of earthly memory were more in evidence early on, certainly exercised less individual choice in their discretionary power over property than where mendicant values dampened any zeal for earthly self-preservation. Far from exemplifying the status of women, Florence, where the cult of remembrance was as strong as anywhere studied in this book, was the worst place to have been born a woman, at least in terms of one's power over property. Fewer Florentine women determined the individual fate of their properties through the instrument of the will, and when they did, the constraints of law—the mundualdus—and their husbands weighed more heavily on them than elsewhere. By contrast, in Pisa, where lineage was weak and the cult of remembrance less pervasive, women redacted wills early on almost as often as men. Moreover, they commonly imposed their choices over property, both dotal and nondotal, while their husbands lived. Unlike women in Florence, where such practice was rare and when it did occur was no less than an instrument by which the husband assumed all the earlier total control over his wife's patrimony, Pisan women customarily gave their husbands only a standard 15 lire. Finally, husbands' property settlements for their future widows were more favorable in the three cities, Assisi, Pisa, and Siena, where the mendicant patterns of self-abnegation were most entrenched. To assume the *usufructus* of the husbands' property in Arezzo, Florence, and Perugia, widows customarily had to relinquish their claims to their dowries, while for the other three towns, the dowry remained inviolable.

The patterns over time traced by testamentary bequests, both quantitatively and qualitatively, emerge in bolder relief than those over geography. Despite the differences among these cities before the recurrence of plague in the 1360s, they all changed along similar paths, so that by the end of this study (1425) the differences in the patterns of bequests had become negligible. This convergence ran beyond the ambit of Florentine or Perugian centralization, indicating that larger forces must have been active. Even where commissions for art and symbols of familial pride had dotted the records earlier, these manifestations of earthly memory multiplied and expanded in complexity after the 1360s. In cities such as Pisa, which earlier extolled the ideals of mendicant humility as fervently as anywhere, the number of pious legacies and the fragmentation of these pious patrimonies fell even below the levels found for the three cities whose more variegated character of piety had shaped the pre–Black Death wills. At the same time, by the 1390s, Pisan testators began to enter the art market for earthly mementos almost as commonly as the Aretines; and, unlike before the plague, native Pisans instead of immigrants commissioned art for shrines, not in distant lands as was earlier the case, but for churches in Pisa proper.

Indeed, these impulses spurred demand for testamentary sacred art in all six city-states, especially in the 1360s and 1370s. Increased demand, however, did not mean (as some historians have assumed) improved craftsmanship or more beautiful works of art. Instead, as can happen to commodities subjected to similar market conditions, the organization of production changed and art cheapened. In this case, what was produced were the simplistic "didactic" themes and "uniform and regimented" figures that Millard Meiss and other art historians have interpreted (I would argue wrongly) as the "recovery" of the ascetic otherworldly values of the Duecento—the very reverse, that is, of the trends uncovered in these thousands of last wills and testaments.

Here, comparative study corroborates the experience of Siena. The long-term changes there were not unique, nor should they be attributed to its remarkable artistic and spiritual development after the Black Death or to a supposed retardation in the Quattrocento. These changes were unlike the late Cinquecento spread of Counter-Reformation spirituality in Siena, which was sharply fragmented by sex, class, status, and residence. The plague, or rather its recurrence and its psychological impact, was more democratic. As with Petrarch's experience of 1348 and his reliving of that trauma when it returned to Milan in 1361, the attitudes toward that "scourge against mankind" changed radically with the plague's recurrence for patricians as well as peasants throughout the regions of central Italy investigated in this book. More than in "the revival of antiquity" or the acting out of antique models of behavior,[18] the cause of the new sensibilities toward the self and "earthly glory" can be located in matters closer to hand and more accessible to wide sectors of the population—the immediate psychological effects of the late Trecento and the double experience of plague.

When pestilence returned, the experience of reliving the trauma was not, at the outset, the same in all six cities. In 1362, Pisa shifted momentarily in the opposite direction from Siena as, with a last gasp of renewed vigor, testators embraced the mendicant patterns that had been more widespread at the turn of the century. In Florence, the statistics on bequests went in both directions. However, soon afterward (in Pisa within a year), the trends began to move decisively along the same track in all six cities, spelling the end of these forms of mendicant piety that had structured last wills and testaments since the last decades of the Duecento.[19] In their place, testators now sought the opposite—the preservation of their memories and the salvation of their souls through human means formerly deemed of only ephemeral value.

Through these statistics buttressed by illustrations, from attitudes about property to commissions for altarpieces, where testators demanded to be painted in their "very likeness" boasting inscriptions and family arms, this book has delved the psychological subsoil of the Renaissance. It has found a more variegated spread and deeper social bed than historians now imagine. A Renaissance mentality penetrated beyond and below the intellectual and social domain of a Francesco Petrarch, a Leonardo Bruni, or a Cosimo de' Medici, and it shook that citadel of Franciscan piety—Assisi—at the same time that it transformed notions of the self and the efficacy of worldly acts in the supposed capital of the Renaissance—Florence.

APPENDIX A

The Sources

For Siena, testaments came from two sources—the notarial protocols housed in the public archives of the city, which became the nucleus of the present Archivio di Stato, Siena,[1] and loose parchment rolls, which formed the Diplomatico. Until the archival centralization initiated by the Lorrainian regime in the last decades of the eighteenth century, these loose parchments had been a part of private (mostly ecclesiastical) archives. For the Sienese sample, I was able to avoid the bias in selection toward a hospital or a particular religious order by utilizing only those parchments contained in the large Archivio Generale, which formed a major collection of parchments within the Sienese Diplomatico and whose records derived from a number of private archives.

These sampling procedures were not possible for the other five cities in this study. While all these cities possess collections of notarial books (protocols and the rougher versions in Umbria called *bastardelli*),[2] and at least half of my sample of testaments comes from these "public" sources, no subarchive comparable to Siena's Archivio Generale exists for the other city-states. In Arezzo, Pisa, and Florence, the collections of parchments bearing the same nomenclature (Archivio Generale) are not the same as the Sienese one. First, these collections are far smaller and do not, by themselves, possess enough wills for the periods before 1426. Second, the Archivio Generale collections in the other Tuscan towns were not general grab bags of documents like the one in Siena, which contained a wide variety of parchments from numerous ecclesiastical collections. Instead, elsewhere these parchments carried a particular connection to matters of state. In Florence, for instance, they include a predominance of wills redacted by those from the old feudal magnate families, such as the Guicciardini and the Tornaquinci, or from new and powerful merchant families, such as the Cerchi, whose familial struggles shaped the political history of the city. The property and behavior of these *ottimati* would have been the concerns of the commune, subject to the Ordinances of Justice (1293) and under the state's scrutiny. This archive, in addition, gathered the wills of exiles or those who left property to those in exile or who were condemned by the Florentine commune. Third, they include those wills, again usually of magnates, who possessed special communal licenses to bear arms, which usually were transmitted to the eldest son or the male next of kin.

Thus, for Florence as well as for Arezzo, Perugia, Pisa, and Assisi, the parchment samples for this study were compiled from a number of archives, which before the centralization of the Hapsburg Pietro Leopoldo in 1784 or, for Perugia, before the unification of Italy were the prized charters of private ecclesiastical holdings. The major archive of individual parchments in Assisi still remains in the hands of an ecclesiastical institution—the Franciscan mother church, the Sacro Convento.[3] For these towns, I therefore could not avoid selecting parchment copies of wills from collections that—whether housed in public archives or not—still pertained to particular religious corporations or families. In all the cities except Florence,[4] I surveyed nearly all these ecclesiastical archives in order to include representative samples from hospitals, Benedictine monasteries, nunneries, and the mendicant orders.

I assembled the parchment samples by selecting testaments that from the inventory descriptions appeared to be complete last wills and tried to avoid codicils and those fragments copied by clerics for the purposes of their institutions. However, on occasion the eighteenth-century inventories incorrectly list fragments as complete testaments. Because of the small numbers of *pergamene* that archives (particularly the Archivio di Stato di Firenze) allow the scholar each day (eight documents at Florence), I nonetheless coded these fragments and entered them into my databank, but I excluded them from the tallies of pious and nonpious bequests as well as from the computations of the values for the legacies.[5]

With a multiple regression model, it is possible to estimate the weight of the selection from the various archives on the trends in the mean number of pious gifts over time and across geography. In these models, the "archive" variable proved significant; those testaments today preserved in vellum or taken from notarial protocols once kept in ecclesiastical archives, such as the *filze* of notarial contracts found in the archives of the hospital of Santa Chiara in Pisa, were redacted by wealthier testators who bequeathed more pious gifts per capita than testaments found scattered through the protocols of the public notaries. The effect of this variable (its beta coefficient) on the number of pious gifts, however, was less than all the other variables considered in the regression model:

gender, status, state of health (whether on deathbed or in good health), whether there were surviving sons, and six time periods.[6]

When the series of pious gifts is drawn from only those testaments once privately kept in ecclesiastical archives, the trends found for the data as a whole are not seriously modified. As in Siena, the numbers of pious bequests become higher than when testaments from the notarial books are included, particularly for the periods of the earliest charters through the Black Death of 1348. In Florence, pious bequests gathered solely from the parchment scrolls reach their apex a quarter-century earlier and are larger, 13.38 gifts as opposed to 9.92. Nonetheless, the trends traced by the records from the Diplomatico are similar: by 1326–47, the number of these gifts fell to 6.77, only slightly higher than that reflected by the data as a whole. Then, as in the overall data, the numbers rebound in the horrific summer months of 1348 to nearly the levels of the earlier part of the century. Immediately following the plague, the trend once again turned downward: those Florentines whose testaments were preserved in ecclesiastical archives gave fewer than six gifts apiece, and for the remainder of the Trecento through the early Quattrocento the numbers continued gradually to decline. Since a greater proportion of the testaments for Florence are taken from these various private ecclesiastical holdings, whose testaments included larger numbers of pious gifts than for any other city with the exception of Assisi, the tables in fact overstate the numbers of pious bequests found in Florence in comparison with the other cities, especially for the periods before the recurrence of pestilence in 1363.

For Arezzo, the parchment scrolls considered alone show some discrepancies. First, testators in the earliest documents for the quarter-century 1301–25 show levels of pious giving that rival even the extremely high figures gathered from Assisi. Since only five documents from the loose charters appear for these figures, their representativeness is highly questionable. For the years 1325–47, the pious bequests from the Diplomatico decline to numbers not out of line with those from testaments taken as a whole, but afterward the more privileged documents preserved in church archives do trace a trend at variance with that shown by the notarial records; the numbers of pious bequests, instead of gradually declining, continue to rise, reaching a peak in the years following the Black Death.

Part of the reason for this deviation results from the rich set of charters preserved in the testamentary collections kept by the confraternity archive of the Misericordia. This archive copied many of the

wills of the most wealthy testators in the territory of Arezzo. In addition
to the Tarlati will of 1348, which conveyed more in terms of the value
of gifts (5,937 florins) than any other testament except for the 1338 will
of the Pisan Donoratico, the Laici transcribed into their testamentary
ledgers the Trecento wills of members of other powerful Aretine lineages:
a nobleman from the Ubertini family, a doctor of canon and civil law
from the Acceptanti family, a widow from the Guasconi family.[7] In the
period after the recurrence of pestilence, 1364–75, the numbers of pious
bequests deviated once more from the trend now traced largely by the
gifts from the *notarile:* they jump to a level reminiscent of the early
Trecento, 11.2 gifts, which was substantially higher for that period than
for any of the other cities in our sample. Again, the Misericordia archives
were the culprit. In the third plague of 1374, a number of wealthy
Aretines deposited their testaments with the Laici. As we have seen,
these testaments from the third wave of pestilence in no way revived
the mendicant disdain for earthly hubris and the consequent desire to
liquidate and proliferate one's pious offerings across the landscape of
ecclesiastical institutions and holy causes.[8]

My regression model has controlled for these deviations in wealth
and status. When the Aretine testaments are regressed alone, the periods
1364–75, 1376–1400, and 1401–25 all show highly significant and strong
negative departures from the patterns of piety before the Black Death.[9]
In fact, the period 1376–1400 explains more of the variance than any
other variable in this model (beta $= -.312$), including wealth (beta
$= +.251$).

A comparison of the pious bequests from the Diplomatico in Pisa
with its total database, as in Siena, presents few deviations or surprises.
For the earliest documents until 1325, however, almost all the testaments
come from either parchment scrolls or notarial protocols kept by Pisa's
megahospital, Santa Chiara. The following period, 1326–47, in contrast,
relied heavily on both sources, and the pious bequests from the notarial
books slightly exceeded those from the more privileged ecclesiastical
archives. For the remainder of the documentation, the public notarial
books supplied the major portion of the testaments found in this sample.
In Pisa, unlike Arezzo, documents that came from the protocols generally
contained more pious gifts than those from the parchment scrolls. For
the latter part of the Trecento, the trends from both sets of documents
followed along similar lines, except for the crucial year of the plague's
return, 1362. Instead of a momentary reaction in the direction of the
ideals of piety held by the Pisan ancestors of the early part of the

century, the pious bequests found in the parchment scrolls continued their downward turn. But here the representativeness of the Diplomatico source should be questioned—for 1362, only five testaments came from these once-private archives.

For Perugia, our glimpse of testamentary piety before the Black Death is afforded almost exclusively by parchments and notarial protocols originally kept by ecclesiastical institutions. With the Black Death of 1348, the sample divides nearly equally between these once-private parchments and the testaments from public sources. In the subsequent periods, while both sources provide substantial numbers of testaments, the notarial records become the major source. The samples for these periods show a remarkable consistency between the two types of documents.[10] In the plague year of 1363, the frequency from the parchment rolls momentarily dipped below that recorded from the notarial sources, then returned to slightly more, winding up almost exactly the same at the end of this analysis.

Assisi is the one town where a comparison between the two sources is impossible. The archives of the Sacro Convento supply almost entirely the remarkable collection of early documents until the Black Death of 1348. Afterward, testaments from this source nearly disappear, while from the 1370s on they begin to appear in the earliest surviving public notarial books.

How, then, can we have confidence in the trends sketched by these two different sources? Could the change in piety—the drastic drop in the number of pious bequests after 1363—have been a fiction produced by the character of these two different samples? First, we have seen from the other cities that the parchment rolls generally do contain wealthier testators, who in fact made more bequests to pious institutions. The differences, however, between the samples compiled from the once-private archives and the total data never exceed three gifts per testator (for samples containing at least five testaments). And on occasion, even before 1348, bequests from the parchment samples could be inferior to those from the public notarial books. Second, although the parchment rolls may overstate the number of pious bequests for the early records from Assisi, these figures nonetheless reach higher frequencies than for any of the other city-states when only parchment rolls from these other places are considered. Third, when the numbers of pious bequests reached their highest point for this city, as well as for any other in this study, the majority of documents come no longer from the Sacro Convento but from other records housed in the cathedral archives.

Although the survival of records from Assisi makes it difficult to pinpoint the collapse in pious giving with the same precision as in the other cities, the handful of testaments that do survive for this plague year hint that the change took place in these summer months of relived trauma. Nonetheless, it is undeniable that at some time closely following the plague of 1363, piety in Assisi, as elsewhere studied in this book, underwent a total transformation. Indeed, what survives from the birthplace of Saint Francis suggests that the transformation there was indeed the most drastic of any found for any of these six city-states.

Catalog Numbers of the ASF, Notarile antecosimiano, Sampled for This Book

Pre-1989 Numbers	New Numbers	Provenance	Pre-1989 Numbers	New Numbers	Provenance
A164 (1414–20)	164	Florence	A981 (1254–75)	995	Florence
A195 (1338–48)	195	Florence	B296 (1421–39)	1,310	Florence
A205 (1363–84)	205	Florence	B516 (1403–23)	1,530	Florence
A775 (1391–1403)	788	Pisa	B744 (1400–1408)	1,758	Florence
A943 bis (1369–73)	957	Arezzo	B787 (1401–47)	1,801	Florence
A959 (1306–8)	973	Arezzo	B354 (1346–48)	1,368	Arezzo
A960 (1308–11)	974	Arezzo	B887 (1353–63)	1,901	Pisa
A961 (1311–12)	975	Arezzo	B902 (1348–60)	1,916	Arezzo
A962 (1312–13)	976	Arezzo	B905 (1375–79)	1,919	Arezzo
A963 (1313)	977	Arezzo	B907 (1392–1404)	1,921	Arezzo
A964 (1318)	978	Arezzo	B1258 (1377–80)	2,272	Arezzo
A965 (1318–19)	979	Arezzo	B1320 (1377–1441)	2,334	Florence
A966 (1320)	980	Arezzo	B1403 (1420–28)	2,417	Florence
A967 (1321)	981	Arezzo	B1607 (1423–26)	2,621	Florence
A968 (1322)	982	Arezzo	B1299 (1333–35)	2,313	Florence
A969 (1323–24)	983	Arezzo	B1955 (1406–7)	2,969	Pisa
A970 (1324)	984	Arezzo	B1340 (1296–1347)	2,354	Florence
A971 (1325)	985	Arezzo	B2568 (1356–63)	3,583	Florence
A972 (1326)	986	Arezzo	B2570 (1364–65)	3,584	Florence
A974 (1327)	988	Arezzo	B2744 (1401–17)	3,758	Pisa
A975 (1331–32)	989	Arezzo	C90 1415–19)	4,064	Florence
A976 (1332)	990	Arezzo	C187 (1406–8)	4,360	Florence
A977 (1332–33)	991	Arezzo	C197 (1362–64)	4,388	Pisa
A976 (1334)	992	Arezzo	C205 (1400–1414)	4,417	Florence
A979 (1328–36)	993	Arezzo	C256 (1416–23)	4,620	Florence
A980 (1331–39)	994	Arezzo	C295 (1347–62)	4,725	Pisa

Pre-1989 Numbers	New Numbers	Provenance	Pre-1989 Numbers	New Numbers	Provenance
C336 (1400–1430)	4,864	Florence	G167 (1326–48)	8,911	Florence
C356 (1331–35)	4,919	Arezzo	G331 (1413–20)	9,405	Pisa
C356 (1338–40)	4,920	Arezzo	G362 (1307–8)	9,483	Florence
C356 (1339–40)	4,921	Arezzo	G362 (1310)	9,484	Florence
C430 (1385–1412)	5,124	Florence	G362 (1313–15)	9,485	Florence
C462 (1301–5)	5,208	Pisa	G362 (1304–17)	9,486	Florence
C571 (1420–21)	5,474	Pisa	G373 (1385–90)	9,515	Arezzo
C605 (1327–30)	5,553	Florence	G374 (1409–19)[a]	9,523	Arezzo
C605 (1330–32)	5,554	Florence	G381 (1358–62)	9,541	Arezzo
C605 (1332–34)	5,555	Florence	G386 (1291–1308)	9,550	Pisa
C733 (1370–72)	5,880	Arezzo	G404 (1371–75)	9,592	Arezzo
C733 (1372–73)	5,881	Arezzo	G449 (1367–76)	9,689	Arezzo
C733 (1373–74)	5,882	Arezzo	G449 (1392–96)	9,690	Arezzo
C733 (1373–77)	5,883	Arezzo	G449 (1396–99)	9,691	Arezzo
C734 (1343–51)	5,884	Arezzo	G553 (1405–12)	9,981	Arezzo
C734 (1350–67)	5,885	Arezzo	G553 (1409–15)	9,982	Arezzo
C734 (1363–64)	5,886	Arezzo	G624 (1349–50)	10,213	Arezzo
C735 (1362–63)	5,891	Arezzo	G779 (1390–97)	10,736	Arezzo
C735 (1363–64)	5,892	Arezzo	G779 (1401–2)	10,738	Arezzo
D121 (1383–86)	6,292	Arezzo	G779 (1403–4)	10,739	Arezzo
F305 (1409–53)	7,401	Florence	G782 (1423–31)	10,747	Arezzo
F374 (1329–37)	7,575	Pisa	G837 (1349)	10,910	Arezzo
F374 (1338–43)	7,576	Pisa	G837 (1350–51)	10,911	Arezzo
F375 (1339–41)	7,577	Pisa	G837 (1352–54)	10,912	Arezzo
F375 (1340–44)	7,578	Pisa	G837 (1360)	10,913	Arezzo
F380 (1382–85)	7,588	Pisa	G837 (1360–61)	10,914	Arezzo
F527 (1401–2)	7,991	Pisa	G837 (1362)[a]	10,915	Arezzo
F527 (1404)	7,992	Pisa	I14 (1348–49)	11,050	Pisa
F556 (1406–24)	8,066	Pisa	I22 (1350–56)	11,063	Pisa
F556 (1407–24)	8,067	Pisa	I22 (1358–61)	11,064	Pisa
F556 (1411–16)	8,068	Pisa	I22 (1361–71)	11,065	Pisa
F557 (1417–21)	8,069	Pisa	I23 (1369–75)	11,066	Pisa
F557 (1419–46)	8,070	Pisa	I23 (1376–80)	11,067	Pisa
F558 (1422–27)	8,071	Pisa	I52 (1376–1426)	11,127	Arezzo
F565 (1320–22)	8,097	Pisa	I52 (1398–1412)	11,128	Arezzo
F569 (1360–64)	8,105	Pisa	I102 (1368–70)	11,247	Arezzo
F570 (1356–78)	8,110	Pisa	I102 (1371–76)	11,248	Arezzo
F598 (1421)	8,189	Pisa	I104 (1276–1311)	11,250	Florence
G167 (1303–34)	8,910	Florence	L76 (1298–1327)	11,484	Florence

Pre-1989 Numbers	New Numbers	Provenance	Pre-1989 Numbers	New Numbers	Provenance
L256 (1378–92)	12,063	Florence	N160 (1382)	15,219	Florence
L256 (1392–1411)	12,064	Florence	N160 (1385)	15,220	Florence
L256 (1411–25)	12,065	Florence	N174 (1339–59)	15,256	Pisa
L384 (1356–59)	12,392	Pisa	P228 (1374–83)	16,489	Arezzo
L384 (1359–62)	12,393	Pisa	R40 (1268–78)	17,563	Florence
L384 (1359–63)	12,394	Pisa	R206 (1385–1416)	18,041	Arezzo
M293 (1294–96)	13,363	Florence	T179 (1338–48)	20,307	Florence
M293 (1300–1314)	13,364	Florence	U122 (1360–82)	20,729	Pisa
N160 (1372)	15,217	Florence	V67 (1328–49)	20,833	Arezzo
N160 (1377)	15,218	Florence			

[a]Booklet composed solely of testaments.

A Gazetteer of Villages and Provincial Towns Mentioned in the Text

Agnano (Aretine): In the Val d'Ambra, 21 km west of Arezzo; Repetti, 1: 56–57.

Agnano (Pisan): In the Pian di Pisa to the west of the Monte Pisano, 6 km northeast of Pisa.

Allimite: Limite, Limiti, in the Valdarno inferiore, in the diocese of Pistoia; Repetti, 2: 698.

Ascagnano: An abandoned castle village in a dominant position above the Val Teverino, 15 km from Perugia, 7 km from Umbertide; Grohmann, 2: 983–84.

Asciano: A walled town in the Val d'Ombrone, 24 km southeast of Siena; Repetti, 1: 151–56.

Bibbiena: In the diocese of Arezzo, 5.5 km south of Poppi, 31.7 km north of Arezzo in the Valdarno casentinese; Repetti, 1: 310–14.

Bonèggio (Castello di poggio): about 8 km south of Perugia; Grohmann, 2: 917, 973.

Buti: In the Valdarno inferiore, in the diocese of Pisa, 6 km north of Vicopisano; Repetti, 1: 376.

Calci: 13 km east of Pisa, the site of the Certosa di Pisa, founded in 1366; Repetti, 1: 384–85.

Calcinaria, Calcinaja: in the Valdarno pisano 4.5 km southeast of Vicopisano, 19 km west of Pisa; Repetti, 1: 386–88.

Campora: In the southern suburbs of Florence attached to an Augustinian monastery which Pope Eugenio IV suppressed in 1434; Repetti, 1: 432.

Capolona: In the Valdarno aretino, 10 km northeast of Arezzo; Repetti, 1: 459–60.

Cappaja: Probably Capraja in the Valdarno inferiore, less than 1 km northeast of Montelupo, 21 km east of Florence; Repetti, 1: 462–64.

Cappiani, Cappiano: In the Valdarno superiore in the parish of Incisa, 6 km southeast of Rignano; Repetti, 1: 462.

Careggi: 3 km northwest of Florence; Repetti, 1: 474.

Casalina: On the road to Todi, near the Tiber River, about 3 km south of Deruta, it was the seat of one of the oldest and most important possessions of the monastery of San Pietro in Perugia; Grohmann, 2: 919.

Cascia: In the Valdarno superiore, the diocese of Fiesole, 3 km southeast of Regello.

Casciana: In the Pisan hills of the Val d'Era, 4 km west of Lari; Repetti, 1: 500.

Cascina: A walled village in the Valdarno pisano, 8 km west of Pontedra; Repetti, 1: 503–6.

Castelfiorentino: A principal market town in the Valdelsa, 39 km north of Volterra, 36 km southwest of Florence; Repetti, 1: 535–39.

Castel Focognano: In the Valdarno casentinese, 10 km miles west of Poppi, 24 km north-northeast of Arezzo; Repetti, 1: 540–41.

Castel Leone: In the hills about 2.75 km southeast of Deruta; Grohmann, 2: 921–22.

Castelnuovo: Castelnuovo d'Avane, in the diocese of Fiesole, on the eastern slopes of the hills that separate the Chianti and the Valle superiore of the Pesa from the Arno; Repetti, 1: 171.

Castro Casalalte: In the hills above the Val Teverino, about 2 km from Castelleone.

Castro Sieci: Castel-Secco or Poggio di S. Cornelio in the southern suburbs of Arezzo; Repetti, 1: 585.

Catignano: In the Valdarbia, about 6 km northeast of Siena; Repetti, 1: 622.

Celaria (Cegliuolo): In the diocese of Arezzo, Val di Chiana (S. Pietro); Repetti, 1: 641.

Chiana: At the northernmost tip of the Val di Chiana, 7 km west of Arezzo.

Chianciano (Clancianum): In the Val di Chiara, 12 km northeast of Chiusi; Repetti, 1: 687–91.

Chiusi: Possibly the Etruscan metropolis in the Val di Chiana, 60 km south-southeast of Arezzo, but more likely Chiusi (del Casentino) in the Valdarno casentinese 16 km east of Poppi; Repetti, 1: 725–29.

Cisanello: In the eastern suburbs of Pisa on the right bank of the Arno, reputedly the birthplace of Pisa's patron saint, Ranieri; Repetti, 1: 740.

Citerna: In the hills above the Val di Sovara on the border of Tuscany and Umbria, about 30 km east of Arezzo.

Collinis (Colline Pisane): In the Pisan Maremma, bordered to the southeast by the Cascina River, about 110 square miles; Repetti, 1: 776–77.

Colonica: In the Valle dell'Ombrone pistoiese, the diocese of Pistoia, 3 km west of the city.

Corciano: A well-preserved castle town about 13 km east-northeast of Perugia, admirably portrayed in Bonfigli's painting of the plague in 1472; Grohmann, 2: 932–33.

Cordigliano: Above the Tiber River, about 7 km north-northeast of Perugia.

Cortina: In the Valdelsa, 4.5 km east-southeast of Barberino Valdelsa; Repetti, 1: 810–11.

Empoli: A major market town along the Arno, 30 km west of Florence; Repetti, 2: 55–68.

Falcona: Most likely, Faltona in the Valdarno casentinese in the jurisdiction of Castel-Focognano and the diocese of Arezzo; Repetti, 2: 92.

Faltone: High in the southern part of the Pratomagna Mountains (722 meters in altitude), in the Valdarno casentinese about 25 km north of Arezzo; Repetti, 2: 92.

Foiano: The principal market town of the Val di Chiana, about 28 km south of Arezzo; Repetti, 2: 312–18; Neretti, *Foiano della chiana.*

Fontigiano: Presently an abandoned castle without traces of its village walls, 17 km southeast of Perugia; Grohmann, 2: 655, 962.

Forgone: *See* Lippiano.

Fronzola, Frongola, Frònzola, Fonzano: About 2 km south of Poppi in the Valdarno casentinese; Repetti, 2: 347.

Gangalandi: About 14 km west of Florence, near Lastra a Signa; see Repetti, 2: 396–97.

Giampareto: Giampereta, in the Valdarno casentinese, in the diocese of Bibbiena and the diocese of Arezzo; Repetti, 2: 443.

Giovo: Borgo a Giovi, on the Arno in the Valdarno aretino, 7.5 km north of Arezzo; Repetti, 2: 450.

Lari: A diocese in the Colline superiori pisane, 30 km southeast of Pisa; Repetti, 2: 644–49.

Legoli: In the Val d'Era in the diocese of Volterra; at the beginning of the Trecento, the Pisan republic occupied its castle and destroyed it in 1336; Repetti, 2: 675–77.

Lignano (Poggio di): In the Val di Chiana in the parish of Bagnolo; the hermitage was dedicated to Saint Martin; Repetti, 2: 696.

Lippiano: In the Val Tiberina, near Monte S. Maria, about 30 km west of Arezzo; Repetti, 2: 702–3.

Lorenzano: Also called Zenna, in the Valdarno casentinese, north of Arezzo; Repetti, 2: 806.

Maiano: A village in the hills beneath Fiesole, 7 km from the center of Florence.

Marcena: About 10 km north of Arezzo in the Valdarno aretino; Repetti, 3: 52.

Marignolla: Marignolle, in the Valdarno fiorentino in the southwest rural suburbs of Florence; Repetti, 3: 79–80.

Marti: A fortified village in the Valdarno inferiore, 6 km north of Palaia, in the jurisdiction of Pontedra; Repetti, 3: 101–2.

Massa (di Carrara): seat of the princes of its territory, 39 km northwest of Pisa; Repetti, 3: 115–56.

Massargia: Possibly Collemassari in the Valle d'Ombrone in the diocese of Grosseto 4.5 km east of Cinigiano; Repetti, 1: 767–68.

Mezzano: 16 km south of Florence.

Montaguto Barbolanarum: In the Valdarno superiore, in the casentino near Castel S. Niccolò; Repetti, 3: 270.

Monte Calvi: Perhaps the deserted village of Calbi in the hills 9 km southeast of Arezzo.

Montecchio: In the Val di Chiana, 6 km southwest of Cortona; Repetti, 3: 367–68.

Monte Feyche: Probably Fexhe (or Fech) haut Clocher, about 14 km west of Liège; Graesse, Benedict, and Plechl, Orbis Latinus, 2: 374; Carte Topographique de la Belgique, no. 41 (Waremme); Friex, Tables des cartes des Pays Bas; de Lat, Reis -en handatlas.

Montelupo: In the Valdarno inferiore, about 24 km west of Florence; Repetti, 3: 412–16.

Monte Pacciano: About 10 km north-northwest of Perugia. The nearest village is the parish of S. Orfito, which possessed only 9 hearths in the Estimo of 1282; Grohmann, 2: 665.

Monterone: Montarone, Montirone di Sestino, in the Valle della Foglia, the diocese of Borgo San Sepolcro and the territory of Arezzo; Repetti, 3: 322–23.

Monte San Savino: The principal market town of the Val di Chiana, within the diocese of Arezzo, 26 km to the city's west; Repetti, 3: 519–26.

Monte Ugo: Montughi, 1 km outside of Florence to the northwest, in the Commune of Fiesole; Repetti, 3: 604.

Montozzi: In the foothills of the Chianti (404 meters) in the Val d'Ambra Arno, about 18 km west of Arezzo; Repetti, 3, 603–4.

Morniano: In the Valdarno superiore, the diocese of Incisa, 10.5 km northeast of Figline. In 1833, the parish numbered 111; Repetti, 1: 612.

Mucciano: In the Val di Sieve, 4.5 km north-northeast of Borgo San Lorenzo; Repetti, 3: 625.

Navacchio: In the Valdarno pisano, 8 km east of Pisa; Repetti, 3: 638.

Novoli: Nuovoli, in the Valdarno fiorentino, 3 km west of Florence; Repetti, 3: 648–49.

Palaia: A village southeast of San Miniato.

Papiano: A castle in the Val Teverino, about 23 km south of Perugia, 5 km north of Marsciano; Grohmann, 2: 969.

Parrano: South of Pisa in the Monte Livornesi; see Repetti, 4: 61.

Peretola: In the western suburbs of Florence, 3.75 km from the center of Florence; Repetti, 4: 101–2.

Pesciola: A hamlet in the Vald'Elsa, near Castel Fiorentino; Repetti, 4: 138.

Petriolo: In the Valdarno fiorentino, between Sesto and Florence, 5 km west of the latter; Repetti, 4: 144–45.

Pietramala: In the Valdarno aretino, now the site of ruins of the medieval castle of the Tarlati, 6 km northeast of Arezzo; Repetti, 4: 211–12.

Pilonico: Pilonico Paterno, about 10 km northwest of Perugia in the Chiasco River valley; Grohmann, 2: 932, 970.

Poggibonsi: In the Valdelsa, on the border between the territories of Florence and Siena; Repetti, 4: 480–87.

Pontedera: A major market town on the Arno, 26 km east of Pisa; Repetti, 5: 526–32.

Poppi: In the Valdarno casentinese, in the diocese of Arezzo; earlier the resident castle of the counts Guidi da Battifolle, whom Henry VI in 1191 made counts of "all of Tuscany"; 39 km north-northwest of Arezzo; Repetti, 4: 565–77.

Poppiano: In the Val di Pesa, 2.5 km northeast of Montespértoli; Repetti, 4: 577–78.

Pratovecchio: In the Valdarno casentino, 10 km north of Poppi.

Pupigliano: In the Valle dell'ombrone pistojese, in the district of Florence; Repetti, 4: 687.

Quarata: 6 km northwest of Arezzo in the Valdarno aretino; Repetti, 4: 688.

Sallecti: Collis Salvecti, Colle-Salvetti, 10 km southeast of Pisa; Repetti, 1: 770.

San Casciano: 20 km south of Florence on the via Cassia in the Val di Pesa.

San Genesio: Borgo San Genesio. The original settlement of San Miniato, 3 km east of San Miniato; Repetti, 1: 352.

San Gervasio: In the eastern suburbs of Florence, 2 km from the city; Repetti, 2: 433–34.

San Gimignano: In the Valdelsa, 33 km northwest of Siena. An independent city-state until Florentine conquest in 1354; Repetti, 5: 35–60; Fiumi, San Gimignano.

San Lorenzo (Aretine): A village of that name lies 10 km south of Cortona; another S. Lorenzo, closer to Arezzo, lies about 3 km south of Anghiari and by road about 30 km from Arezzo.

San Marco: San Marco al Mugnone, in the rural suburbs 4 km north of Florence; Repetti, 1: 64.

San Martino de Colle: In the diocese of Lucca but in the contado of Pistoia, located on the border between the two city-states. The church was a dependency of the Benedictine abbey of S. Benedetto a Polirone sul Pò; Repetti, 1: 761.

San Piero ad Maccadium (Macadio): In the Val di Serchio, in the Commune of Bagni a San Giuliano, the diocese of Pisa; Repetti, 3: 5.

San Pietro a Monticelli: In the southwest suburbs of Florence, near Legnaia.

Sanpolo: Pieve in the Valdarno aretino, 3 km north-northeast of Arezzo; Repetti, 4: 499–500.

San Salvatore a Pilli: Val d'Arbia, 7.5 km southeast of Sovicille and about 16 km south of Siena; Repetti, 4: 264.

Santa Fiora: The ancestral castle town of the counts Aldobrandeschi, on the slopes of Monte Amiata, 7.4 km southeast of Arcidosso and 82 km southeast of Siena; Repetti, 5: 143–59.

Santa Fiora (Aretine): In the Valdarno casentinese, the diocese of Arezzo, 4.5 km east of Castel Focognano; Repetti, 1: 473.

Santa Maria alla Torre: 400 meters from Poppiano; see above.

Santa Maria Castello: A Santa Maria de Castellis or de Castro Castellis existed in the diocese of Amelia (Rationes Decimarum, vol. 161, nos. 567, 569), but it was most likely Castelleone, whose plebis church was named Santa Maria and was in the contado of Perugia.

Sant'Anastasio a Quarto: In the Val di Chiana, 6 km southwest of Arezzo; Repetti, 1: 83.

Scarperia (Castro di): In the Val di Sieve (Mugello), 34 km north of Florence; Repetti, 5: 221–29.

Serra: Villa della Serra or Seravalle, in the Valdarno casentinese, a castle village 10 km north of Bibbiena, in the diocese of Arezzo; Repetti, 5: 245–46.

Stalla, Montaguto or Montagutello di Talla: In the Valdarno casentinese, site of a castle in ruins, near Bibbiena in the diocese of Arezzo; Repetti, 3: 272.

Torciana: In the curia of Parrano and diocese of Pisa; Rationes Decimarum, vol. 98, p. 244, n. 3752.

Torre Classeris (Chiassa): In the Valdarno aretino, along the torrente Chiassa; two pievi and a destroyed castle; Repetti, 1: 699–700.

Vecchiano: In the Valle inferiore of the Serchio, 6.75 km north of Pisa;

Repetti, 5: 681–84.

Veruta: Verruca del Monte Pisano in the Vladarno northeast of Pisa; Repetti, 5: 701.

Vicchio: In the Val di Sieve, 29 km northeast of Florence; Repetti, 5: 748–51.

Vico: Vico Fiorentino, in the Valdelsa 6 km southwest of Barberino; Repetti, 5: 753–54.

Vico: Vicopisano, in the valdarno about 18 km east of Pisa; Repetti, 5: 757–66.

Vignale: Vignale di Agazzi, the curia of Santa Fiora, in the Valdarno aretino, 3.75 km southwest of Arezzo; Repetti, 5: 768.

Villa Ama: Hamlet near Camaldoli, the diocese of Fiesole, 3 km northeast of Pratovecchio; Repetti, 1: 78.

Villa Fratte di Sant'Andrea: small village 7 km southwest of Perugia. In the Estimo of 1282 it registered only 19 hearths; Grohmann, 2: 655, 971–72.

Villalba: In the Valdarno aretino, 6 km north of Arezzo; Repetti, 5: 773.

Villa Mori: In the diocese of Arezzo, listed in the Rationes Decimarum of 1302–3, vol. 98, p. 129, n. 2317, under "Ecclesia S. Blaxii."

Villa Plancarpinis: In the Estimo of 1282, the villa Plani Carpinis of the Porta S. Susanna, which lay beneath the Castle of Monte Colognole in the mountains above Lake Trasimeno, had 180 hearths. By the next surviving tax register (1438), the village no longer existed; Grohmann, 2: 636, 652, 779.

Villa San Sisto: Castle village on Monte Lacugnano about 4 km southeast of Perugia; Grohmann, 2: 999.

Vinci: In the Valdarno inferiore, 11 km north of Empoli; Repetti, 5: 785–90.

Vitiano: In the hills above the Val di Chiana, north of Castiglion Fiorentino and about 10 km south of Arezzo; Repetti, 5: 793.

The principal sources for these listings are the Carte d'Italia 1:25,000; the Rationes Decimarum; Repetti, Dizionario geografico fiscio e storico della Toscana; and Grohmann, Città e territorio, vol. 2. Larger towns mentioned in the text—Borgo San Sepolcro, Cortona, Pistoia, and San Miniato al Tedesco—can easily be spotted on any general map of Italy.

Notes

1. Introduction

1. See Mundy, "Charity and Social Work," 203–87, and Trexler, "The Bishop's Portion," 408: "The church lived first of all off its landed investment, and it ever reinvigorated this investment through testamentary charity." For confraternities in Borgo San Sepolcro, Banker, *Death in the Community*, chapter 3, argues that pious bequests from last wills became their mainstay by the early fourteenth century. On the other hand, Gavitt, *Charity and Children*, 109, finds that income from testaments, 1448–59, constituted only 4 percent of the annual income of the Florentine Ospedale degli Innocenti. But, in surveying the account books of numerous minor hospitals in the *contado* of Siena, Balestracci, "Per una storia degli ospedali," 41, finds that testamentary legacies constituted their principal source of income.

2. Tetel, Witt, and Goffen, *Life and Death in Fifteenth-Century Florence*, vii.

3. Martines, "The Uses of Mortality," 956.

4. For instance, see Herlihy, *Pistoia*; Herlihy and Klapisch-Zuber, *Les Toscans*; Weissman, *Ritual Brotherhood*; and Molho and Kirshner, "The Dowry Fund."

5. *The Civilization of the Renaissance in Italy*, first published in 1860.

6. Elio Conti, *La formazione*; Cherubini, *Signori, Contadini, Borghesi*; Herlihy and Klapisch-Zuber, *Les Toscans*; Imberciadori, *Mezzadria classica toscana*; Pinto, *La Toscana*; Pinto and Pirillo, *Il contratto di mezzadria*; Balestracci, *La zappa e la retorica*; Piccini, *"Seminare, fruttare, raccogliere"*; *Contadini e proprietari*; Sereni, *Storia del paesaggio*; Mazzi and Raveggi, *Gli uomini e le cose*.

7. See Brucker, *Giovanni and Lusanna*; Bizzocchi, *Chiesa e potere*; Trexler, *Synodal Law*; and Peterson, "Conciliarism, Republicanism, and Corporatism," "An Episcopal Election," and work in progress on Archbishop Antoninus.

8. Cohn, *The Laboring Classes*.

9. See Maier, "La storia comparata," 1395; Cohn, "La 'nuova storia sociale,'" 370–71; and Pastore, *Crimine e giustizia*, vii–xvi.

10. Dale Kent, *The Rise of the Medici*; Francis W. Kent, *Household and Lineage*; Kent and Kent, *Neighbours and Neighbourhood*.

11. In addition to the Kents, cited in n. 10, Cohn, *The Laboring Classes*, Weissman, *Ritual Brotherhood*, and Goldthwaite, *Private Wealth* and *The Building of Renaissance Florence*, consider questions of neighborhood and family almost exclusively within the Florentine context.

12. *The Crisis of the Early Italian Renaissance.* More recently, Burke, *Culture and Society,* 268–72, has tempered Baron's interpretations but nonetheless argues for the centrality of Florence in the formation of an Italian Renaissance culture until the Peace of Lodi (1454).

13. See *L'Umanesimo italiano* and *Portraits from the Quattrocento,* as well as Gilmore, *The World of Italian Humanism.* For a fundamental work of the nineteenth century that singled out Florence as "the highest expression of Italian genius offered to Europe in its transition towards the modern world," see Leo, *Entwicklung der Verfassung.*

14. See Goldberg, *After Vasari,* 3–14, and *Patterns in Late Medici Art Patronage,* 5–20; also Rearick, *Dynasty and Destiny.* For more recent examples of Florence's crucial role in the formation of Renaissance culture, see Wackernagel, *The Florentine Artist,* and Goldthwaite, *The Building of Renaissance Florence.*

15. The anthropological works of Pitt-Rivers, "Honour and Social Status"; Schneider, "Of Vigilance and Virgins"; Campbell, *Honour, Family, and Patronage;* and Davis, *Land and Family* and *People of the Mediterranean,* now resonate through numerous works on Renaissance Florence.

16. While the use of anthropology has opened new vistas for historians, certain key concepts such as honor and shame have been borrowed as though they were transhistorical. See, for example, Kirshner, *Pursuing Honor;* Trexler, *Public Life;* Kuehn, " 'Cum Consensu mundualdi' "; Molho, "Visions of the Florentine Family"; Rosenthal, "The Position of Women"; Weissman, *Ritual Brotherhood* and "Taking Patronage Seriously"; Gavitt, *Charity and Children,* 79, 84, 279; and most objectionably, Burke, *Historical Anthropology,* where the use of "pop" anthropology verges on Mediterranean racism. See my review in *American Historical Review.* For a criticism within the anthropological literature of the unity of a Mediterranean world, see Goody, *The Development of the Family and Kinship,* 6–7. Goitein's *A Mediterranean Society* begins with a Braudelian view of the Mediterranean, at least for the period 969–1250 (vol. 1, chap. 1), but departs from it by the end of this multivolume study of Jews reflected in the Cairo documents (vol. 5).

17. Curiously, Edwardian historians in the early twentieth century, who made no pretense to interdisciplinary history, were more comparative in their narratives of individual city-states than most social historians of Florence of the late twentieth century. See, in particular, the studies of Heywood, *A History of Perugia* and *Palio and Ponte;* Douglas, *A History of Siena;* and Schevill, *Siena.*

18. For a defense of this "Annaliste" approach, see Le Goff and Toubert, "Une histoire totale," 37, and Tabacco's criticisms of "total history" in *The Struggle for Power,* 34–35.

19. See Heywood, *Perugia,* and degli Azzi Vitelleschi, *Le Relazioni.*

20. I use the term *city-state* loosely. The testaments derive predominantly from those who resided in the cities (78.42 percent) as opposed to the surrounding territories. All of these cities were bishoprics or archbishoprics; those

testaments from the surrounding countryside tended to fall within the confines of the dioceses of these towns.

21. For an excellent survey of published collections of testaments and interpretative materials for late medieval and early modern Italy, see Bertram, "Mittelalterliche Testamente."

22. For Bologna, see Bertram, "Hundert Bologneser Testamente" and "Bologneser Testamente." For Orvieto, see Riccetti, "Orvieto" and *Il duomo di Orvieto;* Caponeri, "Nota su alcuni testamenti"; and Caponeri and Riccetti, *Chiese e conventi degli ordini mendicanti in Umbria nei secoli XII–XIV.* For Borgo, see Banker, *Death in the Community.*

23. See Grohmann, *Città e territorio* and *Perugia.*

24. For example, see the surveys in D'Angiolini and Pavone, *Guida generale;* Mazzatinti, *Gli Archivi;* and Mazzatinti, Pulignani, and Santoni, *Archivio storico.*

25. Bowsky, "The Impact of the Black Death," 6, 9. Bartolotti, *Siena,* 19, questions this figure and argues that the city in 1328 numbered no more than 25,000.

26. Tangheroni, *Politica, commercio, agricoltura,* 77; Rossi, "Lo sviluppo demografico."

27. Cristiani, *Nobiltà e popolo,* 166–68.

28. Grohmann, *Perugia,* 20–21. Mira, "L'estimo di Perugia," 397–400, estimated the population to be between 27,600 and 38,700. According to Mira, "Il fabbisogno dei cereali," 505–17, the population remained at this level through the early fourteenth century: 28,000 in the city; 45,000 in the *contado.*

29. Black, *Benedetto Accolti,* 17. Dini, "Lineamenti per la storia," 7, describes the precarious nature of population figures for Arezzo before the end of the fourteenth century but speculates that the city population ranged between 18,000 and 20,000, and that the population of the territory "certainly surpassed 100,000." The figure—18,000—supposedly comes from a census of 1321 (see Aldinucci, "Economia aretina," 8). Based on Varese, "Condizioni economiche," Cherubini, "Schede per uno studio," 6, puts the figure for the city population at 13,000.

30. Grohmann, *Assisi,* 35. Mira, "Aspetti di vita economica," 130–31, puts it between 11,300 and 15,800. Fortini, *Nova vita di s. Francesco,* has published the tax record. According to Grohmann, *Assisi,* 49, the city must have grown beyond this point, since two new circuits of city walls were constructed afterward, one in 1260 and the other in 1316.

31. For Florence, see Herlihy and Klapisch-Zuber, *Les Toscans,* 181, and Pampaloni, "Popolazione e società," 361–93.

32. Herlihy and Klapisch-Zuber, *Les Toscans,* 348.

33. For the period after the plague, 1427–29, Luzzati, "I registri notarili," 19, estimates the population of the city to have been around 7,500 and the *contado,* 15,000. In the second half of the fourteenth century, della Pina, "Andamento e distribuzione," 25–27, estimates that the population of city and

contado was around 35,000. By the end of the fifteenth century, he finds little difference: 10,000 for the city and 20,000 for its countryside.

34. Dini, *Arezzo intorno al 1400*, v. According to Varese, "Condizioni economiche," the city population numbered circa 9,000 in 1389, 7,000 after the plague in 1393, and between 5,500 and 6,000 from 1403 to 1468.

35. Herlihy, "The Distribution of Wealth," 133. Dini, *Arezzo intorno al 1400*, v, puts it at 4,152 and estimates the population of its territory at 19,397 ("Lineamenti per la storia," 7). Arezzo's decline between the Estimo of 1390 and the Catasto of 1427 was less drastic than for Pisa and Pistoia, which were also of middling size; see Varese, "Condizioni economiche," 17, and Herlihy and Klapisch-Zuber, *Les Toscans*, 180.

36. Based on the statistics presented in Pardi, "La popolazione di Siena."

37. Grohmann, *Perugia*, 60–61.

38. Based on the statistics presented in Ottolenghi, "Studi demografici," and Pardi, "La popolazione di Siena."

39. Beloch, *Bevölkerungsgeschichte Italiens*, 1: 74.

40. Herlihy, *Pisa*, 185–86.

41. The son of the former, hereafter abbreviated f.q.

42. Archivio di Stato di Firenze (hereafter abbreviated ASF), Diplomatico (hereafter abbreviated Dipl.), S.M. Novella, 1396.vi.24.

43. ASF, Dipl., S.M. Novella, 1351.iv.2.

44. On Pisan long-distance emigration, see Petralia, "Per la storia dell'emigrazione."

45. Archivio di Stato di Pisa (hereafter ASPi), Osp. di S. Chiara, no. 2070, 343ᵛ–345ʳ, 1285.v.5; 23r–25v, 1285.xii.10.

46. Ibid., no. 2071, 23r–25v, 1285.xii.10.

47. ASPi, Dipl., Primaziale, 1386.ix.12.

48. Ibid., S. Marta, 1324.vii.23.

49. Only two examples appear in the Florentine samples: ASF, Dipl., S.M. Novella, 1371.ii.3; idem, Arch. Gen., 1413.iv.12.

50. On the slave trade in Pisa, see Ashtor, *Levant Trade;* for Tuscany, see Origio, "The Domestic Enemy"; and on slavery more generally during the Middle Ages in Europe, see Verlinden, *L'esclavage*, and Heers, *Esclaves et domestiques.*

51. On the various cycles and relative values of slaves of different origins, see Bresc, *Un monde méditerranéen*, 1: 439–54. The Tartars, particularly women, were highly valued in the slave trade of the second half of the fourteenth century.

52. In Pisa, the parish was called a *cappella.*

53. ASF, Not. antecos., no. 11,065, 46r, 1360.vi.4.

54. See Herlihy, *Pistoia*, 155–60, "The Distribution of Wealth"; Malanima, "L'attività industriali," 217–80; Tangheroni, "Il sistema economico della toscana," 57–62; Melis, "Lazzaro Bracci," "Momenti dell'economia del Casentino"; and Grohmann, *Perugia*, 23–24, *Città e territorio*, 2: 609–79.

55. Lopez and Miskimin, "The Economic Depression of the Renaissance," 408–27; Lopez, "Hard Times and Investment in Culture." For a review of this literature, see Brown, "Prosperity or Hard Times?" Sapori, *Le marchand italien*, lvii, also stressed the relative decline of Italy after the Black Death. For the development of this thesis in Italian historiography, see Romano, *Tra due crisi*.

56. See Cohn, "Florentine Insurrections," 160–62.

57. Banti, *D'Appiano*, 9, 59, 71–93.

58. Herlihy, *Pistoia*, 155–60, "The Distribution of Wealth," 137ff.; Herlihy and Klapisch-Zuber, *Les Toscans*, 291–300.

59. Goldthwaite, *The Building of Renaissance Florence*, "The Medici Bank," "The Empire of Things."

60. For the earlier view, see Mengozzi, *Il monte dei Paschi;* Heywood, *Perugia;* Ross and Erichsen, *The Story of Pisa;* Silva, *Pisa sotto Firenze;* Rossi Sabatini, *L'espansione;* and, more recently, Herlihy, *Pisa;* Hook, *Siena;* and Ginatempo, *Crisi di un territorio*, especially 58off.

61. Hicks, "Sources of Wealth."

62. Mira, "Aspetti dell'organizzazione corporativa," "Aspetti di vita economica," 152–53.

63. Pierotti, "Aspetti del mercato."

64. Grohmann, *Perugia*, 23–24, *Città e territorio*, 609–79; for the countryside, see Desplanques, *Campagnes ombriennes*.

65. Tangheroni, *Politica, commercio, agricoltura*, 79, 103–7.

66. Historians have seen this event as the turning point in Pisan history; see, most recently, Caleca, "Profilo dell'arte pisana," 9; Baldelli, "La letteratura volgare," 73.

67. Melis, "L'economia delle città minori," goes the farthest of these authors, claiming that "in 1406 nothing changed." See Tangheroni's criticism in the introduction to Melis's *Industria e commercio*, xxiv–xxv.

68. *Politica, commercio, agricoltura*.

69. Mallett, *The Florentine Galleys*, 3–20, "Pisa and Florence."

70. Silva, *Pisa sotto Firenze*, 19ff.; Ross and Erichsen, *The Story of Pisa*, 68–87.

71. See Melis, "Lazzaro Bracci"; Cherubini, "Schede per uno studio"; Aldinucci, "Economia aretina"; and Pardo, *Arezzo*. For a negative picture of the Aretine economy by the third decade of the Quattrocento, see Dini, "Lineamenti per la storia"; Black, *Benedetto Accolti*, 11.

72. "Schede per uno studio," 3. See also Aldinucci's comments in "Economia aretina": "Nei trattati di storia economica l'importanza di Arezzo è sottovalutata e se ne parla indirettamente e solo per esultare Firenze alla quale Arezzo fu sottomessa" (3).

73. Wieruszowski, "Arezzo as a Center of Learning," and Lazzeri, *Guglielmino Ubertini*, 110, claim that the university was in serious decline by the beginning of the fourteenth century and had ceased to exist by 1327.

74. See Luzzati, *Firenze e la Toscana,* 128; Aldinucci, "Economia aretina," 3; and Black, *Benedetto Accolti,* 5–12, "Humanism and Education." In the last-named, Black states, "Under Florentine rule after 1384, Arezzo was a decaying city with a falling population, growing impoverishment and a depressed economy" (214). However, Black's evidence for decline, like Dini's in "Lineamenti per la storia," comes from the 1420s and 1430s. For a similar trajectory of economic stability and decline, see Cassandro's evidence for Prato in "Commercio, manifatture, e industrie," 418–19.

75. The first historian to argue against the view that cultural and economic decline accelerated after the loss of independence was Pasqui, *Documenti,* 1: xv. See also Melis, "Lazzaro Bracci," 175–91. Aldinucci, "Economia aretina," 13ff., closely follows Melis's interpretation, much of which is based on the career of Arezzo's premier merchant, Lazzaro Bracci. On the other hand, Dini, "Lineamenti per la storia," 16, interprets the changes in Bracci's career around 1390 as a sign of "difficulties" in the Aretine wool industry. According to Nicolaj [Petronio], "Notariato aretino," 635–36, both the earlier *"campanilistiche"* views of economic decline with the political loss of independence and the "optimistic" view of "progress" under the dominance of Florence are "simplistic and schematic." She fails, however, to offer any new interpretations.

76. See note 35.

77. Dini, "Lineamenti per la storia," 15.

78. Ibid., 15, 19. Cherubini, "Schede per uno studio," draws a "fragmentary and incomplete" (p. 19) picture of the social and occupational structure of the city from its earliest surviving tax survey, the Estimo (or Lira) of 1390. While Cherubini points to "a group of important men of affairs" in the city, he comments that "the city in its entirety did not present a striking mercantile complexion" (8). He does not compare these data with earlier evidence, however, to speculate whether the mercantile sector grew or declined in importance during the Trecento.

79. Ibid., 16–20.

80. Mira, "Aspetti di vita economica," 153–55; Fortini, *Nova vita di s. Francesco,* 2: 101–2.

81. Zaccaria, "L'Arte dei Guarnellari e dei Bambagiari," 2ff. Cristofani, *Assisi,* 201, notes that in 1377 305 masters were matriculated in the shoemakers' guild.

82. The terms for these noble factions originated in Germany with the imperial struggle between Frederick II and Otto IV of Saxony. Initially, the Guelphs were associated with the papacy and the Ghibellines with the "imperial party." But adherence to these broad ideological causes soon dissipated in the realpolitik of local factional strife. By 1355, the famous jurist Bartolo de Sassoferrato, writing in *Tractus de guelfis et gebellinis,* had already demystified these conflicts: their names had no relation "either to the church or to the Empire, but only to those factions which exist in a city or in a province." For these

events and their impact on thirteenth-century Italian politics, see Tabacco, *The Struggle for Power*, 256–57, and Waley, *The Italian City-Republics*, 200. The oldest evidence of a division in the nobility into factions bearing these names and their respective alliances to church and empire comes from Florence in the 1230s and 1240s. The most detailed treatment of these factions for Florence or for any other city remains Davidsohn, *Storia di Firenze*, vols. 2, 3.

83. Recently, Tabacco has suggested that these alliances may have played a more important cultural role in the late medieval history of Italian city-states than historians have envisioned—"types of behavior which tended to persist over time and to be transmitted from one generation to the next with a progressive enrichment of language and myth" (*The Struggle for Power*, 256–57). On differences in the mentality, sensibilities, and *linguaggio* of Guelphs and Ghibellines in Pisa, see Luzzati, "Le origini di una famiglia nobile pisana," 73–75, 60–118. On the Ghibelline influence on poetry and language, see Davidsohn, *Storia di Firenze*, 5: 41–48.

84. Heywood, *Perugia*, 61–66; Tabacco, *The Struggle for Power*, 317. Perhaps Assisi was also a member: see Waley, "Le istituzioni communali," *The Papal States*, 31–36.

85. Tabacco, "Nobiltà e potere ad Arezzo," 22–23.

86. The city did not pass formally under the Signoria of Bishop Guido until 1321. He ruled until his death in 1327, when communal control passed to his brother Piero Saccone, who was ousted by a coup in 1337. The city then passed for a brief period under the control of Florence, which lasted until Florence's *signore*, the duke of Athens, was ousted in 1343. See Nicolaj [Petronio], "Notariato aretino," 633–60.

87. Cristiani, *Nobiltà e popolo;* Banti, *Breve storia di Pisa,* 50–54.

88. See Cristofani, *Assisi.* Earlier with the papacy of Innocent III, Assisi had submitted to papal suzerainty, but, according to Waley, "questo trasferimento legale non ebbe consequenze pratiche" ("Le istituzioni communali," 56).

89. Fasoli's definition, in "Ricerche sulla legislazione antimagnatizia," 91. Since Salvemini, *Magnati e popolani,* and Volpe, *Studi sulle istituzioni comunali a Pisa,* historians have questioned these terms and the utility of a class analysis for the late thirteenth and the fourteenth centuries. Among these historians are Ottokar, *Il Comune di Firenze;* Rubinstein, "La lotta contro i magnati"; Cristiani, *Nobiltà e popolo,* "Sul valore politico del cavaliere," "Il ceto dirigente," 27–40; Tabacco, "Nobiltà e potere ad Arezzo," "Interpretazioni e ricerche"; and Maire-Vigneur, "Les institutions communales." Recently, Tabacco, *The Struggle for Power,* 231, 234, has reopened the question of the struggle between the *popolo* and the *magnati,* arguing that these forces represented class and economic interests. See also Martines, *Power and Imagination,* 45–61, and Capitani, "Città e comuni," 34.

90. See Ardito, *Nobiltà, popolo e Signoria,* 57–58; *Statuti di Pisa,* vol. 1.

91. Cristiani, *Nobiltà e popolo;* Tangheroni, *Politica, commercio, agricoltura;* Ai-

dito, *Nobiltà, popolo e Signoria;* Fasoli, "Ricerche sulla legislazione antimagnatizia," 116–17.

92. For Florence the literature is vast; see note 89. Antimagnate laws in Florence originated in 1281, followed by acts in 1284, 1286, and 1289.

93. Fasoli, "Ricerche sulla legislazione antimagnatizia," 115–16. Here, the *popolo* appeared as early as 1201, and its first antimagnate laws were enacted in 1271, when the *popolo grasso* succeeded in barring from government both the *grandi* and the *popolo minuto*.

94. Heywood, *A History of Perugia,* 38; Fasoli, "Ricerche sulla legislazione antimagnatizia," 122–23. The first antimagnate movement, however, dates to 1275, and antimagnate laws appear as early as 19 July 1312. The "Red Book" listed all the noble and magnate families of the city and *contado* against whom the commune imposed "the most severe regulations," which appear in statutes of 1342 but were probably promulgated in 1322. For the rise of the *popolo* and the "subjugation" and decline of the nobility, see Salvatorelli, "La política interna." For him, the turning point came with the insurrections of 1302, which he asserts left the nobility thereafter hopelessly divided.

95. With "the peace of 1203," Assisi may have been the first of these city-states to exclude its local nobility from communal government: see Waley, "Istituzioni comunali," 67–68. But, according to Bartoli Langeli, "La realtà sociale," 309, the Peace established the commune on a firmer footing and gave both groups equal rights under the laws of the commune.

96. Bowsky, *A Medieval Commune.* Even in Florence, where the Ordinances of Justice have been seen as the most thoroughgoing of antimagnate legislation, noblemen of the old lineages still enjoyed privileges and exemptions from sumptuary laws: see ASF, Statuti del Comune di Firenze, no. 11, rub. lxxviii, 150r–153v, "Ordinamenta Mortuorum."

97. Grohmann, *Perugia,* 54. For a contrary view, see Salvatorelli, "La politica interna," 81.

98. Cristiani, *Nobiltà e popolo,* 133–34, has stressed the intermingling and loss of distinctive behavior and interests between the *magnati* and the *popolani* during the Trecento. For a different view that stresses the distinctiveness of a noble ethos in Pisa and its ability to retain power in certain niches, such as in the Cathedral's College of Canons, see Luzzati, "Le origini di una famiglia nobile pisana," 97, 118. The case of Pisa is further complicated by a distinction between the consular-maritime and the landed nobilities, though Luzzati maintains that by the thirteenth century the two had assumed common characteristics (66).

99. Fasoli, "Ricerche sulla legislazione antimagnatizia," 118. Nonetheless armed societies appear as early as 1196, and the first Capitano del Popolo came into existence in 1243. Fasoli speculates that antimagnate laws may have appeared in 1287, the year of insurrection, but are missing in the

earliest surviving communal statutues of 1327. They appear in those of 1337 and disappear at the time of the Signoria of the duke of Athens in 1342.

100. See Luzzati, *Firenze e la Toscana*, 125, and Tabacco, "Nobiltà e potere ad Arezzo."

101. Cohn, "Florentine Insurrections."

102. Douglas, *A History of Siena*, 153–63; Wainwright, "Conflict and Popular Government," 57–80, "The Testing of a Popular Sienese Regime."

103. D'Ajano, "Lotte sociali"; Grohmann, *Perugia*, 55. Again, Salvatorelli, in "La politica interna," 85–108, draws contrasting conclusions. For him the Statuto del 1342 in Perugia was parallel to the Ordinamenti sacrati e sacratissimi in Bologna and to the Ordinamenti di giustizia in Florence; it created a new alliance between the disenfranchized nobility and the *popolo minuto* against the merchant elites (Raspanti), leading to the *"tumulti"* of 1371, 1382, 1389, 1392, and 1393. He draws parallels, moreover, in the social and economic character of the *popolo minuto* between Perugia and Florence. The Statutes of 1342 abolished the "new guilds," subjected the artisans in these trades to the authority of other guilds, and, similar to the early fourteenth-century statutes of Florence, prohibited the workers subject to guilds to form any associations or to congregate for any purpose.

104. Tangheroni, *Politica, commercio, agricoltura*, 42–43.

105. *Cronaca Pisana di Ranieri Sardo*, 132, [1356] chap. 108, "Gran novità di Pisa"; 170, [1369] chap. 153, "Dello rumore che si levoe in Pisa." For 1392, see Banti, *D'Appiano*, 71–72.

106. For a succinct synopsis of Florentine-Aretine relations, see Black, *Benedetto Accolti*, 1–6.

107. On the juridical character of the will, pious bequests, executors, and *fideicommissarii*, see Gatti, "Antonomia privata."

108. Pasqui, *Documenti*, no. 325, pp. 283–85, dated 1068, from the chartulary of SS. Flora and Lucilla; the other, no. 289, pp. 395–96, dated 1098.

109. The city's subjugation to Perugian lordship should not have affected the recordkeeping of the principal repository of Assisani testaments—the Sacro Convento of San Francesco. No surviving *fondo* of Assisani *pergamene* or notarial protocols exist from this date in the State Archives of Perugia. According to Cenci, *Documentazione*, 1: 12–14, only one protocol of acts from Assisi exists there. Curiously, this protocol (from the village of Bettona, 1381–84) comes after the period of Perugian suzerainty, when Assisi had become a part of the Papal States.

110. See Bonanno, Bonanno, and Pellegrini, "I Legati *pro anima*"; Nicolaj [Petronio], "Storia di vescovi," "Notariato aretino"; Mosiici, "Note sul più antico protocollo"; Era, *Ricerche sul Formularium Florentinum;* Rodulphi, *Summa totius artis notariae; Formularium Florentinorum;* Raniero da Perugia, *Ars notaria; Summa notariae Aretii.* Orlandelli, "Genesi dell' 'ars notariae,'" identified the

formula book of Raniero as the prototype for the diffusion of many others in the thirteenth century, including the one by Martino da Fano and the *Summa notariae* for Arezzo. For the origins of the Studio aretino and the presence in Arezzo of *"maestri"* such as Martino da Fano and Raniero da Perugia, see Nicolaj [Petronio], "Notariato aretino," 637.

111. The standard article of clothing donated to the poor—the *tunica*—generally exceeded this amount. The first statutory evidence that I have found for this canonical portion comes only in 1389, when the commune demanded it for the hospital of Santa Maria della Scala: see Morandi, *Cattedrale di Siena*. But well before this date, such formulaic bequests initiated the lists of testamentary gifts.

112. According to Cristofani, *Assisi*, 207, the city statutes did not require testators to give a customary sum to the communal hospital until 1469, when the rubric (n. 162) required a legacy of 20 soldi.

113. See Haines, "Brunelleschi and Bureaucracy."

114. *Statuto di Arezzo*, bk. 2, no. 33, "De Relictis faciendis operi ecclesie Episcopatus."

115. Strocchia, "Burials in Renaissance Florence."

116. In 1384, the commune began selling exemptions from the sumptuary restrictions on funerary display. Strocchia, "Death Rites," 130, 120–45, has tabulated these appeals. From 1384 to 1392 the commune sold 233 such licenses—a minuscule portion of those buried in the territory of Florence. Florentines bearing family names, moreover, purchased the lion's share of these funerary permits (83%). The absence of specific stipulations for funerary expenses may have resulted from a reliance on other organizations to assume these responsibilities. Confraternal membership and communal statutory provisions are discussed in Chapter 4.

117. The earliest such "mundium" recorded in Florence by Mosiici, "Note sul più antico protocollo," 215, was dated 12 March 1264: Mundium domine Sobile, ASF, Not. antecos., A. 981, c.25v. The earliest Florentine testament of a woman redacted with the consent of a *mundualdus*, 228, is the Testamentum domine Romee, 17 November 1260, ASF, Not. antecos., A. 981, c.7r. See *Statuto del Podestà* (1325), bk. 2, rub. lxx, 141–42: "Quod conservetur in successione et de mundualdis et etate legittima;" and *Statuta Florentiae* (1415), I, lib. II, rub. cxii, 204–5: "De mundualdis, et quis possit tutores, vel curatores, et mundualdos dare."

118. Kuehn, *Emancipation in Late Medieval Florence,* "'Cum consensu mundaldi,'" "Women, Marriage, and *Patria Potestas";* Bellomo, *La condizione qiuridica;* Giardina," 'Advocatus' e 'mundualdus' "; *Formularium Florentinum,* 28–29.

119. On the rights and treatment of patrician women principally in Florence, see Klapisch-Zuber, *La famiglia e le donne;* Rosenthal, "The Position of Women"; and Kirshner, "Wives' Claims."

120. An illustrative exception is found in an early Quattrocento testament

from Florence, ASF, Not. antecos., no. 7401, n.p., 1417.vii.18: "Io albizo di charlo dalla piaza del popolo di Sto Friano di Firenze ho scritto di mia propria mano questo mio testamento e questo voglio che sia ultima mia volonta in domenicha mattina 18 Luglio 1417."

121. Valeri, *La fraternità dell'Ospedale*, 25.

122. Antoniella, *L'Archivio della Fraternità*, xv.

123. Catoni, "Gli oblati della Misericordia," 15.

124. See Pullan, "Support and Redeem," 200, and *Rich and Poor in Renaissance Venice*, 213, 415–16.

125. Beyond such formulaic practices, communal statutes could govern the will's form and certain rights of inheritance, even with a written will. See, for example, *Statuti di Perugia*, bk. 2, rub. 10, 302: "Quante testemonia basteno en glie testamente e altre ulteme volentade"; rub. 36, 336: "De l'ulteme volontà da osservare le figliuole e nepote"; rub. 37, 336–37: "Che 'l pate possa lassare al figliuolo spurio de gle bien suoie"; *Breve Pisani Communis*, rub. CXXXVI, "De testamentis executioni mandandis, et quod notarii non faciant testamenta ignotorum; vol. 2: *Constituta legis et usus*, XXXI, 756–65: "De ultimis voluntatibus;" XXXVIIII, 782–85: "Qualiter mulieribus permissum est alienare, vel in ultima voluntate relinquere; XLI, 786–87: "De his que a viro in uxorem dantur vel relinquuntur"; *Il constituto del Comune di Siena*, Distinctio II, XXI, 214: "Quod mulieres non possint relinquere alii, quam filiis, ultra quartam;" XXXIII, 214: "De tertia parte apud maritum retinenda."

126. "Nota introduttiva," xiii.

127. Bertram, "Mittelalterliche Testamente," 528.

128. *Statuti di Pisa*, vol. 2: *Constitutum*, XXXV, 768–76: "De successionibus ab intestato"; *Statuto del Podestà dell'anno 1325*, bk. 2, rub. LXVIIII: "De modo successionis mulierum ab intestato et de ipsorum materia"; *Statuta populi et communis Florentiae (a. 1415)*, vol. 1, bk. 2, rub. CXXVI, 218–19: "De successione communis Florentiae ab intestato, et de haeredibus naturalium, et bastardorum"; CXXX, 223–24: "Qualiter mulier ab intestato succedat"; *Statuto di Arezzo (1327)*, bk. 3, rub. LVII, 169-70: "De Successionibus ab intestato"; *Il constituto del Comune di Siena*, Distinctio II, rub. XXXIII, 214: De tertia parte dotis apud maritum retinenda"; XXXIIII, 214–15: "Ut mulier non succedat, si fuerit a patre vel fratre dotata"; XXXVII, 215: "De testamentis firmis tenendis, Et si ab intestato decesserit." On the differences between customary or Lombard and Roman principles of property succession, see Hughes, "Struttura familiare e sistemi di successione ereditaria."

129. According to Leonij, "La peste," this pestilence first struck Todi and then was spread "throughout Italy" by the military company of the Whites, organized by Giovanni di Monferrato against Bernabò Visconti. This claim, however, needs modification, since the plague struck Pisa earlier in 1362, and chroniclers such as Stefani and Matteo Villani saw the plague arriving in Florence from the west instead of the east. This plague lacks recent analysis

and commentary. Klapisch-Zuber, "Déclin démographique," 259, claims that this plague, similar to that of 1361, which struck large parts of northern Europe, disproportionately afflicted infants in the city of Prato. On the other hand, del Panta, *Le epidemie,* does not even enumerate 1363 among the plague years; his "Dalla mortalità epidemica" (68) and "Cronologia e diffusione" (304) give it only passing notice as a year within the second wave of pestilence, 1360–63. By contrast, contemporary chroniclers and later medical historians viewed it as a significant scourge against humanity. *Cronaca Senese di Donato di Neri,* 599–605, reports that this plague killed off an inordinate number of members of the ruling elite in Siena; Fra Filippo degli Agazzari, *Gli "Assempi,"* 41 (VII), 57 (XII), 135 (XXXVII), 200 (LVII), recalls the plague of 1363 in a number of his moral lessons. For Pisa, see *Chronica Antiqua,* 554; Roncioni, *Delle Istorie Pisane,* 860; and *Cronica di Matteo Villani,* vol. 2, 395, bk. 10, chap. 103. For Perugia, *Cronaca del Graziani;* and Massari, *Saggio sulle pestilenze,* based on chronicles. For Florence, *Cronaca Stefani,* rub. 691, 261, and *Cronica di Matteo Villani,* vol. 2, 446, bk. 11, chap. 57.

130. See Cohn, *Death and Property,* chap. 5; for a similar observation from the early Trecento testaments of the Bardi family, see Sapori, "La beneficenza delle compagnie mercantili": "appare evidente e drammatico il contrasto tra la pratica della vita di quegli uomini audaci e tenaci, costruttori di fortune immense, e il terrore della punizione eterna per aver creato la loro richezza con mezzi poco scrupolosi" (251). Sapori does not, however, attempt to generalize beyond the Bardi or to look for modifications in this contradiction between belief and action over time. See also his *Le marchand italien,* xvii–xxi, on the religion of merchants.

131. For an analysis of asceticism and the "imitation of Christ" from the perspective of women saints and blessed ones, see Bynum, *Holy Feast and Holy Fast.*

132. On this pessimistic view, see Huizinga, *The Waning of the Middle Ages,* and Delumeau, *Le peur en Occident* and *Le pèché et la peur.*

133. For a similar view drawn from literary sources, see the pioneering work of Tenenti, *Il senso della morte,* and its recapitulations in "Processi formativi," and Mollat, "Le sentiment de la mort."

134. For shifts in the directions of charity in late medieval and Renaissance Tuscany, see Herlihy, *Pistoia,* 241–58; Brucker, *Renaissance Florence,* 172–212; Becker, "Aspects of Lay Piety," *Medieval Italy;* and Gavitt, *Charity and Children,* 8, 33. For cities outside Tuscany, see Brentano, "Death in Gualdo Tadino."

135. Cohn, *Death and Property,* 90. Watkins, in "Petrarch and the Black Death," finds similarly that 1348 did not mark a change in Petrarch's mentality, but she argues that Petrarch's asceticism and otherworldly stoicism began to intensify by 1350.

136. According to Pasqui, "La biblioteca," Symoneus was born around 1280,

was a notary and either a judge or a lawyer, and taught at the university (Studio aretino) as a Maestro.

137. Some of these volumes held as many as 16 titles. While some bound the works of Cicero together, others appear as more haphazard miscellanea, such as the volume containing "Esopes' fabules" and a "Tractatum" of Thomas Aquinas on the reasons of faith against the Antiocenum. Wieruszowski, in "Arezzo as a Center of Learning," has pointed to this library as "another important contribution to the new [humanist] movement in Arezzo" (382–83), but no one has commented on the testator's passion and the measures he took to preserve his library after his death.

138. ASF, Dipl., Domenicani d'Arezzo, 1338.viii.12. According to Pasqui, "La biblioteca," Symoneus's desires for the perpetual preservation of his library were thwarted: his library was dispersed in the campaigns of 1381 and 1384, when marauding bands of French and Italian soldiers "barbarously" sacked churches, monasteries, and private residences, "robbing books and furnishings of every sort" (251).

From the perspective of the testaments of cardinals in late Duecento Rome, Symoneus's preoccupation with the survival of his library might not seem as striking as it does from the context of Sienese wills: see Paravicini Bagliani, *I Testamenti dei Cardinali*. Of these, the will that most closely resembles Symoneus's is Conte Casati's, redacted in 1287: "quod omnes libri sui theologie . . . assignentur et deponantur apud priorem et conventum fratrum Predicatorem et apud guardianum et conventum fratrum Minorum [both in Milan]." But none of the wills in this collection took the measures detailed in Symoneus's will for his library's perpetual preservation or attached these worldly objects so explicitly to earthly memory.

139. Archivio di Stato, Siena (ASS), Not. 1457, 1512.xi.30.

140. Wieruszowski, "Arezzo as a Center of Learning"; Black, *Benedetto Accolti,* chapter 1.

141. Arch. dei Laici, 34v–37r.

142. Wackernagel, *The Florentine Artist,* 136; Hills, "The Renaissance Altarpiece," 39; and Chapter 7 of this book.

143. ASF, Dipl., Olivetani d'Arezzo, 1348.———.

144. Arch. Capitolare, Arezzo, Notarile, no. 57 (Pace Pucci), 143r–151r, 1348.ix.21.

145. ASF, Dipl., S.M. Novella, 1312.vi.15.

146. Ibid., 1348.vii. 22; for a partial transcription of this document and discussion, see Orlandi, *"Necrologio,"* 1: 457; 2: app. 2, doc. 24, 436–37. For a more recent discussion, see Lunardi, *Arte e Storia,* 31.

147. ASF, Dipl., S.M. Nuova, 1343.iv.25.

148. Ibid., 1323.ix.21.

149. Ibid., 1368.viii.24.

150. Since Lanzi, *Storia pittorica,* Umbrian art and the spiritual values art historians have interpreted from it have been seen as forming a distinctive regional school. See, among many others, Berenson, *Italian Painters.* On Lanzi and Italian schools of painting, see Castelnuovo and Ginzburg, "Centro e periferia," 287–94. On such regional distinctions drawn from saints' lives and spirituality, see Fumi, *Eretici e ribelli,* and Salvatorelli, "Spiritualità umbra." More recently, the authors contributing to *Convegno di studi umbri* carefully skirted conclusions pointing to a distinctive Umbrian culture.

151. Tateo, "I Toscani e gli altri," 14.

152. See Lesnick, *Preaching in Medieval Florence,* 257–58; Delcorno, *Giordano da Pisa;* and Murray, "Piety and Impiety," 86ff.

153. See *Bibliotheca Sanctorum,* 1:1294–1321, and Origo, *San Bernardino.*

154. In Pisa, the plague arrived a year earlier: see Chap. 3, n. 13.

155. Tateo, "I Toscani e gli altri," 26, has recently argued from vernacular literary chronicles and mercantile tracts that a new Florentine *"civiltà"* began to dominate Tuscany toward the end of the fourteenth century, distinguishing it from other regions.

156. The most extensive study to date of the Black Death remains Biraben, *Les hommes et la peste.* For a global interpretation of plagues in history, see McNeill, *Plagues and Peoples.*

157. Saltmarsh, "Plague and Economic Decline"; Shrewsbury, *A History of Bubonic Plague;* Gottfried, *The Black Death* and *Doctors and Medicine in Medieval England;* Carmichael, *Plague and the Poor.*

158. Carpentier, *Une ville devant la peste.*

159. Postan, *The Medieval Economy;* Genicot, "Crisis"; Bridbury, *Economic Growth;* Herlihy, *Pistoia;* and, for the 1970s, see Aston and Philpin, *The Brenner Debate.*

160. See William Langer's presidential address to the American Historical Association in 1957, "The Next Assignment," and McNeill, *Plagues and Peoples.*

161. Williman, *The Black Death.*

162. The exception to this rule is the work of Chiffoleau, "Perché cambia la morte" and *La comptabilité de l'au-delà.*

163. Williman, *The Black Death,* 19. For another example of discounting the cultural and psychological importance of the plague, see the introductory remarks on page 17: "Perhaps the truth of the matter is that both the harsher realities of medieval life, even in such relatively good times as the 12th and 13th centuries—high infant mortality, extensive malnutrition among the poor, ineffective therapeutics—and the teaching of Christian tradition on the transitoriness of human life had combined long before 1347 to provide people with very adequate psychological and cultural mechanisms for dealing with the shock and horror." And Lerner, "The Black Death": "Mentalities, like Mediterranean sailing routes, have their *longues durées"* (94); and even more transhistorical, Polzer, "Fourteenth-Century Iconography": "Death is a perpetual

human dilemma . . . it must be kept in mind that dying is a constant human concern which does not wait for epidemics" (123–26).

164. See Appendix A.

165. See, for example, Panofsky, *Tomb Sculpture;* Herklotz, *"Sepulcro" e "Monumenta";* Kristeller, "The Immortality of the Soul"; Greenblatt, *Renaissance Self-Fashioning,* 1–9; Baron, "Franciscan Poverty"; Becker, "Individualism," "Aspects of Lay Piety"; and Goldthwaite, *The Building of Renaissance Florence.*

2. Pious Choices

1. Vovelle, *Piété baroque, La mort et l'occident;* Chaunu, *La mort à Paris;* Lebrun, *Les hommes et la mort en Anjou;* Chiffoleau, *La comptabilité de l'au-dela,* "Perché cambia la morte." Historians such as Croix, *La Bretagne aux 16e et 17e siècles;* Hoffman, *Church and Community;* and Norberg, *Rich and Poor in Grenoble,* have looked more closely at the mix of pious choices but do not place their findings in the full contexts of testamentary bequests, both pious and nonpious, or within traditions of property descent. For a discussion of the historiography on death, mentality, and testaments, see Le Roy Ladurie, "The New History of Death," and Cohn, *Death and Property,* 2–5.

2. Becker, *Medieval Italy.*

3. Becker, "Aspects of Lay Piety."

4. Herlihy, *Pistoia,* 241–58; Brucker, *Renaissance Florence,* 172-212. For areas outside of Tuscany, see Brentano, "Death in Gualdo Tadino": he adopts Herlihy's notion of "civic Christianity" in describing a shift in piety, which he labels "modernist piety," but he applies it to the period preceding the Black Death (99).

5. Gavitt, *Charity and Children:* cf. pp. 8 and 33.

6. See Brucker, *Renaissance Florence,* 210–11; Origo, *The Merchant of Prato;* and Herlihy, *Pistoia,* 240 and 249: "Francesco di Marco Datini, the rich merchant of Prato, while urged to give his wealth to a monastery, chose rather to endow a hospital, and the choice was characteristic of his age" (249). In a chapter devoted exclusively to an analysis of Datini's testaments, Gavitt, *Charity and Children,* 33–59, argues: "This spiritualization of the secular was central to the shifting territories of human and divine that so characterized the cultural history of early Renaissance Florence. . . . Datini's anxiety that the Ceppo should not in any way be considered an ecclesiastical institution reflects his confidence in the ability of the Commune to distribute his patrimony according to his best intentions" (56). However, from the thirty-four hundred testaments I have coded, Datini's reliance on a communal government as the guarantor of an estate, far from being the norm, appears extraordinary.

7. See, for example, Herlihy, *Pistoia,* 254–58, and Brucker, *Renaissance Florence:* "Elio Conti's researches into the patterns of land ownership in the Florentine *contado* reveal that Bonifazio's foundation, the hospital of S. Maria Nuova, and

the Foundling Home of the Innocenti significantly increased their real estate holdings in the fifteenth century" (210).

8. Cohn, *Death and Property,* 36.

9. For Florence, see Wackernagel, *The Florentine Artist,* 38-53.

10. Through the period under study, San Marco housed the Silvestrini monks of Vallambrosa, and it did not become the seat of the reformed Dominicans until 1436: see Hood, "Fra Angelico at San Marco," 109ff.

11. There were 294 gifts for Santa Maria Novella and 28 for San Pietro Murrone, out of a total for the city mendicants of 745. On the other hand, Santa Croce received 205 bequests. Mendicants from the territory attracted an additional 91 gifts. These figures give credence to Antal's claims, in *Florentine Painting,* that, in the course of the fourteenth century, the Dominicans managed "to get the upper hand and to drive the Franciscans from the strong position they still had at the beginning of the century" (74). See also Brucker, *Renaissance Florence:* "Of the religious orders in Florence, the Dominicans were the most active and distinguished in the late Trecento and early Quattrocento" (199).

12. There were 91, 77, and 50 legacies respectively.

13. Before the Black Death, 40 percent of bequests to city mendicants went to the Dominicans (117 of 289) and 24 percent to Franciscans (70).

14. On the Dominican influence on the culture of Pisa, see Meiss, "An Illuminated *Inferno,"* 33; Hinnebusch, *The History of the Dominican Order,* 1: 317-18, 2: 200 and Banti, *Breve storia di Pisa,* 48-49. For the Franciscans, see Ronzani, "Il francescanismo a Pisa."

15. These four categories received 439, 382, 261, and 222 bequests out of 1,314 pious legacies to mendicants within the city walls. Houses in the countryside attracted an additional 74 gifts.

16. They received 277 bequests of 803; in addition, testators made 57 legacies to mendicant houses in the countryside.

17. There were 174 bequests for the Augustinians, 173 for the Dominicans, 114 for the Servites, and 65 for the Carmelites.

18. Salmi, *San Domenico and San Francesco,* 23.

19. S. Maria degli Angeli received 159 pious legacies out of 637.

20. San Damiano received 63 gifts. In 1260, the Clarissians moved to the convent of Santa Chiara in town; afterwards, the church became a Franciscan friary: see Moorman, *The Franciscan Order,* 372.

21. These hermits drew 40 bequests; later, with the schism that divided the order into the conventuals and observants, they were called the observants.

22. These Franciscan houses received 51 gifts.

23. Davis, "Ubertino da Casale," and Monfasani, "The Fraticelli and Clerical Wealth"; for the impact of these changes on Florence, see Trexler, "The Bishop's Portion" and "Death and Testament."

24. The Dominicans received 277 of a total of 637 legacies destined for mendicant houses or individual friars within Perugia and the surrounding

suburbs. If the mendicant houses from the territory are added, the denominator rises to 672; the Franciscans in the city received 221 between the two houses, San Francesco al Prato and Monte. (Often it is impossible to know for which house the legacy was intended, since the bequest stated only the "house of San Francesco.") These figures, however, underestimate the importance of the Dominicans. Their new church, Santo Stefano, built over the course of my analysis and whose *opera* received numerous building funds, also served as a parish church and was tallied consistently under the latter rubric.

25. The number of legacies is as follows: Augustinians, 71; Servites, 59; Carmelites, 9.

26. While only two convents appear in the itemized legacies of early Quattrocento wills in Siena, 15 different nunneries appear in the Florentine samples between 1400 and 1425.

27. Herlihy, *Pistoia*, 55–77; Herlihy and Klapisch-Zuber, *Les Toscans*, 165–81.

28. See Henderson, "The Hospitals of Late-Medieval and Renaissance Florence."

29. For a recent bibliography on religious confraternities, see Banker, *Death in the Community*, 1–10. He finds a chronological transition in the types of confraternal organization in Borgo San Sepolcro from the all-embracing, citywide society of San Bartolomeo in the late thirteenth century to *laudesi* groups in the early fourteenth century to a predominance of *disciplinati* groups after the Black Death. The evidence from testamentary gifts suggest a similar pattern for Arezzo but not a general developmental trend for all the six cities studied here.

30. On the political and economic history of this powerful interregional institution, see Epstein, *Alle origini della fattoria toscana,* and Redon, "Autour de l'Hôpital."

31. See Catoni, *Le pergamene dell'università di Siena,* and Catoni, "Gli oblati della Misericordia.

32. Pullan, in "Support and Redeem," states that the concentration and monopolization of single hospitals in cities such as Milan followed the spread of preaching by Franciscan observants in the mid-fifteenth century, who argued that "to rescue the poor from the possibility of corruption and fraud, large centralised hospitals should be established. . . . By practising what in modern terms might be called 'economies of scale,' hospitals would be able to spend more on the wellbeing of inmates, and less on the emoluments of their staff" (190–91). Pullan recognizes that this process may have been anticipated earlier in Tuscany, but comments that they "seem to have been luxuriant natural growths, rather than amalgamations brought about by statutes and blessed by papal bulls" (192). On the "organizational transformation" of health services and the rise of the *"ospedale grande"* in southern Tuscany, see Balestracci, "Per una storia degli ospedali."

33. Passerini, *Storia degli stabilmenti,* 284–395; Henderson, "The Hospitals of Late-Medieval and Renaissance Florence," 69; Pampaloni, *L'ospedale di Santa Maria Nuova;* Park, *Doctors and Medicine.*

34. Pinto, *La società del bisogno,* x.

35. Passerini, *Storia degli stabilmenti,* 659–75; Henderson, "The Hospitals of Late-Medieval and Renaissance Florence," 69; Trexler, "The Foundlings of Florence."

36. See Cohn, *The Laboring Classes,* 115–28.

37. See Goldthwaite and Rearick, "Michelozzo and the Ospedale di San Paolo," 222–23.

38. On San Matteo, see Sandri, "Ospedali e utenti,"

39. ASF, Not. antecos., no. 4064, 58r–v, 1417.viii.27; see Brucker, *Renaissance Florence,* 210; Passerini, *Storia degli stabilmenti,* 216–41; and Coturri, "L'Ospedale così detto 'di Bonifazio.'"

40. Not. antecos., no. 4064, 58r–v, 1417.viii.27. Legacies to the "societas" of San Paolo appeared earlier. For a history of the hospital, see Goldthwaite and Rearick, "Michelozzo and the Ospedale di San Paolo," and Passerini, *Storia degli stabilmenti,* 163–88.

41. ASF, Dipl., S.M. Nuova, 1422.i.22; see Passerini, *Storia degli stabilmenti,* 685, 704, and Gavitt, *Charity and Children.* Francesco Datini initiated the project with a one thousand-florin bequest in his will of 1411, and in 1421 the silk guild Por Santa Maria assumed the patronage of the hospital.

42. Before and after the plague, the figures for Santa Maria Nuova were 84 of 238 bequests and 185 of 236 bequests.

43. Seventy testaments are dated before 1363 and 104 after. The selection was made by a systematic sampling.

44. Thirty-four of 140 legacies come from before 1363, 88 of 132 after.

45. Santa Maria Nuova received 14 legacies out of 91 to hospitals; San Gallo, 29, and hospitals from the territory, 16.

46. The Z-score is highly significant: $z = 245$; $n = 95$; hypothesized proportion $= 56.5$ percent; observed proportion $= 44$ percent.

47. Santa Maria Nuova received 29 of 66 bequests in 1348; 20 of 29 bequests in the 1349–62 period; 20 of 29 bequests in 1363; 90 of 105 in the 1364–1400 period and 44 of 59 between 1401 and 1425.

48. Cohn, *Death and Property,* 120.

49. The cathedral collections of *Pergamene* dell'archivio Capitolare hold five pre-1300 wills (see Cristiani, "Un inventario"). In addition, my sample might have been supplanted by a few testaments in a handful of pre-fourteenth-century notarial books to be found in the archives of L'Opera del Duomo (one protocol), Fondi vari (3), Archivio Capitolare (3), and Archivio della Mensa Arcivescovile (7). See Luzzati, "I registri notarili," 23.

50. See del Guerre, *L'Ospedale pisano;* Casini, *Il fondo degli ospedali riuniti;* and Ronzani, "Gli Ordini Mendicanti." Because they had followed the orders of

the Holy Roman Emperor, Frederick II, to attack Genoese ships off the coast of the Island of Giglio and had captured prelates coming to attend a church council in Rome, Pope Gregory IX excommunicated the Pisans. In 1257 the commune agreed to put up ten thousand lire within five years for the foundation of a hospital to care for the sick. The hospital was governed by Augustinian friars, who elected its rector.

51. The 18 percent figure represents 64 testaments out of 354.

52. As reported in Chapter 1, even if the notary did not begin a fragmentary testament with the formula "est particula testamenti" or similar phraseology, the fragment can be readily detected by the copiers' habits of recording mostly those legacies pertaining to the ecclesiastical institution that ordered and preserved the copy. The other itemized gifts would then bear only the word "Item" followed by a dash or wavy line; or the copyist would simply neglect to copy whole sections of the will, such as the portions pertaining to the choice of nonpious universal heirs.

53. Luzzati, "I registri notarili," 14.

54. The archive of the hospital of Santa Chiara was assembled in the modern period, after this hospital had incorporated a number of smaller hospitals, such as those of the trovatelli of San Domenico and Santo Spirito, which in the late Middle Ages and Renaissance had been administered separately.

55. There were 790 bequests to hospitals of a total of 3,356 from the protocols of Santa Chiara, and 42 out of 340 from the other testaments.

56. The number of bequests was 262 out of a total of 2,467.

57. Santa Chiara received 356 bequests of 832.

58. The hospital of Santo Spirito was the second orphanage founded in Pisa (it was established in 1192 by Lotterio and Grotto, the sons of the deceased Lamberto) and was administered by the church of San Martino in Chinzica. The earliest, San Frediano, does not appear in these documents. The hospital of San Domenico became the third orphanage: it was founded in 1218 by the blessed Domenico Vernagalli and was governed by the monastic church of San Michele in Borgo.

59. The numbers for these three periods are 81 of 155, 67 of 111, and 17 of 53.

60. The figures for these last-cited two periods are 17 of 26 and 50 of 65; of the same sample provided by the first years of the Quattrocento (17 bequests to hospitals), Santa Chiara's percentage of all hospital bequests fell insignificantly to 65 (11 out of 17).

61. Santa Chiara's ability to attract greater concentrations of pious bequests in the first quarter of the fifteenth century seems to run counter to Casini's argument in Il fondo degli ospedali riunite: "La perdita della libertà e la sotto-missione della Repubblica ai Fiorentini [1406] fu anche per l'Ospedale l'inizio di un triste periodo di decadenza economica" (13).

62. These figures are 10 of 33 and 22 of 77.

63. Herlihy, *Pistoia*, 248; Goldthwaite and Rearick, "Michelozzo and the Ospedale di San Paolo," 286; Becker, "Aspects of Lay Piety," 186 and 189. According to Becker, "In the decades immediately thereafter [the Revolt of the Ciompi, 1378] we note the founding of great hospitals, hospices, and orphanages in greater numbers than ever before" (189).

64. On "the close connection between confraternities and hospitals," see Vauchez and Manselli, "'Ordo fraternitatis,'" and Pullan, "Support and Redeem." Pullan draws the following distinction: "In principle the hospital, dedicated to hospitality, differed from the confraternity, whose concerns were often with outdoor relief, practised either in the recipient's home or under some inhospitable roof, such as a debtor's prison" (188). In practice, however, such a distinction was not always so simple. For instance, the center of the religious life of the confraternity of Santo Stefano in Assisi became its hospital: see Meloni, "Per la storia delle confraternite disciplinate," 566–67, who argues more generally: "Originato dalla confraternita, l'ospedale diviene subito non soltanto il logico centro gravitazionale della sua attività assistenziale e caritativa, ma spesso finisce per diventare il pernio della vita economica del sodalizio" (584).

65. Two hundred seventy of 320 legacies were designated for the Misericordia as a confraternity.

66. Antoniella, *L'Archivio della Fraternità*, vii–viii, and Moriani, "Assistenza e beneficenza ad Arezzo."

67. Between 1301 and 1325 the bishop's hospital took 23 percent of hospital bequests (14 legacies); the Ponte, 27 percent (16); the Misericordia, 18 percent (11): and the Oriente, 8 percent (5). In the next 25 years the Oriente led with 27 percent (36); followed closely by the Ponte, 25 percent (33); the Bishop's hospital, 22 percent (29); and the Misericordia, 15 percent (19).

68. For 1348, the Oriente received 29 of 60 legacies; for 1349–62, 15 of 37; for 1363, 23 of 42.

69. At the end of the century, the Oriente received only 14 of 49 legacies.

70. The Annunciation received 14 of 42 bequests.

71. The Misericordia's figures during the early Trecento were 38 of 60 bequests.

72. For 1325–47, the Misericordia received 75 of 131 bequests (46 percent); in 1348, 54 of 114 (47 percent); for 1349–62, 23 of 60 (45 percent); in 1363, 23 of 65 (35 percent); for 1364–75, 26 of 75 (35 percent); and for 1375–1400, 6 of 30 (20 percent). In 1384, with the incorporation of Arezzo into the district of Florence, the Misericordia lost its autonomy and thereafter was governed by the priors and *gonfalonieri di giustizia* of the Commune of Arezzo; see Antoniella, *L'Archivio della Fraternità*, xix.

73. In the early Quattrocento, the Misericordia received 22 of 64 bequests.

74. According to Bellucci, "Notizie storiche," and Valeri, *La fraternità dell'Ospedale di S. Maria*, 17, this was the moment when a "great number" of small hospitals "for the poor, pilgrims and the injured" arose in Perugia.

75. Grohmann, *Perugia,* 66, maintains that the Misericordia was the most important of the "enti assistenziali" of the city. It was located in the *rione* of the Porta S. Pietro in the *piazza centrale* of the *sopramuro:* see fig. 50, p. 68.

76. See Bellucci, "Notizie storiche"; Guêze, "Le origini dell'ospedale"; and Valeri, *La fraternità dell'Ospedale di S. Maria,* 17. The hospital was "confirmed" by the Bishop of Perugia on 11 March 1305, under the protection of the commune.

77. The Misericordia gained 9 of 14 gifts. The high proportion may have resulted from a bias in the documentation: several notarial protocols kept by the Misericordia as well as a handful of this hospital's *pergamene* supplied most of the testaments of the early Trecento.

78. A meeting of the congregation of the hospital on 13 July 1363 gives evidence of severe financial and administrative difficulties: see Valeri, *La fraternità dell'Ospedale di S. Maria,* 20, and document 3, 43–49.

79. By that time (1389), the Commune of Perugia had directly intervened in the administration of the hospital, and the fraternity had lost its previous autonomy and responsibility for the assistance of the poor and infirm: see Valeri, *La fraternità dell'Ospedale di S. Maria,* 22.

80. The Misericordia received 11 out of 21 gifts in the early Quattrocento.

81. Valeri, *La fraternità dell'Ospedale di S. Maria,* 27.

82. Cristofani, *Assisi,* 207.

83. Ibid., 207. This hospital, founded by Vanni di Bonamico in 1337, was initially a hospice, giving lodging to German pilgrims who came to Assisi for indulgences.

84. Note that the period 1349–62 provides insufficient data.

85. As mentioned in Chapter 1, Cristofani, in *Assisi,* 207, finds this legislation promulgated only by 1446; yet the testaments give testimony of earlier such regulations.

86. See Herlihy, *Pistoia,* 248.

87. ASPi, Dipl., Primaziale, 1374.i.18.

88. Cohn, *Death and Property,* 22.

89. ASPi, Aquisto Cappelli, 1325.xii.9.

90. ASF, Dipl., S.M. Novella, 1374.iii.4.

91. Ibid., Arch. Gen., 1382.vii. 29.

92. Ibid., S.M. Novella, 1348.iv.7.

93. In 1310, the widow donna Fighinensis left as her universal heir a hospital to be constructed in the "district and Borgo" of Policiano, Arch. dei Laici, no. 726, 1v–2v.

94. ASA, Antichi notari, no. 12, 23v–24r, 1424.iv.24.

95. ASPr, Perg., Mt. Morcino, no. 79, 1361.vi.27.

96. Ibid., no. 228, 1389.iii.4.

97. ASPi, Dipl., Primiziale, 1374.i.18.

98. A cleric who could not be brought before, tried in, or sentenced by a

lay court of law: see *Dictionnaire de théologie catholique,* vol. 6, "For (Privilège Du)," 526–37.

99. ASPi, Dipl., Misericordia, 1328.xi.14.

100. Ibid., 1343.vi.12.

101. ASPr, Not. Prot., no. 7, 55v–56v, 1390.viii.16.

102. Arch. dei Laici, reg. 726, 60r–61r, 1374.vi.2.

103. Arch. Capitolare, Assisi, Co. S. Stefano (perg. numerata), no. 34, 5r–11r, 1362.———. This confraternity already possessed a hospital, which Meloni, "Per la storia delle confraternite disciplinate," 566–67, argues became the center of its activities. Pope John XXII confirmed the hospital with a bull of 22 April 1327.

104. Arch. Capitolare, Assisi, Co. S. Stefano (perg. numerata), no. 29, 1362.x.30.

105. For bibliographies on confraternities, see Weissman, *Ritual Brotherhood;* Henderson, "Charity in Late-Medieval Florence," "Le Confraternite religiose," and *Piety and Charity* (forthcoming); Banker, *Death in the Community,* 1–14; Casagrande, "La recente storiografia umbra"; Papi, "Le Confraternite fiorentine," "Confraternite ed ordine mendicanti"; Monti, *Le confraternite medievali;* and, most recently, Little, *Liberty, Charity, Fraternity.* The classic work on religious companies remains Meersseman, *Ordo Fraternitatis.*

106. For Borgo San Sepolcro, see Banker, *Death in the Community,* 145–73; for Florence, Weissman, *Ritual Brotherhood,* 43–58; Papi, "Le Confraternite fiorentine"; and Henderson, *Piety and Charity* and "Religious Confraternities and Death"; and for Umbria, Meloni, "Per la storia delle confraternite disciplinate," 540.

107. Banker, *Death in the Community,* posits for Borgo San Sepolcro that a general loosely structured confraternity comprising nearly all adults in the community antedated the *laudesi* and *disciplinati* organizations. See note 29.

108. For a summary of the various forms of assistance provided by confraternities, see Pullan, "Poveri, mendicanti, e vagabondi."

109. Sacro Convento, I, 46, 1267.viii.7.

110. Ibid., I, 58, 1278.x.14; II, 30, 1273.ix.20; II, 34, 1277.ii.17; II, 37, 1278.v.29; II, 39, 1278.v.31; II, 46, 1282.x.20; V, 14, 1283.ii.8; V, 18, 1284.ix.13; V, 24, 1286.viii.28.

111. On this confraternity's role in poor relief, see Henderson, "The Parish and the Poor." Saint Peter Martyr founded it in 1244; it was merged with the Misericordia in 1425. See Gavitt, *Charity and Children,* 11, 14–15; Saalman, *The Bigallo;* and Passerini, *Storia degli stabilimenti,* 1–60.

112. ASF, Dipl., S.M. Novella, 1261.ix.14.

113. See La Sorsa, *La compagnia d'Or S. Michele;* Zervas, *The Parte Guelfa;* and Gavitt, *Charity and Children,* 15–16. These bequests appear to have defied communal custom: Florence authorized the Society of Orsanmichele to receive bequests only in 1318.

114. ASF, Not. antecos., no. 2354, 90r, 1299.iii.16.

115. The earliest testament published by Pasqui, *Documenti,* vol. 1, no. 199, pp. 283–85, redacted in 1068, bequeathed three lire to a "Fraternitas huius plebis Sancte Marie in gradis," which Pasqui claims was the Fraternitas Clericorum.

116. ASF, Dipl., Domenicani d'Arezzo, 1305.iv.13.

117. According to Antoniella, *L'Archivio della Fraternità,* viii–ix, the Misericordia was already active by the beginning of the thirteenth century. Pope Alexander IV confirmed it with a bull dated 9 December 1257.

118. ASF, Dipl., Domenicani d'Arezzo, 1305.iv.13; Not. antecos., no. 977, 47r–v, 1313.iv.14; 57v–58v, 1313.vii.15; no. 984, 115r–v, 1324.viii.15; no. 985, 114r, 1325.ix.8.

119. For 1260 in Perugia, see Nicolini, "Nuove testimonianze su fra Raniero Fasani" and "Ricerche sulla sede di Fra Raniero Fasani"; and Frugoni, "Sui flagellanti del 1260." For the movement through Italy and an extensive bibliography, see Dickson, "The Flagellants of 1260."

120. With its statutes of 1262, all inhabitants of Arezzo were considered ipso facto members of the fraternity, "sine alia scriptura facienda de receptione personarum." Its rolls recorded 1,700 members for that year and about the same in 1299: see Antoniella, *L'Archivio della Fraternità,* xv, xvii. The popularity of this citywide organization may have run parallel to the development of confraternal life that Banker has found for Borgo San Sepolcro, but from the testaments surviving after 1304, this development cannot be determined with certainty. The Misericordia's predominance in the testaments did not antedate the growth in importance of a multitude of *laudesi* and *disciplinati* societies; rather, the vitality of these various types of lay society remained vigorous throughout the Aretine documentation.

121. On the role of the Florentine state after the Black Death in regulating charity through tighter control of organizations such as Orsanmichele, see Becker, "Lay Piety," 177, 185, and Gavitt, *Charity and Children,* 33ff.

122. The first documentary evidence for this confraternity comes from its commission (12 April 1285) to Duccio di Buoninsegna to paint what later was called the *Rucellai Madonna* for the confraternity's altar in Santa Maria Novella. White, *Duccio,* 32, speculates that this company arose at the same time as the Bigallo in 1244. See also Weissman, *Ritual Brotherhood,* 46.

123. Gavitt, *Charity and Children,* 14.

124. See Henderson's acute remark in "Religious Confraternities and Death": "Although many flagellant companies in Florence showed a marked reluctance to accept legacies, we must not fall into the trap of assuming that these organizations remained static—an error which is only too easy to commit if one follows the common practice of relying on statute books. There is no doubt that bequests were an important factor in influencing the way many companies developed. The duties which were performed under the terms of bequests often themselves became one of the main features of the company's

reputation. This was particularly true during the 150 years following the Black Death" (390).

125. Banker, *Death in the Community,* 77–78. For Borgo San Sepolcro's principal confraternity, "legacies outpaced income from incoming members"; but after the Black Death, the confraternity, according to Banker, entered a "second phase" in which the religious company's prime objective became the administration of pious legacies—"the property of the dead."

126. Henderson, "Religious Confraternities and Death," 390.

127. The rarity of gifts to confraternities in all six cities from the earliest documents until the early fourteenth century may support Banker's conclusions in *Death in the Community.* Before the fourteenth century in Borgo San Sepolcro, the principal confraternity, San Bartolommeo, which had citywide participation, was funded by annual dues and burial fees and not by bequests from last wills and testaments. These came later, in the early fourteenth century, when the confraternity had changed its membership and its pious objectives. Perhaps the rarity of legacies to religious confraternities in the cities studied here underlies such a transition in the development of lay religious life, at least, for the first transition sketched by Banker for Borgo San Sepolcro.

128. At first glance, this trend appears to run counter to the statistics on the growth in the number of confraternities after the Black Death, especially given the tendency of confraternities at that time to draw support more from pious legacies than from dues. See Papi, "Confraternite ed ordine mendicanti"; Henderson, "Religious Confraternities and Death"; and Meloni, "Per la storia delle confraternite disciplinate," who finds 150 confraternities, of which only one-third date from the fourteenth century (521). But the number of confraternities, many of which were small and appear for only short periods, may not be an adequate gauge for judging membership, popularity, or success. The rapid appearance and turnover of many such societies, like the effects of bankruptcy on the appearance of new business companies, may indeed suggest the opposite.

129. For theories of who constituted the "poor of Christ" and the now enormous literature on the poor in preindustrial societies, see Cohn, *Death and Property,* 25–28; Pullan, "Poveri, mendicanti, e vagabondi," especially 985ff. and 997ff., where the terms *paupertas, miserabile o egens,* and *I poveri di Cristo* are discussed; and Murray, "Religion among the Poor," 285–324.

130. Cohn, *Death and Property,* 28–32.

131. On the dowry in Renaissance society, see, most recently, Molho and Kirshner, "Dowry Fund."

132. ASF, Dipl., S. Croce, 1279.iv.5.

133. ASPi, Osp. di S. Chiara, no. 2075, 46r–v, 1301.x.14.

134. ASPr, Osp. di Misericordia, no. 1, 43r, 1333.iv.19.

135. ASF, Not. antecos., no. 993, 172r–173v, 1329.iv.1.

136. Henderson, "The Parish and the Poor," 259, argues that the period

after the Black Death witnessed a general shift in poor relief, which had "come to concentrate much of its attention on women."

137. For a recent depiction of mendicant saints in the Trecento, see Holmes, *Florence, Rome, and the Origins of the Renaissance.*

3. The Structure of Pious Bequests

1. See the letters of Saint Catherine of Siena: *I, Catherine, The Letters of St. Catherine,* and *Epistolario di Santa Caterina da Siena.*

2. See Cohn, *Death and Property,* 37–45.

3. la Roncière, "L'influence des franciscains," "Aspects de la religiosité populaire en toscane," 354ff.

4. The two eleventh-century Aretine testaments published by Pasqui, *Documenti,* no. 199, 283–85, 1068.viii, and no. 289, 1098.x, evoke a different epoch from the long lists of itemized pious bequests found in the Aretine testaments of the early Trecento. The earliest of these, a joint husband-wife testament, made seven pious bequests of landed property and money. The second, the will of Heinricus f. Ugonis et nepos Henrici, divided an extraordinary territory including "churches, manses, villages, cultivated and barren lands, vineyards, woodlands, swamps, ponds, rivers, fountains," identified by at least ten castles accompanied with their seignorial territories (*curtes*) that extended from "the city of Arezzo" to the Castello of Montevarchi. (On the *curtis,* see Tabacco, *The Struggle for Power,* 194.) The *usufructus* of these estates were divided among the church of San Benedetto, the nunnery of Santa Maria de Petroio, and the monastery of SS. Fiora et Lucilla. Heinricus freed all his serfs (*servos suos et ancilles*) but required "these men" to make various monetary gifts for his soul. On the strategies of pious giving for the eleventh century, see Wickham, *The Mountains and the City.*

5. Similarly, Rigon, "Influssi francescani nei testamenti," finds the first decade of the fourteenth century to be the pinnacle of mendicant success in influencing the laity of Padua through their testamentary bequests.

6. I found more than 196 different pious institutions in these legacies. (To ease the task of coding, I created several residual categories; thus, this number understates the exact number of different institutions found in these samples.)

7. These numbers do not include each individual parish church; instead, the parish or the *plebis* was coded as a single generic category.

8. *Rationes Decimarum,* vols. 58, 98, 161, 162.

9. Giusti, *Tuscia,* vol. 98 of *Rationes Decimarum,* vii, has calculated and compared the number of ecclesiastical entities appearing in both volumes of the *Rationes.* He finds the following increases from the last quarter of the thirteenth through the first third of the fourteenth centuries. Parish and canonical churches varied from 68 to 75 percent of the entities.

City	vol. 1	vol. 2
Florence	595	748
Arezzo	602	734
Siena	190	259
Pisa	242	423

10. By a T-test: F = 2.08; t = .81, degrees of freedom (df) = 44; probability = .423.

11. See *Cronaca Pisana di Ranieri Sardo*, 114. Chap. 82: "La mortalità grande universalmente."

"In del milletrecento quarantotto, alla intrata di gennaio venneno a Pisa due galee di Genovesi che veniano di Romania; e come funno giunti alla piassa dei pesci, chiunqua favellò con loro, di subbito sue amalato e morto; e chiunqua favellava loro, a quelli malati, e toccasse di quelli morti altresí, tosto amalavano e morivano; e cusí fu sparta la grande corruzione in tanto che ogni persona moria. E fue si grande la paura, che nimo volea l'un l'altro vedere . . . E ogni persona fuggiva la morte; ma pogo li valea, chè chiunqua dovea morire si moria; e non si trovava persona che li volesse portare a fossa. Ma quello Signore che fece lo cielo e la terra, provvide bene ogni cosa, che lo padre, vedendo morto lo suo figliuolo e abbandonato da ogni persona (chè nimo lo volea toccare, nè cucire, nè portare), egli si recusava morto e poi faceva egli stesso lo meglio che potea, egli lo cucia e poi lo mettea in della cascia, e con aiuto lo portava alla fossa, e egli stesso lo sotterrava. . . . nondimeno non ne rimase in nessuna casa nè in sul letto nessuno a sotterrare, che egli non fosse onorevilmente sotterrato secondo la sua qualità: tanta carità diede Dio all'uno coll'altro, recusandosi ciascuno morto. E dicea: *aiutiamo, e portianli a fossa, acciocchè noi ancora siamo portati*. E chi per amore e chi per denari. E duroe questa mortalità infine al maggio: ciò fue cinque mesi. E morinno molta gente; delli cinque li quattro."

A number of chronicles and histories repeated the same story. See, for example, *Storie Pistoresi*, 235–36, which also estimated that 25,000 "Christians" died in less than three months in Pisa; and Roncioni, *Delle Istorie Pisane*, 807–8, who reports that 70 percent of the Pisan population died over the course of nine months.

12. Even the principal chronicler of Perugia pointed to Pisa as the gateway to pestilence and the place of "maximum" mortality: "[1348] Adi 8 de aprile nel dicto millesimo comenzò in Peroscia una grande mortalità de pestilenzia . . . Comenzò la dicta mortalità in Toscana, et maxime in Pisa . . . et fu si terrible che non bastavano li cimiterii" (*Cronaca . . . Diario del Graziani*, 148–49).

13. Again, the plague struck Pisa before the other five cities; this second time, an entire year earlier. For evidence on the Pisan plague of 1362, see *Chronica Antiqua*, 554; *Le Croniche di Giovanni Sercambi*, 117–18: "CLII Come Idio mandò una moría e maximamente per tucto Ytalia (1362). Idio, il quale tucto

cognoscie, vedendo la querra cruda & aspra, & acta a crescere più tosto che mancare, dispuose la sua providensa mandare una moría per la quale si rifrenasse la furia della guerra. E cosí la dicta moría mandò in Luccha e im Pisa & per le parti di Toscana; ma principiò im Pisa & im Lucca, chè molti ne morinno & maximamente i più fanciulli da .xv. anni in giù, & durò questa moria quazi uno anno." See also *Cronica di Matteo Villani,* vol. 2, 395, bk. x, chap. 103: "Della mortalità dell'anguinaia . . . a' Pisani tolse molti cittadini . . . nel 1362," and Banti, *D'Appiano,* 90.

On the wave of pestilence in 1363, Villani reports: chap. 57, 446: "Della mortalità dell'anguinaia. Anche gravemente ritoccò nelle terre di Toscana, e quasi tutte comprese, e in Firenze, già stata generale tre mesi per tutto giugno con fracasso d'ogni maniera di gente."

14. Using a multivariate regression model, the dummy variables for the time brackets in the plague years 1362–63, 1364–1375, 1376–1400, and 1401–25 all showed strong and significant differences from the periods before the Black Death of 1348. The model controlled for type of document (parchment or notarial protocol), status of testator (noble or nonnoble), whether or not he or she lay on the deathbed at the time of redaction, gender, city or country residence, wealth, and whether the testator had living sons to inherit the patrimony. The adjusted R-square of the model (2,533 cases) is .19657. The weights or beta coefficients for these time periods were the highest of all the variables entered into the model with the exception of wealth, which registered a beta coefficient of +.2563, but was followed closely in its impact by the period 1376–1400, −.2335, and the period 1401–25, −.2252. If the time bracket includes the years after the recurrence of plague, then time becomes the strongest variable in the regression model in the determination of the number of pious bequests for all six cities (beta = −.3045; the R-square for the model remains the same).

As one might expect, wealth, nobility, city residence, and lying on one's deathbed at the time of the testament's redaction correlated positively with the number of pious bequests a testator made. Perhaps counterintuitively (see criticisms of *Death and Property* by Banker and by Kuehn), those with surviving sons ready to inherit the patrimony gave fewer pious bequests than those without surviving male heirs: the beta coefficient for this dummy variable was .1175, and its T-score was highly significant, 6.049.

15. With a multivariate regression model, this convergence can be shown not to have resulted from differences in the survival of documents or from possible changes in the characteristics of the testators. The model controls for differences in wealth, the source of the document, the occupational status of the testator, gender, whether the testator was on the deathbed at the time of redaction, and whether he or she had surviving sons. When only those testaments through the recurrence of the plague in 1362–63 are considered, the two sets of cities show a high degree of resemblance—Assisi, Pisa, and Siena,

on the one hand, and Arezzo, Florence, and Perugia, on the other—and a high degree of dissimilarity when the two groups are compared. (The T-score is 2.9, which is significant at .0037: 1,566 cases.) When the period from the second plague onward is examined, the difference between the two groups of cities loses all its significance. (The T-score equals .198, which is insignificant at even .84, and its determinancy in the regression model is minuscule; the beta coefficient equals .0056.)

16. Moorman, *The Franciscan Order,* 62–65; Little, *Religious Poverty,* 146–52; Brooke, "La prima espansione francescana in Europa"; Cresi, "Statistica dell'ordine minoritico," 157–62; Le Goff, "Ordres mendicants et urbanisation," 924–46. By 1282, the order numbered 1,224 houses. According to Emery, *The Friars in Medieval France,* 4–5, the mendicants numbered over 10,000 in France circa 1300, most of whom were Franciscans. Similarly, the number of Dominican friaries expanded rapidly in the latter half of the thirteenth century. According to Murray, "Religion among the Poor," 287, by 1277 the order probably numbered some 5,000 to 10,000 members and possessed 414 male Dominican convents. On Franciscan foundations in rural Tuscany and the pace of Franciscan popularity, see la Roncière, "L'influence des franciscains," especially 43–47.

17. Cohn, *Death and Property,* 37–45.

18. By a T-test, this change is, however, insignificant at .05: t = −1.35; df = 101; probability = .182.

19. ASF, Not. antecos., no. 12394, 156 bis r–159r, 1363.vi.21.

20. Ibid., no. 4388, 166r–167v, 1363.viii.6. Little has been written on these hermits who walked the streets; see Ronzani, "Penitenti e ordini mendicanti a Pisa": "ermiti cellati e indipendenti che venivano lungo la via di San Piero a Grado e in altri punti della città nel Due e Trecento, era entrato nello 'stato' canonico della penitenza. Alcuni di costoro, a loro volta, poterano nominare loro rappresentante, per riscuotere legati testamentari, un terziario francescano" (740–41).

21. ASF, Not. antecos. no. 4388, 160r–161v, 1363.vii.15.

22. On the possibility of multiple and illogical reactions to relived trauma, see Langer, "The Next Assignment," 291; Binion, *Hitler among the Germans,* xv–xvii, *Soundings,* 15–61, 62–96, *Introduction à la psychohistoire,* 25–42, and "Corrigenda," 69–79.

23. For 1363 the documentation is only suggestive; four Pisan testators can be found for this year, in which a mere nine pious gifts were granted.

24. ASPi, Dipl., Primaziale, 1393.viii.6.

25. Arch. Capitolare, Assisi, Co. S. Stefano (perg. numerate), no. 34, 1362.———.

26. Ibid., no. 29, 1362.x.30.

27. In the diocese of Assisi, the site of a *plebis* church (plebe Podii Morici); *Rationes Decimarum,* vol. 161, no. 3347, p. 223.

28. Sacro Convento, Instr. IV, no. 22, 1363.viii.23.

29. According to Massari, *Saggio sulle pestilenze,* the plague of 1363 was virulent and spread through the *contado* of Perugia, of which Assisi was then a part.

30. Cenci, *Documentazione,* 1:143−48; including busta Z would not have increased the Assisi sample size beyond these 1363 testaments. These are the earliest testaments found in this bundle; the next testaments jump to the 1420s.

31. Sacro Convento, Archivi amministrativi, no. 371, 150r, 1363.———.

32. Sacro Convento, busta Z, no. 3 (1363−1543), 1363.———.

33. Ibid., 1363.vi.15.

34. I was able to uncover only four testaments redacted before 1301 from the *pergamene* and notarial protocol collections housed in the Archivio di Stato and the archives of the monastery of San Pietro (one from the Dominican charters; the other three from the Franciscan house of Santa Maria di Monteluce). Once the rich charter collection of Perugia's principal hospital, the Misericordia, becomes open to the public, the sample for these early documents should increase. Still, this archive may not produce an ample sample size for the analysis of testaments drafted before the fourteenth century. By special permission, I was able to consult the Misericordia's *pergamene* for the years 1300 to 1315, when testaments become available in large numbers for other monastic archives in Perugia. I found only seven testaments from the Misericordia's *pergamene.* (I thank the archivists at the ASPr for this privilege.)

35. On the flagellant movement of 1260 and the importance of *disciplinati* confraternities of fourteenth-century Perugia and Umbria, see Chapter 2, n.108.

36. By a T-test: T value $= -.01$, df $= 135$, probability $= .991$.

37. T-test: t $= 1.58$, df $= 77$, probability $= .119$.

38. T-test: t $= .81$, df $= 128$, probability $= .419$.

39. T-test: t $= .83$, df $= 90$, probability $= .410$.

40. Arch. S. Lorenzo, no. 868, 1348.ix.19.

41. ASF, Dipl., Cestello, 1278.

42. ASF, Not. antecos., no. 205, 15v−17v, 1363.vi.21.

43. Arch. dei Laici, reg. 726, 48v−50v, 1348.ix.27. According to the Lira del 1390 (Cherubini, "Schede per uno studio," 8), the Tarlati and the noble family of the Ubertini (also bishops and rulers of Arezzo) were the richest families of the city and district, on a plane far apart from even the wealthiest merchants of the city, such as the famous Lazzaro Bracci (see Chapter 7).

44. See Lensi, *La Verna;* da Caprese, *Guida Illustrata della Verna,* 209−11; Moorman, *The Franciscan Order,* 62.

45. A *staio* was a unit of dry measure varying slightly in quantity from one commune to another. In Pistoia it was equivalent to about 0.73 bushels or 25.92 liters (Herlihy, *Pistoia,* xix); in Siena, 22.78 liters (Epstein, *Alle origini della fattoria toscana,* 6); and in Florence, 24.36 liters (*Tavole di Riduzione delle misure e pesi,* 21). For slight variations in this and other measurements from place to place in Tuscany during the period of the Grand Dukes, see *Tavole di Ragguaglio . . . del granducato di Toscana.*

46. Arch. dei Laici, reg. 726, 34v−37r, 1348.vi.30.

47. ASF, Not. antecos., no. 10915, 79v−80v, 1363.vii.25.

48. For the general model, the beta coefficient for wealth is $+.258$.

49. The adjusted R-squares for three of the six cities considered singly were higher than that found in the general model, despite the smaller sample sizes:

City	Number of Cases	adj. R-Square	Beta for Wealth
Arezzo	534	.199	+.251
Assisi	210	.284	+.335
Florence	442	.116	+.192
Perugia	397	.165	+.362
Pisa	577	.350	+.496
Siena	390	.135	+.149

50. See, for example, Lane and Mueller, *Money and Banking;* for differences in monies of account over time and place, see Cipolla, *Studi di storia della moneta;* Goldthwaite, "I prezzi del grano"; and Repetti, *Dizionario,* 4: 395. I have used the tables contained in these studies to create constant florins for the analysis that follows.

51. Cohn, *Death and Property,* 127.

52. Mazzi and Raveggi, *Gli uomini e le cose,* 104; see, moreover, their portrait of the peasant Nanni di Bernardo, "La storia di un'eredità 'inutile e dannosa,' " 307–15.

53. This case concerned Pope John XXIII's executors' efforts to secure 800 florins on deposit with the Arte di Calimala in order to complete work on his tomb in the baptistry of Florence: see Lightbown, *Donatello & Michelozzo,* 1–23. I wish to thank John Paoletti for this reference.

54. Tenenti, *Il senso della morte;* see Camporeale's critical review essay, "Senso della morte." While Ariès, in *Western Attitudes toward Death,* 40, originally agreed with Tenenti's analysis, in *The Hour of Our Death,* 128–29, he returned to the traditional interpretation, viewing the danse macabre and Renaissance obsessions with death as evidence for a general sense of pessimism and revulsion toward worldly concerns.

55. This figure is most likely biased downward by a heavy reliance on the single notarial protocol of Pietro di Lippolo for the period of the Black Death (1348). According to Ricci, "Il notaio perugino," this notary worked one of the poorest quarters of the city: "abbracciava quasi esclusivamente la parte del rione situata fuori delle antiche mura della città, il cosidetto borgo; qui abitavano quegli strati sociali costituiti da piccoli artigiani e commerciali . . . per il momento può essi costituivano gli strati più poveri della popolazione" (379).

56. Herlihy, "The Distribution of Wealth," 133.

57. See Herlihy, *Pistoia,* 155ff.; Melis, "Lazzaro Bracci," "Momenti dell'economia del Casentino"; and Tangheroni, "Il sistema economico della toscana," 57–62.

58. Banti, *D'Appiano,* 65, 71–93.

59. Ibid., 90–91.

60. ASF, Not. antecos., no. 8066, 14r–16r, 1406.vi.18.

61. In constant florins (determined by grain prices), testamentary legacies slipped in price from 265.85 florins to 84.75 florins.

62. The values of legacies in constant florins were 95.77 at the beginning of the Trecento and 44.51 a century later.

63. See Coulton, *The Black Death,* 66–67, and *Cronaca senese . . . Agnolo di Tura,* 556, 560.

64. In the 1301–25 period, the values of legacies per testator were 332.53 florins; for 1401–25, they amounted to 1183.98 in nominal values and 763.48 in constant florins.

65. In criticizing the work of Postan and Le Roy Ladurie, Brenner has argued that the Black Death and its ensuing demographic effects did not reproduce the same social and economic consequences in France, England, and Germany east of the Elbe River: see "Agrarian Class Structure" and "The Agrarian Roots of European Capitalism," in Aston and Philpin, *The Brenner Debate.* The results from the comparison of these six cities show that the researcher need not look so far afield to find variations in social and economic consequences of the plague; they might vary radically among cities and territories within the same province.

66. See Genicot, "Crisis," 672–73; Bridbury, *Economic Growth;* Bois, *Crise du féodalisme;* Le Roy Ladurie, *Les paysans du Languedoc;* Herlihy, *Pistoia;* Goldthwaite, "I prezzi del grano"; and la Roncière, *Florence.*

67. For the rationalization of economies in Tuscany, see Chapter 1, note 53; for Umbria, see Grohmann, *Perugia,* 23–24, and *Città e territorio,* 2: 609–79.

68. Herlihy, *Pisa:* "By the early 1300's she [Pisa] found that she was coming to stand vis-à-vis Florence in the same way that, fifty years before her own contado had stood vis-à-vis her. Urbanization and concentration continued, but Pisa was forced from the center. She abandoned forever her historic position as 'head of the Tuscan province,' and, a second-rate city surrounded by greater powers, waited on issues not hers to decide" (185–86).

69. Herlihy, *Pistoia,* 155–79, "The Distribution of Wealth"; Goldthwaite, *The Building of Renaissance Florence.*

70. Mallett, "Pisa and Florence," argues against the imperialist claims of early twentieth-century historians such as Pietro Silva, who stressed the destitution of the Pisan state and economy after its defeat and domination by the Florentines. Mallett's evidence of Pisan recovery comes, however, after my analysis, in the second half of the Quattrocento.

71. See Chapter 1, note 51; and, most recently, Black, *Accolti,* 5–12.

72. Brown, *In the Shadow of Florence.*

73. Mallett, "Pisa and Florence."

74. Melis, "Lazzaro Bracci," 175–191: "La sottomissione di Arezzo a Firenze— o meglio, la congiunzione fra questi due stati cittadini—non segna, dunque, un periodo di decadenza per l'economia aretina: questa, al contrario, si innesta regolarmente nel sistema di relazioni dominato da Firenze, come nucleo, come nudo principale, di un ampio settore circolare (il ricordato arco tra Forlí e Terni), nel quale ritrasmette la straordinaria vitalità e gli incessanti impulsi che provengono da Firenze" (178). See also "Momenti dell'economia del Casentino."

75. In addition to Melis, see Cherubini on Simo d'Umberto, "La proprietà fondiaria," in *Signori, Contadini, Borghesi,* 313–92.

76. Melis, "Lazzaro Bracci," "L'economia delle città minori," and "Momenti dell'economia del Casentino," 193.

77. For the wool industry, see Dini, "Lineamenti per la storia;" for tax law and the Catasto of 1427, see Black, *Benedetto Accolti,* 5–12.

78. ASF, Dipl., Cestello, 1278.ii.18.

79. Ibid., S. Croce, 1279.iv.5.

80. ASF, Not. antecos., no. 13364, 27r, 1301.v.16.

81. ASF, Dipl., S.M. Novella, 1300.ii.9.

82. See ASF, Statuti del Comune di Firenze, no. 11, rub. lxxviii, 150r–153v, "Ordinamenta Mortuorum," which granted the nobility special funerary and burial privileges, such as draping the coffin and garbing the pallbearers in furs.

83. See White, *Duccio,* 32–33 and doc. 5, 185–87; Gardner, "Andrea Di Bonaiuto"; and Orlandi, "Il VII centanario," 111.

84. Orlandi, *"Necrologia,"* 2: 111, reported that this section of Ricchuccius's will incorrectly called the artwork at Prato a crucifix; the document reads, "Conventui fratrum predicatorum de Prato XX soldi f.p. solvendos prope temporis sepulture corporis ipsius testatoris ut expendantur in dicto pro il-luminanda pulcra tabula existens in ecclesia ipsius conventus qua ipse Ric-chuccius fecit pingi per egregium pictorem nomine Giottum bondonis de florentie." This painting is believed to have been destroyed in a fire in 1647. See Bellosi, Angelini, and Ragionieri, "Le arti figurative," 914.

85. Ibid., "Et allegatur et ad memoriam reducatur dicto Guardiano quod ipse Ricchuccius cum fecit executionem testamenti dudum conditi per dictum Ricchum olim Avunculum suum honoravit dictum conventum florentinum et totam eorum provinciam in largitione elymosinarum." For other long-list tes-taments of 40 or more pious bequests, see the will of the cleric Ser Grimaldus f.q. Campagni, who served as the *familiaris* at the hospitals of the clergy in Florence, ASF, Dipl., S.M. Nuova, 1320.ix.25 (52 pious bequests); the notary Ser Gullielmus f.q. Ser Johannis from Castro Fiorentino, who resided in the Florentine parish of San Lorenzo, Arch. S. Lorenzo, no. 868, 1348.ix.19 (63 gifts); and domina Elisabetta, the widow of Michaelis Uberti degli Albizzis and the daughter of the former Batis de Boscicis, ASF, Not. antecos., no. 205, 1363.vi.21, 15v–18r (78 gifts).

86. *Il Canzoniere,* 129, sonnet 99: "S'i' fossi."

87. ASF, Not. antecos., no. 974, 13r–v, 1308.v.1.

88. Ibid., 145r–46r, 1310.iv.2; *Petrarch's Testament,* 75; for other Aretine testaments of this character, see ASF, Dipl., Domenicani d'Arezzo, 1305.iv.13 (42 pious gifts); ASF, Not. antecos., no. 974, 13r–v, 1308.v.1 (35 pious gifts); no. 976, 123r–v, 1312.vi.26 (27 pious gifts), no. 982, 3r–v, 1322.xii.31 (30 pious gifts); no. 984, 115r–v, 1324.viii.15 (30 pious gifts); Arch. dei Laici, reg. 726, 1345.ii.27 (30 pious gifts); and idem, 37v, 1348.vii.29 (35 pious gifts).

89. *I, Catherine,* 133.

90. See Cohn, *Death and Property,* chapter 5, for numerous examples from the lives of late thirteenth- and early fourteenth-century *beati* and *beatae;* and see citations at the beginning of this chapter.

91. Lesnick, *Preaching in Medieval Florence,* 96–133.

92. Cited in Murray, "Piety and Impiety," 89.

93. *I, Catherine,* 62.

94. ASF, Dipl., Domenicani d'Arezzo, 1338.viii.12.

95. Cohn, *Death and Property,* 102–13.

96. ASF, Dipl., Domenicani d'Arezzo, 1338.viii.12.

97. White, *Duccio,* 35 and doc. 5, 185–87.

98. ASF, Dipl., Olivetani d'Arezzo, 1348.————.

99. ASPr, Osp. di Misericordia, no. 3, 2v–3r, 1331.ii.27.

100. Arch. S. Pietro, Liber contractuum, no. 495, 203v–204v, 1348.vi.9.

101. ASPr, Perg., S. Domenico, no. 43, 1348.iv.21.

102. Arch. dei Laici, reg. 726, 20v, 1348.vii.17.

103. If the period from the earliest documents through the recurrence of plague in 1362 is considered, the portion increases to one-fifth of the testaments. Only four testaments redacted after this date conveyed 20 or more pious legacies.

104. ASPi, Osp. di S. Chiara, no. 2071, 23r–25v, 1285.xii.10.

105. This sum even outstripped the commission for the *Rucellai Madonna* of the same period, which, according to White, *Duccio,* 39, went to the panel painter whose work "was technically the best and stylistically the most exciting that money could buy."

106. ASPi, Osp. di S. Chiara, no. 2070, 343v–345r, 1285.v.5.

107. See Ardito, *Nobiltà, Popolo e Signoria;* Tangheroni, *Politica, commercio, agricoltura,* 61ff., 174ff.; and Cristiani, *Nobiltà e popolo.*

108. The Palazzo degli Anziani is the present seat of the Scuola Normale of Pisa.

109. It was in fact later constructed; see Tangheroni, *Politica, commercio, agricoltura,* 174.

110. ASPi, Dipl., San Martino, 1338.vii.10.

111. Arch. dei Laici, reg. 726, 48v–50v, 1348.ix.27: "Et etiam voluit et mandavit predictus testator quod ecclesia iam incepta et fundata per eum in sacro loco alaverne predicto fiat et proficiatur ad laudem, reverentiam et honorem omnipotentis dei et beate marie Virginis matris eius et Beati Michaelis Angeli et beati francisci et totius celestis curie in cuius ecclesie laborerio constructione complemento expendantur et dentur de bonis et ex bonis dicti testatoris floreni iiii mille iusti ponendi et lige floreni aurii in qua quidem ecclesia scilicet in capella de medio dicte ecclesie dictus testator elegit sui corporis sepulturam ante et iuxta immediater predellam altaris dicte capelle de medio."

112. Lensi, *La Verna,* 87. According to da Caprese, *Guida Illustrata della Verna,*

209–11, the third church, la Basilica di Santa Maria Maggiore, was initiated in 1348 with these testamentary funds left by Tarlatus and his wife. But, because of the "greedy avarice" of their heirs, La Verna received only 1,500 florins, construction was halted in midstream, and the church was left uncovered for more than 100 years. After a bull of Pope Nicholas V in 1451 requesting funds from the faithful, this church was finally completed in 1457 "through the generosity of the consuls of the Arte della lana."

113. Instead of declining, the number of nuns and nunneries in Florence gradually increased through the second half of the Trecento and more sharply through the second half of the Quattrocento and early Cinquecento. See Bizzocchi, *Chiesa e potere,* 30–31; Trexler, "Le célibat," 1337; and Brucker, "Monasteries, Friaries, and Nunneries," 45–50.

4. *The Body*

1. Hertz, *Death and the Right Hand;* see also Bloch and Perry, *Death and the Regeneration of Life.*

2. La Sorsa, *La compagnia d'Or S. Michele,* 202. See also Henderson, "Religious Confraternities and Death": "The confraternity made an important contribution to the ritual surrounding death: it provided money, more elaborate ceremonial and a throng of mourners that an average member such as an artisan or shopkeeper could not have afforded by himself" (385). Henderson's conclusions regarding the growth of confraternities in general and the flagellant groups more particularly underscore the trends found in these testaments. According to Henderson, the number of these groups grew and their concerns "for commemoration and a decent burial" intensified after the Black Death through the Quattrocento.

3. ASPi, Osp. di S. Chiara, no. 2065, 60r, 1264.x.9; these death-day celebrations, according to Herklotz, *"Sepulcro" e "Monumenta,"* 15, were of paleo-Christian origin and could also include the third and ninth days, depending on local custom.

4. ASPi, Osp. di S. Chiara, no. 2065, 72r–74v, 1264.ii.9.

5. Ibid., no. 2069, 98v–101r, 1279.ix.9.

6. Ibid., no. 2072, 24v, 1314.vi.nonus.

7. ASF, Not. antecos., no. 12394, 159r–161v, 1361.v.7.

8. The altar's "dowry" follows immediately after the archbishop's request for his sculpted effigy and appears as a separate itemized bequest with no reference to his burial or funeral. It becomes clear that the altar expense and the burial are of one piece when the testator provides for the contingencies to this donation, that is, if his burial should not become possible in this selected spot in the cathedral, "in such a case I order my corpse to be buried in the church of San Paolo di Riperarno . . . with the same conditions as above."

9. Archbishop Giovanni (Scarlatti) in fact had recently founded this monastery himself, and a large portion of his patrimony went to building it. The monastery was the first house of the Olivetani to be established in the area of Pisa: Repetti, *Dizionario*, 1: 57; ASF, Not. antecos., no. 12394, 88r–89v, 1362.ii.16.

10. Carrara is the famous quarry where Michelangelo and other sculptors from the late Middle Ages to the present have procured their marble; see Klapisch-Zuber, *Les maîtres du marbre*.

11. ASF, Not. antecos., no. 12394, 103v–104v, 1362.iii.15; for an artistic assessment of this monument, see Burresi, "Andrea, Nino, e Tommaso," 19–36; Kreytenberg, *Andrea Pisano und die toskanische Skulptur*, 127, pls. 228–30; and Moskowitz, *The Sculpture of Andrea and Nino Pisano*, 207–9, who remarks on the humanistic and Renaissance character of the sculpture.

12. ASPi, Osp. di S. Chiara, no. 2078, 192v–194v, 1323.vii.4.

13. ASF, Not. antecos., no. 12392, 45r–48v, 1346.xi.9.

14. ASPi, Dipl., Primaziale, 1347.viii.19.

15. ASF, Not. antecos., no. 12392, 103v–107v, 1348.vii.29.

16. ASPi, Dipl., Misericordia, 1365.vii.10.

17. Ibid., Olivetani, 1381.ix.13.

18. Ibid., Primiziale, 1383.ii.1.

19. ASF, Not. antecos., no. 788, 184r, 1397.i.23.

20. Ibid., no. 8068, 377v–379r, 1416.v.13.

21. Ibid., no. 8069, 75v–76r, 1417.ii.18.

22. Arch. dei Laici, reg. 726, 58r–60r, 1359.ix.13.

23. ASF, Not. antecos., no. 974, 7v–8r, 1308.iii.31.

24. Arch. dei Laici, reg. 726, 22r–23r, 1348.———.

25. ASF, Not. antecos, no. 10914, n.p., 1361.i.24.

26. For his protocols, see Not. antecos. G676 (1300–1303). See also *Il notaio nella civiltà fiorentina*, nos. 231–32, pp. 203–5. I wish to thank William Bowsky for this reference.

27. ASF, Dipl., S.M. Nuova, 1320.xi.25.

28. Ibid., 1378.v.27.

29. ASF, Dipl., S.M. Novella, 1396.vi.24.

30. Arch. S. Lorenzo, no. 809, 1369.xi.3.

31. A *salumen* is equivalent to 116.91 liters of wine: *Tavole di Ragguaglio . . . dello Stato Pontifico*, 54-55.

32. Sacro Convento, Instr. X, 30, 1348.vi.28; see also the 1415 testament of Bettus Ciccoli de Simonis, who asked for two torches, two barrels of wine, one *raseum* of grain, and three pounds of candles to be carried behind his corpse, and that each priest who accompanied his body be given five soldi: Bibl. Com., Notarile, C.21. (Francesco di Benvenuto di Stefano, 1399–1424), n.p., 1415.xii.30.

33. The parish church was the predominant place (or at least choice) of burial in all these cities except Assisi, where the Basilica of San Francesco

reigned supreme, as in so much of the religious and social life of this new Christian mecca. Elsewhere, the second choice after the parish was burial with the Franciscans, either in their church or "among" (*apud*) its grounds, except in Pisa, where burial choices in the cemetery of the major hospital, Santa Chiara, and thirdly in the cathedral or in its special mausoleum, the Campo Santo, predominated. Next came the Dominicans and then the other mendicant houses. Nunneries and confraternal churches or their collective graves within other churches remained rare for the entire period under study in all six cities and their territories.

34. For Perugia, 100 percent of those testaments redacted before 1276 indicated the place for burial, but the minute sample size (2) gives no confidence in this figure. In the last quarter of the Duecento, only half the testators "elected" their graves; again, this portion comes from an inadequate sample size (4). On the other hand, the Pisan figure for this period had sprung to 100 percent based on 42 testaments.

35. ASF, Not. antecos., no. 20833, n.p., 1348.vii.14.

36. Arch. Capitolare, Arezzo, Not. no. 57, 143r–145r, 1348.ix.21. Wackernagel, *The Florentine Artist,* comments that such practices were widespread in the Quattrocento, although they began to die out toward the end of the century: "All manner of trophies and personal memorabilia of famous ancestors were freely hung there on the family tombs: armor and other military apparatus, festive clothes, coats of arms, banners and the like" (243).

37. The privilege of laymen specifying burial sites inside churches and constructing burial chapels (previously reserved for monarchs and princes of the Church) may have been of recent foundation. "The *Decretum Gratiani* of c. 1140 reputedly reaffirmed the decision of the Synod of Tours that burial inside of the church was to be limited to the high clergy and 'digni presbiteri vel fideles laici'—a conveniently ambiguous phrase. During the thirteenth century with the cult of relics and popular pilgrimage churches, this policy was greatly relaxed. Important Bulls implementing lay burial within the cloisters and churches of the Mendicant Orders are those of Gregory IX in 1229, of Alexander IV in 1255" (Borsook, *The Mural Painters of Tuscany,* xviii, based on Hoger's dissertation, "Studien zur Entstehung der Familienkapelle," 20–54). For conflicts between the mendicant orders and the cathedral in Pisa during the 1230s to the 1260s, see Ronzani, "Gli ordini mendicanti."

For new strictures against lay burials in the new mendicant churches in the latter half of the thirteenth century, see Gardner, "Arnolfo di Cambio," 432–35: "The two great mendicant orders, the Franciscans and Dominicans, had gone to considerable trouble to legislate about tombs in their churches. . . . At the General Chapter of Bologna the Dominicans had forbidden the erection of prominent tombs. Those already admitted were to be removed. . . . Yet by 1274 the Dominican General Chapter had been reduced to prohibiting friars from enticing people who had chosen to be buried in their own parish churches to change their minds. . . . . The Franciscan Order can be seen yielding to similar pressures in the Statutes of the General Chapter from Narbonne in 1260 to those of Paris in 1292, but the first securely datable sculpted tomb in a Franciscan church is much later than the Dominican examples." See also Trexler, "Death and Testament," "Bishop's Portion"; Rigon, "Influssi francescani nei testamenti," 106ff.; and Pellegrini, "Mendicanti e parroci."

38. Sacro Convento, Instr. VIII, no. 55, 1348.viii.7.

39. Ibid., Instr. VIII, no. 44, 1348.vi.26.

40. Ibid., Instr. IX, no. 44, 1360.viii.2.

41. Bibl. Com., C.21, 5r–6v, 1399.iv.17.

42. Ibid., 15v–17r, 1400.v.31.

43. Arch. Capitolare, Assisi, no. 34, 5r–11r, 1362.———.

44. Another lawyer, the pettifogger Nicholas Magistrello, a citizen of Siena, ordered a tombstone in 1484—the first to appear in the samples selected for Siena; see Cohn, *Death and Property*, 61.

45. Ibid., 105.

46. ASF, Dipl., S.M. Novella, 1334.iv.6.

47. Ibid., S.M. Nuova, 1340.x.14.

48. *Diario del Graziani*, 148–49, cited by Grohmann in *Perugia*, 56: "[1348] Adí 8 de aprile nel dicto millesimo comenzò in Peroscia una grande mortalità de pestilenzia [. . .] che per fino al mese de agosto proximo fuoro numerati esser morti in dicta città cento migliaia de persone, cioè fra la città et el contado [. . .] et fu la magiore mortalità che se recorasse mai; et fu sí terribile che non bastavano li cimiteri nè sepolture de le chiese per sepelire gli morti; et per gli cimiterii fuoro fatte pozze molto cupe, et tutte se repivano de corpi morti, et ad ogni modo non bastavano" (56).

Cronaca Pisana di Ranieri Sardo, 114; *Storie Pistoresi*, 235, 148: "Grandissime e pericolose novità furono in quello anno 1347 e 1348 di fame e di pestilenziosa mortalitade per tutto lo mondo . . . e in Toscana e massimamente in Pisa: dove lo padre abbandonava li figliuoli, e' figliuoli lo padre e la madre, e l'uno fratello l'altro; e che non si tro'vava chi volesse servire nullo malato nè portare morto a sepoltura nè frate nè prete che andare vi volesse, perche' la 'nfertà s'appiccava dallo 'nfermo al sano: e durò la 'nfertà piú di iiij° mesi continui."

Cronaca fiorentina di Stefani, 230, rub. 634: "D'una mortalità la quale fu nella città di Firenze, dove morirono molte persone [1348] Lo figliuolo abbandonava il padre, lo marito la moglie, la moglie il marito, l'uno fratello l'altro, l'una sirocchia l'altra. Tutta la città non avea a fare altro che a portare morti a seppellire; molti ne morirono, che non ebbono alla lor fine nè confessione ed altri sacramenti; e moltissimi ne morirono, che non fu chi li vedesse, e molti ne morirono di fame, imperocchè come uno si ponea in sul letto malato. . . . 'Io vo per lo medico' e serravano pianamente l'uscio da via, e non vi tornavano piú. Costui abbandonato dalle persone e poi da cibo. . . . (p. 231) E quando s'addormentava l'ammalato, se n'andava via, e non tornava."

See also the famous passage from Boccaccio's *Decameron:* "they dug for each graveyard a huge trench, in which they laid the corpses as they arrived by hundreds at a time, piling them up tier upon tier as merchandise is stowed on a ship (cited in Meiss, *Painting in Florence and Siena,* 65). And see Petrarch's poem "Ad seipsum," cited at the beginning of this chapter. Tripet, *Pétrarque,* 110–111; Watkins, "Petrarch and the Black Death"; and others have assumed that the plague of 1348 spawned these fears. The editors of the most recent edition of *Rime, Trionfi, Poesie latine,* in which "Ad seipsum" appears, argue, based on a codice in the Biblioteca Laurenziana, which contains a marginal note in Boccaccio's hand, that the poem arose from the mass deaths in 1340.

49. Not. antecos., no. 195, 1348.vii.4.

50. ASF, Dipl., S.M. Nuova, 1348.vii.16.

51. Ibid., S. Croce, 1348.vii.9.

52. Moisé, *Santa Croce,* transcribed this will (appendix 5). The Alberti attempt to preserve their ancestral graves against the restructuring of Santa Croce was a *cause célèbre* in 1566 over patronage rights. While they managed to retain their graves intact, they lost all previous rights to their chapel: see pp. 126–28. See also Hall, *Renovation and Counter Reformation,* (22–24).

53. For the Dominicans' reception of a chapel named after their rival saint, see Chapter 7, note 59.

54. ASF, Dipl., S.M. Novella, 1363.vi.16.

55. ASF, Not. antecos., no. 3570, 80r–, 1363.v.21.

56. Ibid., no. 205, 23v–, 1363.vii.8.

57. ASF, Dipl., S.M. Novella, 1363.vi.3.

58. Of 20 rural testators for this period, 1401–25, only three (15 percent) specified the exact location of their graves.

59. Arch. S. Lorenzo, no. 899, 1371.ix.1.

60. ASF, Dipl., S.M. Novella, 1375.v.17.

61. On the Monte, see Becker, *Florence in Transition,* and Molho, *Florentine Public Finances.*

62. On stained-glass windows in the Renaissance, see Luchs, "Stained Glass above Renaissance Altars."

63. ASF, Dipl., S.M. Novella, 1411.iv.17.

64. Goldthwaite has continued to argue that the patrician Florentines of the fifteenth century shunned notions of lineage and behaved as individuals unencumbered by the constraints and psychology of lineage; see, most recently, "The Empire of Things," where he makes the extraordinary claim that entail or *fidecommissum* did not exist in fifteenth-century Florence. In addition to Kent's criticisms in *Household and Lineage,* see, more recently, those of Hughes, "Representing the Family," 23.

65. ASF, Not. antecos., no. 1758, n.p., 1405.i.15.

66. ASF, Dipl., S.M. Nuova, 1422.i.22.

67. Ibid., 1417.vi.19.

68. ASF, Arch. Gen., 1417.x.27.

69. ASF, Not. antecos., no. 1758, n.p., 1407.x.28.

70. In Florence, 72 of 134 specified sepulchers (54 percent) had already been planned or built.

71. In Florence, 72 of 320 testators chose burial places.

72. ASF, Not. antecos., no. 974, 7v–8r, 1308.iii.31.

73. Manente degli Uberti, called Farinata, died in 1264: Dante Alighieri, *La Divina Commedia, Inferno,* Canto VI, 79 and X, 32. See *Enciclopedia Dantesca,* 804–8.

74. Du Cange, *Glossarium Mediae et Infimae,* 3: 260.

75. Arch. dei Laici, no. 726, 3r–v, 1325.x.1.

76. Arch. Capitolare, Arezzo, no. 57 (Ser Pace Puccii), 110r–v, 1345.ix.4.

77. Ibid., 135r–v, 1348.ix.15.

78. ASF, Not. antecos., no. 994, n.p., 1348.viii.7. The Dominicans preserved a parchment copy of this testament with a slightly different wording: ASF, Domenicani d'Arezzo, 1348.viii.7.

79. Arch. dei Laici, reg. 726, 47v–50v, 1348.ix.27.

80. Ibid., 58r–, 1359.ix.13.

81. Ibid., 61r–61v, 1362.viii.6; a parchment copy is preserved in the Diplomatico of the Olivetani in the Archivio di Stato, Florence, same date.

82. ASF, Not. antecos., no. 10915, 81r–, 1363.vii.26.

83. The likelihood of finding funerary or artistic remains in this early medieval church, whose earliest documentary reference is dated 1009, is slight, because of the Counter Reformation renovations directed by Giorgio Vasari between 1560 and 1564 and, after that, the mid-nineteenth century restoration: see Mercantini, *La pieve di S. Maria ad Arezzo.*

84. *Congios* is also spelled *concios* and is a liquid measure; see Du Cange, *Glossarium Mediae et Infimae,* 2: 481. It was equivalent to 10 barrels of wine, or 456 liters; see Mazzi and Raveggi, *Gli uomini e le cose,* 11.

85. A *quartum* is one-fourth of an *emina* or *staio,* which would be equivalent to 6.09 liters.

86. Arch. dei Laici, reg. 726, 52v–55r, 1374.v.18.

87. According to Salmi, *San Domenico e San Francesco,* 26, this was the funding to complete the major chapel of San Francesco.

88. Arch. dei Laici, reg. 726, 50v–51r, 1374.vi.24.

89. Ibid., 10v, 1374.vi.9.

90. ASF, Not. antecos., no. 9523, 59r–60r, 1419.ix.23.

91. ASF, Dipl., Domenicani d'Arezzo, 1377.v.22.

92. On the career of this exceptional merchant, manufacturer, banker, and landowner, whose business enterprises can be traced throughout northern and central Italy as well as in other parts of Europe and the Near East, see Melis,

"Lazzaro Bracci"; Aldinucci, "Economia aretina," 13–22; and Lazzeri, *Aspetti e figure di vita medievale*. On the plans for his chapel construction, see Borsook, *The Mural Painters of Tuscany,* 92–93.

93. Vasari, *Le Vite,* vol. 3 (*Testo*), "La vita di Parri Spinelli, aretino": "e fra essi uno chiamato Braccio, che oggi quando si parla di lui é chiamato Lazzaro Ricco, il quale morí l'anno 1422, e lasciò tutte le sue ricchezze e facultà a quel luogo che le dispensa in servigio de' poveri di Dio, essercitando con molto carità" (119). According to Aldinucci, Lazzaro died on 2 September 1425.

94. ASA, Perg., no. 12, 1410.xi.10, and Arch. dei Laici, reg. 727, 8v–9r. According to Aldinucci, "Economia aretina," the original of this testament is conserved in the archivio dell'Ospedale di Santa Maria Nuova in Florence.

95. Melis, "Lazzaro Bracci," 179.

96. See Salmi, "I Bacci di Arezzo," which includes excerpts from a transcribed 1417 will translated in a fifteenth-century *ricordanze*.

97. ASF, Not. antecos., no. 9982, 38v–42v.

98. Borsook, *The Mural Painters,* 92–93. According to Aldinucci, "Economia aretina," 21, the monks of the Pieve di Santa Maria and the friars of San Francesco fought for centuries ("per qualche secolo liti atroci") over the rights to celebrate the two offices stipulated in his will—one on his death day, the other to commemorate his patron saint, Lazarus.

99. Arch. dei Laici, reg. 727, 6r–v, 1419.viii.30.

100. ASF, Dipl., Olivetani d'Arezzo, 1328.x.16.

101. ASF, Not. antecos., no. 5884, 49v–50v, 1348.ix.3.

102. ASF, Dipl., Misericordia di Arezzo, 1362.v.28.

103. ASF, Not. antecos., no. 5882, 83v, 1374.vi.14.

104. ASPr, Not. Prot., no. 7, 18v–20v, 1385.xii.22. Ten years later, Finus drafted another will making the same provisions for his burial in the church of the minor friars with the construction of a chapel above it (ASPr, Perg., S. Francesco al Prato, 1395.xii.22).

105. ASPr, Not. Prot., no. 22, 18r–19v, 1390.x.21.

106. ASPr, Perg., San Francesco al Prato, nos. 151, 152, 1399.iii.14.

107. Arch. di S. Pietro, Liber contractuum, no. 495, 203v–204v, 1348.vi.9.

108. A *mezzolino,* or 24.57 liters of olive oil. *Tavole di Raggluaglio . . . dello Stato Pontifico,* 54–55.

109. ASPr, Not. Bast., no. 39, 60v–67v, 1348.vii.1.

110. ASPr, Perg., Mt. Morcino, no. 78, 1362.iii.23.

111. Ibid., S. Maria di Monte Luce, 1367.xi.12.

112. ASPr, Not. Bast., no. 4, 32r–33v, 1383.viii.11.

113. ASPr, Perg., S. Domenico, no. 90, 1383.viii.14.

114. ASPr, Not. Prot., no. 22, 79r–80r, 1400.i.27.

115. ASPr, Not. Bast., no. 11, 74v–77r, 1390.vii.13.

116. See Arias, Cristiani, and Gabba, *Camposanto monumentale di Pisa;* Carli, *Il Camposanto di Pisa;* Bucci, *Campo Santo Monumentale;* and Caleca, "Profilo dell'arte

pisana," 9-18. According to *Cronaca Pisana di Ranieri Sardo,* Archbishop Ubaldi (ob. 1208) purchased the properties for the new mausoleum earlier in the century: "Cap XXXII. Come la Teranaia di Pisa e lo Camposanto s'incominciò. In milleduegento anni, fue incominciata la Tersanaia di Pisa, e lo Camposanto fondato per lo arcivescovo Ubaldo, e comprato al Capitolo lo terreno assegnato. Ed é detto Camposanto, perché si recoe della terra del Camposanto d'Oltremare, quando tornonno dal passaggio preditto, e sparsesi in quello luogo" (86).

117. In these samples, the earliest will that specified burial in the *"campum Sanctum,"* as opposed to *"apud cimiterium maioris ecclesiae Pisis,"* was redacted in 1309: ASPi, Osp. di S. Chiara, no. 2079, 236r–v, 1310.vii.11.

118. ASF, Not. antecos., no. 11050, 7r–9r, 1349.iv.1.

119. Ibid., no. 8066, 268r–v, 1410.ii.16.

120. ASPi, Dipl., Primaziale, 1422.x.9.

121. ASF, Not. antecos., no. 11064, 101v, 1364.viii.4.

122. ASPi, Dipl., Primaziale, 1391.vi.13.

123. Ibid., 1411.viii. 14.

124. ASF, Not. antecos., no. 8069, 83r–84v, 1417.iii.23.

125. Ibid., no. 8069, 22r–23v, 1417.vii.12.

126. Ibid., no. 7588, 204r–205r, 1384.i.3; see also the testament of Ninus f.q. Borghini Federigi, ASPi, Dipl., Primiziale, 1343.vi.22.

127. See ASPi, Osp. di S. Chiara, no. 2077, 87v–88r, 1309.v.Idus; no. 2078, 11r–v, 1308.ii.7; no. 2078, 188r–v, 1321.iii.pridie.

128. Ibid., no. 2077, 87v–88r, 1309.v.Idus; ASF, Not. antecos., no. 8071, 166v–167v, 1424.ii.6; ASPi, Osp. di S. Chiara, no. 2078, 74r–v, 1313.x.15, no. 2079, 97r, 1309.x.13; ASPi, Dipl., Primaziale, 1284.vii.15, 1412.iv.5, 1411.viii.14.

129. In Giovanni's progression through the ecclesiastical hierarchy, he crossed much of late-medieval Christendom. From being a subdeacon in Armenia, he became an archdeacon in Spain, then the bishop of Coron (Greece) before becoming archbishop of Pisa in 1349, see Eubel, *Hierarchia Catholica,* 1: 212, 399.

130. ASPi, Dipl., S. Martino, 1382.viii.13.

131. Ibid., 1391.viii.24.

132. ASF, Not. antecos., no. 11067, 173v–175r, 1378.viii.pridie. In his testament, the merchant and citizen of Pisa Pierus f.q. Ser Vanni Sciorta allocated between 10 and 12 florins for his sepulcher and "Emonumentum" with his coat of arms.

133. Herklotz, *"Sepulcra" e "Monumenta,"* 24–25; moreover, he argues (pp. 36–39) that Roman burial practices and ideology disappeared in the fifth century, and that with the exception of Ravenna, monumental graves remained rare everywhere in the West until their revival by the early Normans in the eleventh century.

134. See Baron, *The Crisis of the Early Italian Renaissance.* In an earlier, seminal essay, "Franciscan Poverty," he defined the Renaissance by contrasting Franciscan and stoic values of poverty with a new justification and praise of "civic"

wealth. For him, the transition comes well into the fifteenth century: "Civic funeral orations of that time breathe the same spirit. They praise the deceased no longer on account of his renunciation of vain worldly goods, but rather for his acquisition of wealth by labor and industry, and for the praise-worthy use he made of his possessions" (22). Baron then goes on to describe the funeral oration for Leonardo Bruni (d. 1444) and Alamanno Rinuccini's for Matteo Palmeri (d. 1474).

135. From his Burckhardtian frame of reference regarding celebrated tombs and funerary works of art, Panofsky, in *Tomb Sculpture,* stridently emphasizes the change wrought by the Renaissance, which he saw as a mid-fifteenth-century movement: "And it is precisely in its attitude toward the dead that the new epoch most vigorously asserted its "modernity" (67). . . . Here we have indeed a complete reversal of the medieval attitude. Glorification of intellectual achievements and academic honors has taken the place of pious expectations for the future of the soul" (69). More recently, from an in-depth survey of epitaphs and monumental tombs, Herklotz, in *"Sepulcra" e "Monumenta,"* has delivered the same message. This time, however, the break occurs two centuries earlier: "In brief, the content of funeral inscriptions of the high middle ages, the hope for another life after death, requests for the intercession from saints and survivors—*topos* of the *contemptus mundi*—have practically disappeared by the second half of the thirteenth century, at least from monumental tombs . . . which accentuate that *Ruhmsinn* Jacob Burckhardt theorized for the Renaissance" (199).

5. Property

1. Tenenti, *Il senso della morte,* has drawn similar conclusions for the fifteenth century from literature and art.

2. See Catoni, *Le pergamene dell'università di Siena,* 27–35, and "Gli oblati della Misericordia."

3. See La Sorsa, *La compagnia d'Or S. Michele,* 56–65, and Gavitt, *Charity and Children,* 14–16. The Misericordia of Perugia also experienced a financial crisis— in its case, in the year of the plague's return, 1363. See Chapter 2, note 78.

4. *Cronica di Matteo Villani,* vol. 1, chap. 6; Gavitt, *Charity and Children,* 15; Becker, "Aspects of Lay Piety," 177.

5. Arch. dei Laici, reg. 726, 60r–61r, 1374.vi.2.

6. *Stioro, staio,* or *stario:* a unit of surface area equivalent to about 12.65 ares, or 0.313 acres, in Pistoia, but like the unit of dry measure bearing the same name, it varied slightly from commune to commune: see Herlihy, *Pistoia,* xix, and *Tavole di Ragguaglio per la riduzione . . . del granducato di Toscana.*

7. ASF, Not. antecos., no. 975, 36r–37r, 1311.iii.17.

8. See for instance, ASPi, Dipl., Aquisto Cappelli, 1357.xi.9.

9. ASPi, Osp. di S. Chiara, no. 2078, 185r–186v, 1321.v.4.

10. Ibid., no. 2070, 200r–201v, 1303.x.9.

11. Ibid., no. 2079, 233r–34r, 1310.vi.2.

12. ASF, Not. antecos., no. 12394, 159r–161v, 1361.v.7.

13. On the legal distinctions of women's property, see Ercole, "L'istituto dotale"; Kirshner and Pluss, "Two Fourteenth-Century Opinions on Dowries"; Kirshner, "Non-Dotal Assets"; Izbichi, " 'Ista questio est antiqua' "; Bellomo, *Ricerche sui rapporti patrimoniali fra coniugi;* and Klapisch-Zuber, *La famiglia e le donne,* especially "Il complesso di Griselda," 154–91, and "La 'madre crudele,' " 285–303.

14. ASPi, Dipl., Aquisto Cappelli, 1382.iv.10.

15. Ibid., Primaziale, 1392.vi.1.

16. Ibid., S. Domenico, 1383.viii.13.

17. ASF, Not. antecos., no. 8068, 2330v–231v, 1414.vi.27: "Et non possit vel debeat illam vendere vel alienare sive suppignerare vel baractere et aliter non."

18. ASPi, Dipl., Primaziale, 1402.i.25.

19. ASF, Not. antecos., no. 8066, 14r–16r, 1406.vi.18.

20. ASPi, Dipl., Olivetani, 1420.viii.13.

21. Sacro Convento, instr. x, no. 36, 1348.vii.13.

22. Bibl. Com., Not., A.I., Ser Giovanni di Giacomo, 20r–21v, 1400.ix.8.

23. Ibid., 23r–25r, "Ymmo semper et in perpetuum remaneat comunem et comunia dicti heredibus et eorum subcessoribus."

24. Ibid., C.21, Ser Francesco di Benvenuto, 86r–88r, 1415.ix.25.

25. Cohn, *Death and Property,* 146–58.

26. ASF, Dipl., Arch. Gen., 1291.viii.30.

27. On the business affairs and politics of the Cerchi family in the early fourteenth century, see the introduction and text of *Dino Compagni's Chronicle,* and Davidsohn, *Storia di Firenze,* 6: 371–73.

28. ASF, Dipl., S.M. Novella, 1300.ii.9.

29. ASF, Not. antecos., no. 13364, 7v–, 1300.i.4.

30. ASF, Dipl., Arch. Gen., 1313.ii.6.

31. ASF, Dipl., S.M. Novella, 1348.v.11.

32. Ibid., Arch. Gen., 1348.vi.29.

33. Ibid., 1348.vii.9.

34. Ibid., S.M. Novella, 1355.viii.2.

35. ASF, Ibid., 1363.vi.16.

36. Perhaps a marginal branch or a corruption of the noble Guelph family name Tosinghi (or della Tosa), of the parish of San Lorenzo. On the latter family, see Bowsky, *Piety and Property,* 18.

37. ASF, Not. antecos., no. 205, 28r–29v, 1364.vii.20..

38. Ibid., 29v–31r, 1364.vii.20.

39. ASF, Dipl., 1368.viii.24.

40. See Camporeale, "Giovanni Caroli e la 'Vitae fratrum,' " "Giovanni

Caroli: Dal 'Liber dierum,' " "Humanism and the Religious Crisis," and "Giovanni Caroli, 1460–1480."

41. Earlier, in a *causa donationis* of 1367, Friar Alexio had given all of his movable goods (*supellectilia arnesia et masseritias et omnes et singulos pannos lanos et linos*) to his mother. In 1372, through a *donatio inter vivos,* his mother granted him the usufruct of three-quarters of another *podere,* this one in the village of San Giorgio a Colonica, to be distributed to the poor and to pious places after her death. See Orlandi, *"Necrologio,"* vol. 2, doc. 14, p. 462, and vol. 1, p. 636.

42. The case of Alexio's inheritance from his father was a cause célèbre involving a complex and extended litigation between Santa Maria Novella and the Strozzi family. According to Orlandi, *"Necrologio"* (vol. 1, 131 and 623–47), this estate was extraordinarily rich, valued at 20,000 florins. At age 14, the boy entered the Dominican order at Santa Maria Novella and, according to the boy's uncles, was held there "not for reasons of devotional zeal, but for greed and avarice." To free the boy from this alleged captivity, his uncles utilized their connection with the bishop of Città di Castello and the archbishop of Ravenna and appealed directly to Pope Urban V, who ordered Alexio placed in an apartment belonging to the archbishop of Florence. Thus protected and unencumbered by pressures exerted by the friars and his relatives, the boy was to decide for himself whether he would remain a friar or return to lay existence. The case was resolved in favor of Santa Maria Novella, and Alexio flourished as a scholar of philosophy, dying at the age of 33. His body is still preserved intact in the *cappelleta* under the steps of the chapel of Saint Thomas Aquinas.

43. ASF, Dipl., S.M. Novella, 1377.vii.21.

44. Ibid., 1386.i.23.

45. ASF, Dipl., Arch. Gen., 1406.ix.22.

46. Ibid., S.M. Nuova, 1413.v.6.

47. Ibid., S.M. Novella, 1415.vi.9. On women's rights to these properties, see Klapisch-Zuber, "Il complesso di Griselda," in *La famiglia e le donne,* 154–91. In this case, Lady Pellegrina appears to have had more control over what probably was her "corredo" than what Klapisch-Zuber argues was commonly the practice in Quattrocento Florence.

48. ASF, Not. antecos., no. 2417, n.p., 1422.vi.27.

49. Cohn, *The Laboring Classes,* 115–28.

50. ASF, Dipl., Arch. Gen., 1416.x.13.

51. Ibid., S.M. Nuova, 1422.i.22.

52. Ibid., S.M. Novella, 1362.ix.7.

53. Ibid., 1373.iii.6.

54. Ibid., 1373.iii.12 (by its inventory); the testament, however, is dated 1373.iii.6.

55. Ibid., 1393.v.9.

56. ASF, Not. antecos., no. 195 (1338–48), 220v, 1348.vii.4.

57. ASF, Dipl., S. Croce, 1386.iv.7.

58. ASF, Not. antecos., no. 12064, 102r–v, 1397.iii.30.

59. ASF, Dipl., S.M. Nuova, 1313.vi.23. For similar examples, see idem, 1340.x.14, and Arch. Gen., 1346.iii.16, in which the testator demanded that his nephew be "obedient, reverent, loving and attentive" to his uncle, who was given the authority to manage the nephew's affairs while "in his adolescent years."

60. ASF, Not. antecos., no. 13364, 7v, 1300.i.14.

61. ASF, Dipl., S.M. Nuova, 1319.ii.10.

62. Ibid., S.M. Novella, 1351.iv.2.

63. Ibid., 1396.vi.24.

64. ASF, Not. antecos., no. 4417, 133v–134r, 1406.iii.25.

65. ASF, Dipl., S.M. Nuova, 1390.v.4.

66. Ibid., Arch. Gen., 1407.viii.31.

67. Arch. S. Lorenzo, no. 841, 1370.iii.8.

68. There are 20 and 21 instances, respectively, of property having been channeled down a lineage in Arezzo and Florence.

69. ASF, Not. antecos., no. 992, 152v–54v, 1334.xii.8; no. 993, n.p., 1334.———.

70. Arch. Capitolare, no. 57 (Ser Pace Puccii Notario), 102r–, 1344.xi.14.

71. ASF, Not. antecos., no. 9541, n.p., 1358.iii.16.

72. Ibid., no. 5891, 196v–197v, 1362.viii.18.

73. ASA, Antichi notari, no. 14, 10v, 1374.vi.9.

74. Arch. dei Laici, no. 726, 1374.iii.26.

75. Falcidie and trebellianice are terms for the quarter part of the inheritance guaranteed for the universal heir by Roman law: see Du Cange, Glossarium Mediae et Infimae, 3: 400, and 8: 161.

76. Arch. dei Laici, reg. 726, 61v, 1375.x.31.

77. ASF, Not. antecos., no. 9523, 38v–42v, 1416.viii.5.

78. Ibid., no. 992, 152v–54v, 1334.xii.8; no. 990, n.p.

79. Arch. dei Laici, reg. 726, 51r–52r, 1374.v.23.

80. ASF, Not. antecos., no. 9982, 33r–34v, 1415.ii.25.

81. Arch. dei Laici, reg. 726, 60r–61r, 1374.vi.2.

82. ASF, Not. antecos., no. 9982, 16r, 1411.viii.1.

83. Ibid., no. 9981, 38v–42v, 1416.viii.5.

84. Ibid., no. 993, 33r–v, 1328.viii.11.

85. Arch. Capitolare, Arezzo, no. 57, 39r–42r, 1340.vi.24.

86. ASF, Dipl., Misericordia d'Arezzo, 1363.vi.30.

87. ASF, Not. antecos., no. 993, 197r–198r, 1330.xii.9.

88. ASF, Not. antecos., 25r–v, 1350.iii.14.

89. ASF, Not. antecos., no. 5885, 24r, 1358.xi.13.

90. Ibid., 231r–v, 1363.vi.22.

91. Ibid., no. 5882, 22v, 1373.xii.24.

92. Ibid., no. 10747, 93r–v, 1424.x.28.
93. Ibid., no. 974, 163v, 1312.viii.23.
94. Ibid., no. 993, 192r–193r, 1329.x.15.
95. Arch. dei Laici, reg. 726, 65v–66r, 1344.viii.10.
96. Arch. Capitolare, Arezzo, no. 57, 128r–, 1347.xi.2.
97. ASF, Not. antecos., no. 978, 19v–20v, 1318.iv.17.
98. Ibid., no. 988, 154r, 1327.vii.6.
99. Ibid., no. 993, 62v–63r, 1328.ix.15.
100. Ibid., 75r–76r, 1328.x.7.
101. Ibid., 183r–184v, 1329.vi.9.
102. Ibid., no. 5892, 168v–170r, 1363.v.22.
103. Ibid., no. 1921, 85v, 1400.viii.16.
104. Ibid., no. 9523, 27r, 1412.iii.24.
105. Ibid., 49v–50r, 1418.vi.2.
106. Ibid., no. 9982, 7v–8r, 1411.vi.15.
107. Ibid., 9r–v, 1411.vii.1.
108. Ibid., 18v–19r, 1411.viii.10.
109. Ibid., no. 10747, 83v, 1424.viii.9.
110. Ibid., 84r–85r, 1424.viii.23.
111. Arch. di S. Pietro, Liber contractuum, no. 495, 146r, 1332.iii.18.
112. On the political importance of the Oddonis (Degli Oddi) family in late medieval Perugia, see Heywood, *A History of Perugia,* 156–58, 299–309; Salvatorelli, "La politica interna," 66, 92–93; and Grohmann, *Città e territorio,* 1: 529–31.
113. ASPr, Perg., S. Francesco al Prato, no. 94, 1348.iv.15.
114. Ibid., Mt. Morcino, no. 202, 1383.xi.5.
115. Ibid., S. Domenico, no. 177, 1421.xi.19.
116. See Heywood, *A History of Perugia,* 272; Salvatorelli, "La politica interna," 104ff.; and Grohmann, *Città e territorio,* 1: 517–18. On the assassination of Biordo Michelotti, see Pellini, *Dell'historia di Perugia,* 960, 1006. The family was infamous for its treasonous acts against the Raspanti, which restored the nobility to power in 1384.
117. For the Baglioni family, see Salvatorelli, "La politica interna," 92, and Grohmann, *Città e territorio,* 1: 428–45. The Baglioni and the Oddi were the principal rivals in the conflict of 1302, which split the nobility into two factions.
118. See Heywood, *A History of Perugia,* 272; ASPr, Not. Prot., no. 7, 86v–87v, 1395.i.7.
119. ASPr, Not. Prot., no. 7, 44v–47r, 1389.ix.25.
120. See, for instance, the complex restrictions that the widow from Villa Fratta Sant'Andrea placed on her home with its work hut and piece of land. No one—not her son, her executives, or her descendants—was to sell or alienate the property, except to a certain Johannes Andree: ASPr, Not. Bast., no. 11, 149r–150r, 1390.x.28.

121. Ibid., no. 10, 28v–29v, 1389.ii.26.

122. ASPr, Not. Prot., no. 7, 84r–v, 1393.v.26.

123. ASPr, Perg., Mt. Morcino, no. 94, 1363.viii.26.

124. Ibid., no. 131, 1371.xi.3.

125. ASPr, Not. Prot., no. 7, 27v, 1386.ix.29.

126. Ibid., 48r–v, 1390.iii.30.

127. ASPr, Not. Bast., no. 11, 94v–96r, 1390.viii.15.

128. ASPr, Perg., Monteluce, no. 365, 1417.iv.7.

129. ASPr, Not. Prot., no. 2, 71r–v, 1371.viii.28.

130. ASPr, Perg., Mt. Morcino, no. 78, 1362.iii.23.

131. Ibid., no. 202, 1383.xi.5.

132. ASPr, Perg., S. Domenico, no. 81, 1375.vii.20.

133. For Perugia, 397 of these clauses appear out of 524 testaments (76 percent); for Arezzo, 158 of 648 testaments (24 percent); for Florence, 80 of 581 testaments (14 percent); for Siena, 169 of 446 testaments (38 percent); for Assisi, 96 of 292 testaments (33 percent); and for Pisa, 46 of 737 testaments (6 percent).

134. Long ago, writers such as Fustel de Coulanges, *La Cité antique,* and Maine, *Dissertations on Early Law and Custom,* found this same opposition between the property rights of women and the strength of the patrilineal devolution of property. More recently, anthropologists such as Goody, *Death, Property, and the Ancestors,* and Guichard, *Structures sociales "orientales" et "occidentales,"* have stressed the same relationship but have gone further in relating other rites and customs to the systems of property devolution.

135. Goody, "Inheritance, Property, and Women," 10. Herlihy, in *Opera Muliebra,* claims that women in the earlier Middle Ages, before the thirteenth century, had inherited equally with their brothers. Afterward, aristocratic families favored male offspring and reserved "resources primarily for the support of its sons, often only the eldest son" (63). Unfortunately, no note or statistics underlie this claim. Patterns of primogeniture do not emerge in any of the towns examined in my study. In Siena, traces of primogeniture arise only in the sixteenth century.

136. Goody, "Inheritance, Property, and Women," 10.

137. The difference before and after the 1362-63 plague is highly significant at .01, $p = .5172$, $\pi = .4184$, $N = 631$, $z = 5.04$.

138. The choice of daughters as universal heirs over more distant kinsmen was equal to Florence in Perugia, 36 percent (45 of 126). Assisi, Arezzo, and Siena lay in between Florence and Pisa: 45 percent (23 of 51), 50 percent (55 of 110), and 51 percent (38 of 74), respectively.

139. Riemer, "Women, Dowries, and Capital Investment," 59–79, 72; her conclusions are based on a sample of only 24 testaments drawn between 1283 and 1307.

140. In Perugia, in 49 cases out of 93, women named their husbands as universal heirs.

141. Seven of 19 wills from Florentine women named their husbands as universal heirs.

142. ASPi, Osp. di S. Chiara, no. 2078, 80r, 1311.i.6.

143. On the 15-lire customary gift, see *Statuti di Pisa,* vol. 2, *Constitutum,* XLI, 786–87: "De his que a viro in uxorem dantur vel relinquuntur."

144. On the *mundualdus,* see Cortese, "Per la storia del munio"; Bellomo, *La condizione giuridica,* 26–28; and Giardina, " 'Advocatus' e 'mundualdus.' " Kuehn, " 'Cum Consensu mundualdi,' " argues that "the appointment of a *mundualdus* for a woman was decidedly quotidian" (309), and, from sampling one notarial chartulary of 1422–30, finds 179 participating in notarized contracts with the consent of such a male protector. Unfortunately, he fails to report the number of women who drafted notarized documents without a *mundualdus.* On the other hand, Rosenthal, "The Position of Women," argues forcefully that, against the dictates of communal legislation, most patrician women from Quattrocento Florence drew up contracts without the consent of a male protector; the *mundualdus* appears in only 17 percent of the notarized contracts involving the women she examines. From this evidence, she questions the harsher picture of women drawn by Christiane Klapisch-Zuber (*La famiglia e le donne*) and claims that this information about the *mundualdus* "shatters our present view of female behavior and prerogatives" and displays "the independence of women." Rosenthal's study, however, shows the pitfalls of examining a single place without comparative perspectives. As Kuehn points out from an examination of the communal statutes from Pisa and Siena, and as the testaments drawn for my comparative study illustrate, Florence and the towns subject to its law were unusual in their preservation of these Lombard laws restricting the contractual independence of women.

145. As the wide variety of options practiced by husbands in each of these towns indicates, these differences in widows' property settlements were matters of custom and practice rather than dictates established through communal statutes. On the widow's rights to the property of her deceased husband, see Pertile, *Storia del Diritto Italiano,* vol. 3; Bellomo, *La condizione giuridica,* 26–28, *Ricerche sui rapporti patrimoniali fra coniugi;* Klapisch-Zuber, "Il complesso di Griselda," 154–91, "La zane della sposa," and "La 'madre crudele,' " all in *La famiglia e le donne.* On the succession of the dowry, see *Statuti di Pisa,* vol. 2, *Constitutum,* XXIII, 742–45: "De exactione dotis"; XXV, 748–50: "De sacramento manifestationis bonorum quondam mariti ab eius uxore prestando"; XXVI, 750–51: "Quibus mulieribus permissum sit dotem et donamenta suo sacramento probare"; XXVIII, 752: "Quo casu pater de dote filio prestita in solidum teneatur"; XXVIIII, 752–54: "De donatione propter nunptias"; XXX, 754–56: "Quid mariti ex morte uxoris sine pacto lucrantur." *Statuto di Arezzo,* bk. 3, rub. 63, 173–74: "De dotium et donationum propter nuptias restitutione, et qualiter ius reddatur." *Statuta Florentiae (an. 1415),* bk. 2, rub. 61, 156–59: "De dote, et donatione restituendis, et exigendi modo." *Statuti di Perugia,* bk.

2, rub. 35, 334–36: De le dote e le dotate fenmene." *Il constituto del comune di Siena*, Distinctio II, XXXV, 214–15: "Quod mater possit habere expensas a filiis suis, donec steterit cum eis." See also Chapter 1, note 119.

146. Husbands provided their to-be-widows these property arrangements in 19 out of 115 cases in Assisi; 38 of 254 in Arezzo; 41 of 227 in Perugia; 40 of 176 in Siena; and 84 of 217 in Pisa.

147. Kirshner, "Non-Dotal Assets"; Ercole, "L'istituto dotale," 197–211.

148. In Florence, 46 of 247 husbands with surviving wives left their wives with this choice; next in importance but only half as frequent (24 cases) came the standard formula found for the other cities, in which the widow was granted rights to the usufruct of her husband's property, provided she remain chaste and never remarry. For the social and psychological ramifications of this system of widowhood, see Klapisch, "La 'madre crudele.' " To my knowledge, the communal statutes do not encode this dilemma for the wife, where she would lose the rights to her dowry if she chose the usufruct of her husband's property. Nor does Ercole, "L'istituto dotale," 222–57, mention such a settlement in surveying "the restitution of the dowry to widows" in communal statutes across the Italian peninsula. He instead insists that "la restitutione della dote contro gli eredi del marito è infatti universalmente riconosciuta e protetta; tutti gli statuti non potrebbero essere più espliciti in questo senso" (223).

149. In Perugia, 22 of 227 husbands with surviving wives, and in Arezzo, 27 of 254, left their wives with this arrangement. These practices ran beneath the practices encoded by statutory law and cannot be interpreted from a comparison of the published city statutes of the Trecento for the six cities.

150. See, for instance, Rosenthal, "The Position of Women."

151. See Chapter 8: unlike Tuscany, which fell under Lombard control in the seventh century, the duchy of Perugia (which included Assisi) remained under Byzantine suzerainty and thus retained Roman law.

6. Art and Masses

1. Cohn, *Death and Property*, 63–64.

2. In the period 1301–25, the percentage of perpetual masses was lowest for Perugia. These years, however, comprise a negligible sample size of only 10 testaments.

3. Arch. dei Laici, reg. 726, 34v–37r, 1348.vi.30.

4. Arch. S. Lorenzo, no. 899, 1371.ix.1.

5. ASF, Dipl., Olivetani d'Arezzo, 1363.vii.10.

6. Ibid., Domenicani d'Arezzo, 1338.viii.12.

7. Arch. Capitolare, Arezzo, no. 57, 110r–, 1345.x.4.

8. Arch. dei Laici, reg. 727, 47v–50v, 1348.ix.27.

9. Ibid., reg. 726, 45r–46r, 1371.ii.15.

10. ASF, Not. antecos., no. 11248, 60r–61r, 1379.vi.24; Arch. dei Laici, reg. 726, 50v–51r, 1374.vi.24.

11. Her father already possessed a chapel in Santa Maria Novella, which existed as early as 1352, where Margherita's son Silvestro was buried (Orlandi, *"Necrologio,"* 2: 581). According to Orlandi, on 11 September 1365, the *procuratore* of the convent, Friar Zanobi Guasconi, acted on the testamentary concession made by donna Margherita "revindicating the rights of the chapel" located "under the vaults on an angle behind the church of Santa Maria Novella" founded by her father (610). A reference to the chapel is found in a letter from Giovanni Dominici dated 23 December 1400, narrating a dream from the previous night in which he was hearing a confession in the chapel of San Marco ("ove odo confessione, innanzi alla cappella del prezioso evangelista S. Marco, e fui subito addormentato" [Biscioni, *Lettere di Santi e Beati fiorentini,* lett. 13, p. 139]); see Orlandi, *"Necrologio,"* 2: 92.

12. ASF, Dipl., S.M. Novella, 1367.viii.14. No mention of this chapel appears in the references collected by Orlandi, *"Necrologio."*

13. ASF, Dipl., S.M. Novella, 1396.vi.24.

14. ASPi, Osp. di S. Chiara, no. 2078, 128v–130v, 1314.vi.13.

15. The Upezzinghis were a leading Pisan aristocratic family within the Guelph party; see Luzzati, "Le origini di una famiglia nobile pisana," 90–96.

16. ASF, Not. antecos., no. 8066, 121v–127v, 1409.vii.20.

17. Sixty-four of 183 chapel constructions were endowed by those with family names, while 370 of 3,389 testaments were redacted by those with family names.

18. Of 183 chapel constructions, testators evaluated 92 of these projects in monetary terms. These construction prices usually did not include the endowments for the chaplain's living or salary, or the yearly expenses for candles, commemorative meals, and fees paid to other clerics who were to participate in the festivities; nor did they usually include the costs of decorating and ornamenting the chapel with paintings or furnishing it with the missal, vestments, altarcloths, and "other opportunities."

19. Arch. S. Lorenzo, no. 886, 1348.vi.2. Perhaps this bequest was never carried out; 27 years later, a Bencivennes f.q. Turini left property for a chapel dedicated to Santa Caterina in the same church of San Lorenzo. (See page 220.) According to the *Visite* Pastorali of Amerigo Corsini in 1422 (Archivio Arcivescovile, Firenze, 13v), a chapel dedicated to Saint Catherine was then in place.

20. ASF, Not. antecos., no. 8105, n.p., 1363.viii.9. On the practice of commemorative meals and religious confraternities, see Davidsohn, *Storia di Firenze,* vol. 4, pt. 3, 192–94.

21. ASPr, Not. Bast., no. 11, 74v–77r, 1390.vii.13.

22. ASF, Not. antecos., no. 10914, n.p., 1361.i.24.

23. Arch. Capitolare, Arezzo, Testamenta Ser Johanne Cecchi, 3r–, 1389.i.6.

24. ASPr, Perg., Mt. Morcino, no. 335, 1411.vii.29.

25. ASF, Dipl., Arch. Gen., 1416.x.13.

26. ASF, Not. antecos., no. 20833, n.p., 1348.vii.11.

27. Forty-seven testators of 183 who founded chapels lived outside the city or were émigrés. This figure was representative of the proportion of those residing beyond the walls of the cities investigated in this study—25 percent (851 of 3,386).

28. ASA, Antichi notari, no. 14, 1374.iv.30.

29. ASF, Not. antecos., no. 10747, 84r–85r, 1424.viii.23.

30. Ibid., no. 11248, 90r, 1375.xi.10.

31. Arch. dei Laici, reg. 726, 3r–v, 1325.x.1.

32. Nicholas of Tolentino was not canonized until 5 June 1446: *Bibliotheca Sanctorum,* 11: 962.

33. ASS, Not. antecos., no. 23, 39v–40v, 1348.vi.27.

34. Ibid., no. 9541, n.p., 1358.iv.6.

35. Ibid., no. 11247, n.p., 1374.iii.21.

36. Ibid., no. 10736, n.p., 1396.vii.30.

37. ASPi, Dipl., Primiziale, 1401.iv.13.

38. ASPi, Dipl., Olivetani, 1325.xii.9.

39. 48.10 percent, or 10,533 of 21,896 pious bequests, including those from all testaments, codicils, and fragments, come from testaments redacted before 1348.

40. See Brown, *The Cult of the Saints,* and Herklotz, *"Sepulcro" e "Monumenta."* For church ordinances that attempted to block and regulate the construction of such monuments as burial shrines for lay families, see Chapter 4, note 34.

41. "Item iussit et voluit quod capella sive orratorium [sic] qua est in palatio suo in plano Bisastici per dictos suos heredes manuteneantur et in dicta capella stet et moretur unus sacerdos cum uno clericho in perpetuum ad celebrandum ibi pro anima sua et parentum suorum divina ofitia et judicavit dicte capelle et sacerdoti ibi commoranti suum positum ad terrenzanum cum omnibus pertinentibus in quodam podere [quo] dictus dominus Consillius dixit se emisse a Paolo Bonfilliuoli pro expensis et necessitatis dicti presbiteris et clerici et si dicta capella in dicto loco cum modo esse non poterit, voluit quod dicti sui heredes eam sic faciant in suo territorio dicti testatorias in civitate vel in comunitatis florentie et quod in ea perpetuo celebreantur divina offitia et quod presbiter ipse capelle et clerichus qua ibi morabuntur habeant pro eorum necessitatibus dictum podere de terrenzano. Item voluit quod filii sui et descendentes eorum maschili legiptimi per lineam maschulinam in dicta ecclesia habeant omne ius patronatus et in eam presbiterem et rectorem eligant et eam protegant et defendant et omnia faciant qua in ea viderint expedire ad honorem dei et beate Marie semper virgini."

42. ASPi, Osp. di S. Chiara, no. 2076, 206v–207v, 1307.vii.pridie.

43. ASF, Dipl., Domenicani d'Arezzo, 1338.viii.12.

44. ASA, Perg. varie, 1363.vi.16.

45. Arch. dei Laici, reg. 727, 6r–v, 1419.viii.30.

46. Ibid., reg. 726, 52v–55r, 1374.v.18.

47. Arch. S. Lorenzo, no. 928, 1375.xii.11; see note 19.

48. ASF, Not. antecos., no. 11248, 60r–, 1379.vi.24.

49. ASPi, Dipl., S. Martino, 1384.x.16.

50. Arch. S. Lorenzo, no. 1001, 1389.iv.16. Conti, *La Basilica di S. Lorenzo,* 43, cites a copy of this testament held in the Biblioteca Nazionale, Firenze (*Manoscritti,* II, IB, 379, c. 312), adding that the chapel was to be dedicated to San Girolamo. Evidence that the commission was carried out comes from Milanesi's commentaries on Vasari's *Vite,* 1: 611, n. 3: "Nel 1414 i Consoli dell'Arte della Lana gli fecero fare la tavola [attributed to Marioto di Nardo] per l'altare della cappella di San Girolamo nella Chiesa di San Lorenzo, costruita dalla detta Arte co'denari lasciati per testamento a questo effetto da Sandro d'Iacopo di Ghino, chiamato Sandro di monna Balda."

51. ASF, Not. antecos., no. 10736, 200r–202r, 1396.viii.22.

52. Ibid., no. 8066, 121v–127v, 1409.vii.20.

53. For a similar case, see Borsook and Offerhaus, *Francesco Sassetti and Ghirlandaio,* 13. According to a sixteenth-century chronicler, Sassetti's quarrel with the Dominicans resulted from this patron's wish "to have the life of his patron saint [Francis] painted on the walls of the church's chancel." Perhaps Borsook and Offerhaus's dismissal of this story—"The idea of using a Franciscan theme in the main chapel of a rival order seems too unreasonable to believe"—needs reconsidering in light of Alferri's demands a century earlier. In fact, according to the *Libro delle Cappelle e Sepolture* (cited in Orlandi, *"Necrologio,"* 2: 610–11), this chapel was erected. Much confusion has arisen in the later accounts of this chapel, which have mistaken it for the chapel of San Marco founded by the Alfani family and rededicated by donna Margherita, daughter of Vermiglio Alfani and the widow of Ugo Altoviti. Orlandi (611) claims that Francesco was not able to build a chapel and instead was buried in the chapel of San Marco, whose title was then changed to the Stigmata of Saint Francis, and that in return the family of Vermiglio Alfani was conceded the chapel of San Tommaso d'Aquino in Chiesa, which then took the name of San Marco.

According to Lunardi, *Arte e storia,* "la Cappella di San Marco Evangelista . . . essa abbattuta con tutto l'ultimo tratto del corridoio quando fu realizzato piazza della stazione. Sembra che nella Cappella di San Marco ci fosse soltanto un affresco con San Francesco in atto di ricevere le stimmate. Se ne è forse rintracciato un frammento staccato che attualmente nei depositi del Museo" (92). On the conflict in family patronage aroused by this incident, see also Wackernagel, *The Florentine Artist,* 45–46.

54. ASPr, Perg., Mt. Morcino, no. 407, 1425.ix.12.

55. ASF, Dipl., Olivetani d'Arezzo, 1362.viii.6.

56. ASPr, Perg., Mt. Morcino, no. 365, 1417.iv.7.

57. Ibid., no. 374, 1418.vi.30.

58. On this profession in the late medieval period, see Pevsner, "The Term Architect in the Middle Ages."

59. ASF, Dipl., 1348.v.11.

60. ASF, Not. antecos., no. 205, 32v, 1365.vii.1.

61. Arch. S. Lorenzo, no. 899, 1371.ix.1. For a fuller discussion of this commission, see Chapter 7, page 258.

62. Arch. dei Laici, reg. 726, −57r, 1371.ix.26.

63. ASF, Not. antecos., no. 9982, 43r−v, 1416.i.7.

64. Graziani, "one of the most famous aristocratic families of Perugia, whose members resided principally in the porta S. Pietro" (Grohmann, Città e territorio, 1: 500).

65. ASPr, Perg., Mt. Morcino, no. 407, 1425.ix.12.

66. ASF, Dipl., Olivetani d'Arezzo, 1372.i.20; for the fresco series commissioned by this testator, see Chapter 7, pages 258–59.

67. Arch. dei Laici, reg. 726, 52v−55r, 1374.v.18. For the Medicean impositions on the liturgical cycles at San Lorenzo, see Gaston, "Liturgy and Patronage in San Lorenzo," 127.

68. A patena is a plate used during the celebration of the mass to cover the chalice and to hold the host; a turribulo is a covered vase with three small chains for sprinkling incense.

69. ASPr, Perg., Mt. Morcino, no. 228, 1389.iii.4.

70. According to Lane, "Florentine Painted Glass," "Italy had no share in the medieval tradition of glass-painting that had developed continuously in France and Germany from the tenth to the thirteenth century" (44). This assessment may be overstated: for later developments in the Quattrocento, see Luchs, "Stained Glass above Renaissance Altars." On their production, see Cennini, Il libro dell'arte, 111.

71. ASF, Dipl., S.M. Novella, 1411.iv.17.

72. See Friedman, "The Burial Chapel of Filippo Strozzi."

73. Arch. S. Lorenzo, no. 809, 1369.xi.3. She may have been an in-law of Alessandro di Iacobi Gini, who endowed a chapel in the same church in 1389. This chapel was built in San Lorenzo and appears in the 1422 Visite, Amerigo Corsini, 13v, dedicated to SS. Antonio e Bernardo, "donata per dominam Mantem."

74. Arch. dei Laici, reg. 726, 45r−46r, 1371.ii.15.

75. ASF, Not. antecos., no. 11248, 60r−61r, 1379.vi.24.

76. On the physical sense of this term and others regarding domestic architecture, see Sznura, "Edilizia privata."

77. ASF, Dipl., S.M. Novella, 1396.vi.24.

78. ASF, Not. antecos., no. 1758, n.p., 1405.i.15.

79. Cohn, *Death and Property,* 22.

80. ASF, Dipl., Arch. Gen., 1394.ii.19.

81. Arch. dei Laici, reg. 726, 47v–50v, 1348.ix.27.

82. ASPr, Perg., San Domenico, no. 57, 1360.ii.16.

83. Ibid., no. 45, 1348.vii.1.

84. ASPr, San Domenico, no. 94, 1384.xi.6.

85. ASF, Dipl., Arch. Gen., 1413.iv.12.

86. Arch. Capitolare, Assisi, Co. S. Francesco, no. 3, 1340.———. For other contracts of this testator, see Cenci, *Documentazione,* 1: 76, 96, 97.

87. ASF, Dipl., S.M. Novella, 1351.iv.2.

88. Arch. Capitolare, Assisi, Co. S. Stefano, no. 34, 5r–11r, 1362.———. Cenci, *Documentazione,* 1: 140–41, gives a partial transcription of this testament.

89. Arch. Capitolare, Assisi, Co. S. Stefano, no. 29, 1362.x.30. Cenci, *Documentazione,* 1: 142, gives a partial transcription of this testament.

90. ASPr, Perg., Olivetani, no. 83, 1363.ii.8.

91. Ibid., San Domenico, no. 3, 1383.———. In surveying the *catasti* for this *castro,* Grohmann, *Città e territorio,* 2: 969, finds no mention of a church of San Iacopo. If it had been constructed, its duration was short-lived; in 1385 the village was devastated by mercenaries.

92. ASPr, Not. Prot., no. 7, 55v–56v, 1390.viii.16. This commission was in fact executed: Grohmann, *Città e territorio,* 2: 933, under "Corciano": "Fin dal 1397 vi è documentato uno ospedale dedicato a S. Maria (Catasti, I, reg. 74, c. 65r)."

93. Arch. dei Laici, reg. 726, 58r–60r, 1359.ix.13.

94. ASF, Dipl., Arch. Gen., 1291.viii.30: "ut dictum est ex dicta linea succedat in dicto patronatu et ille talis patronatus habeat plenam potestatem in dicto hospitali eligendi ponendi mictendi et extrahendi hospitalarium et familia[rem] et omnia alia faciendi que viderit expedire in dicto hospitali et fore utilius secundum consilium discretorum vivorum sue domus ex descendentibus per dictam lineam."

95. ASF, Not. antecos., no. 13364, 71v–, 1303.xi.12.

96. ASF, Dipl., Arch. Gen., 1396.xii.21.

97. ASF, Dipl., 1312.vi.15.

98. ASPr, Not. Bast., no. 39, 60v–67v, 1348.vii.1.

99. ASPr, Not. Prot., no. 22, 17r–v, 1390.x.18. Meo da Siena painted this fresco of the *Madonna col Bambino in trono e Angeli,* called the *Maestà delle Volte,* around 1329. See Todini, *La pittura umbra,* 1: 222; 2: fig. 225.

100. ASPi, Dipl., Santa Marta, 1348.i.8. This painting may have been the cult image that Pisan soldiers supposedly brought back to Pisa in the thirteenth century and hung from a pilaster *"destro della crociera che immette nel braccio settentrionale del transetto, esattamente sotto l'organo."* According to legend, it was miraculously saved from flames in a fire of 1595, which destroyed parts of the Duomo.

The published inventories for 1314 and 1369 (Barsotti, *Gli antichi inventari*) list a number of paintings (mainly painted crucifixes) possessing jewels, pearls, rings, articles of clothing, and cloth: for example, "Corona pro ymagine beate Marie de argento deaurato cum perllis et lapidibus" (28); "Anello .I. grande con pietra vermiglia entro et otto piccule dintorno" (64); "Fetta una seu ghirlanda de perlis bonis quam dedit uxor Richuchu de Riccucho ad pampinas" (63); "Mantellum unum de gianbello nigro datum illi Domine que est ad Crucifixum vetus in choro Annunciate per quandam dominam que fuit uxor ser Vanis de Perignano" (65); "Mantellum unum novum de panno nigro Virginis Marie de Crocifixo novo" (67).

101. ASF, Not. antecos., L 384, 156 bis r–159r, 1363.vi.21.

102. Ibid., no. 976, 123r–v, 1312.vi.26; the widow of a notary from the Aretine village of Piscaria gave 10 soldi to have a dress (*veste*) made for the Virgin Mary in the convent of Ognissanti: ibid., no. 981, 132v, 1321.xi.10.

103. ASF, Dipl., S.M. Novella, 1348.vii.22. See Meiss, *Painting in Florence and Siena*, 74; di Pierro, "Contributo alla biografia"; and Brown, *The Dominican Church*, 118.

104. ASF, Dipl., S.M. Nuova, 1348.vi.3. In 1363, the year of the plague's return, Ridolfus f.q. Chiarucci, from San Casciano in the Mugello, wished to have wax figures of women made and offered to the "Virgin" of Orsanmichele (*Fiat quandam in ymago mulieris ceree*): ibid., 1363.vi.30.

105. ASF, Not. antecos., no. 980, 96r–97r, 1320.vii.22. In the early 1320s, several other testators made small contributions ranging from 10 soldi to one florin for "work being done" on this panel painting. These included Ranaldus f.q. Alberti, a grain dealer (*bladaiolus*), ibid., 116v, 1320.ix.8; a widow, domina Iacopa, ibid., no. 981, 108r–v, 1321.ix.21; the wife of a notary, domina Deccha, ibid., no. 982, 101r, 1322.vi.25; the citizen Dinus f.q. Cecchi de Lodomeris, ibid., no. 984, 1324.i.20.

106. ASF, Dipl., S.M. Nuova, 1373.i.28. For depictions of such works of art by silver- and goldsmiths, see *L'Oreficeria nella Firenze*, and Wolbach, *Guide del Museo Sacro Vaticano*, vol. 2.

107. On the survival of these works of art from the Quattrocento, see Wackernagel, *The Florentine Artist*, 142–46, and Museo di San Marco, *Mostra del Tesoro*.

108. San Siro in the *plebis* of Cascia, Santa Maria Novella in Florence, the *plebis* church of San Pietro de Cascia in the diocese of Fiesole, and Santa Maria Maggiore in Florence.

109. ASF, Dipl., S.M. Nuova, 1382.xi.26.

110. Giovannini and Vitolo, *Il Convento del Carmine*, 80–82. "Inventario dei beni del Convento" (1391) ASF, Conv. Soppr. 113, vol. 33, 8r–11r. For example, "Item uno calice smaltato sola la-palla con piè-distallo di-rame con patena di-rame coll-arme dè-Manetti senza patena" (82).

111. Giovannini and Vitolo, 82, and in document, 31v.

112. Casalini, *La SS. Annunziata di Firenze,* 71–128: "Un inventario inedito del secolo XV (1422)," for example, "In prima, una pianeta di velluto bianco con due armi, l'una di Neri di Filippo e l'altra de' Pazzi" (89).

113. Ibid., 93–94.

114. Ibid., 94–97.

115. Ibid., 99–101: "Questi sono e calici e l'ariento della sagrestia."

116. Barsotti, *Gli antichi inventari,* 5–29, "L'Inventario di Giovanni Sacrista." The only approximation to coats of arms was the following from an inventory of 1300: "Item unum pluviale rotatum cum leonibus et aliis variis signis et coloribus quod habet dominus Marcheselli" (21).

117. Ibid., 38–39. In one instance, a chalice bore the arms of two noble families: "Calicem unum de argento cum mallo smaltato, cum patenna ponderis unicarum quatuordecim et quatarum trium, in quo malo sculpta sunt arma domus Benignorum et Seccamerenda" (38).

118. Ibid., 45–47, 55–57: "Pluviale unum de vellosso schacato de rubeo et gialo cum fressio ad figuras domini Petri de Gambacorti [Signore di Pisa, 1370 to 1392]" (57).

119. Ibid., 74–82.

120. ASPi, Osp. di S. Chiara, no. 2091, 51r–57r, 94v–102r.

121. Sacchetti, *Il Trecentonovelle,* LXIII: "A Giotto, gran dipintore, è dato uno palvese a dipingere da un uomo di picciolo affare. Egli, faccendosene scherne, lo dipinge per forma che colui rimane confuso." He concludes with the following moral about those who do not know their place: "Così costui, non misurandosi, fu misurato; chè ogni tristo vuol fare arma e far casati; e cotali che li loro padri seranno stati trovati agli ospedali." See also Vasari, *Le Vite,* "Vita di Giotto," text 2, 120–21.

122. ASF, Dipl., S.M. Nuova, 1368.viii.24.

123. In addition to being one of the principal noble families of Borgo, the Carsidoni were important politically at the regional level. They were among the *milites* at the peace of 1203 between the nobles and the *popolo* in Assisi and were among the earliest *podestà* of Assisi (1222–23). See Waley, "Le istituzioni communali," 63, and Banker, *Death in the Community,* 25, who describes the Carsidoni as one of the three great families of Borgo; see also Fanfani, *Un mercante del Trecento.*

124. ASA, Antichi notari, no. 14, 9r–10r, 1374.v.17.

125. ASF, Not. antecos., no. 9982, n.p., 1411.viii.2.

126. Davidsohn, *Storia di Firenze,* 7: 626–27, in discussing the importance of beds as furniture in late medieval Florentine households, mentions painted ones: "Gli italiani del nord nel 1314 rimproveravano ai fiorentini la loro effeminatezza, perché erano avvezzi a portarsi appresso perfino durante le guerre le lettiere dipinte ed i tappeti."

127. ASF, Dipl., S.M. Nuova, 1323.ix.21.

128. Ibid., 1359.ix.11.

129. ASA, Antichi notari, no. 14, 9r–10r, 1374.v.17.

130. On the production of crests and coats of arms, see Cennini, *Il Libro dell'arte*, 108.

131. See Fiorilli, *I dipinti a Firenze*, 23–27: "Per gli stemmi e le insigne dipinte c'era già stato un decreto delle Riformagioni, in data 1 febbraio 1291, il quale vietava "tenere arma picta vel insignia alicuius vel aliquorum, seu alicuius domi vel casati civitatis vel districtus . . . sub pena magnatibus libr. CC, popularibus libr. C"; e soggiungeva: "Nessuno può tenere in casa l'arme dipinta, dei Grandi, salvo quelli che sono veramente famigliari; ma i pittori le possono dipingere, i sarti cucire, i corazzai e fabbri lavorare, i rigattiere tenere ad vendendum, dummodo faciant bona fide" (23).

"Fra le provvisioni dei consigli maggiori ve n'è una . . . del 20 giugno 1329, intitolata: 'Pingendi arma prohibito' [bk. 3, chap. 35, ed. I Del Lungo] . . . La provvisione deliberata in quella solenne adunanza non soltanto proibiva di dipingere e scolpire immagini e stemmi sulle pareti esterne di certi palagi, ma comandava altresì che si togliessero quelle pitture e sculture che già vi fossero."

In their statutes drawn up in 1374, the Hospital of the Innocenti prohibited the painting of family arms on paintings commissioned for the hospital. In the Quattrocento, the hospital's benefactors clearly ignored these strictures: see Gavitt, *Charity and Children*, 64, 118. Other regulations, such as those in the Communal Statutes of the Podestà in 1325, were aimed at protecting the integrity of one's family arms: *Statuto del Podestà*, II, bk. 3, LXX, 229: "Quod nullus pingat arma alterius. Nullus depingat vel depingi faciat arma alterius persone seu ymagines seu signa armorum aliarum personarum, nec pictores pingere debeant nisi arma illius persone cui pinguntur; et intelligatur una eademque pictura gialla et aurea, alba et argentea, plena et levata; et si quis contro fecerit puniatur et condennetur in libris quinquaginta p. f."

For Pisa, see *Statuti di Pisa*, vol. 1, *Breve Pisani Communis*, LXXXVI, 376: "De non permittendo popolares deferre arma picta de armis nobilium." For Siena, the communal statutes of 1309–10 only prohibited the painting of private arms on the Palazzo comunale or on gates, fountains, and other public "works": *Il costituto del comune di Siena*, 1: 334, dist. I, DXXXIV, Che neune arme si possano dipegnere in alcuno palazo, porta o vero fonte, del comune di Siena.

132. Arch. dei Laici, reg. 726, 62v–63r, 1374.iii.26.

133. A *cotta* is "a white overshirt of linen or cotton that reaches the knees cuffed with crenelations and has wide sleeves; worn by priests and clerics for almost all religious functions, except the mass." *Grande Dizionario*, 3: 921.

134. ASA, Perg., no. 85, 1410.xi.10.

135. ASF, Dipl., S.M. Nuova, 1417.vi.19. Moreni, *Notizie Istoriche*, 4: 109–10, transcribes a section of this will in discussing the patrons of S. Maria della Campora. According to the Catasto of 1427 (ASF, Catasto no. 185 [Vescovado di Firenze], 670v, under the debits of the hospital of Santa Maria Nuova), the friars of Campora were still making annual payments for the soul of this

testator: "Perpetui l'anno—I frati di Santa Maria delle champora per agostino di francescho di ser Giovanni fl. quattro——fl. 4."

136. Procacci, "Di Jacopo di Antonio"; for the involvement of important artists in such crafts, see Wackernagel, *The Florentine Artist*, 138–42, and Dunkerton et al., *Giotto to Dürer*, 122.

137. This is Bernardo Daddi's painting commissioned in 1347 to replace an earlier image of the Virgin which had performed many miracles. The Daddi Virgin was placed on the Orcagna altarpiece (commissioned in 1352), where it stands today. On Daddi's image as a cult object for pilgrims and a stimulus for large numbers of gifts and legacies to Orsanmichele after the Black Death of 1348, see Fabbri and Rutenburg, "The Tabernacle of Orsanmichele," 390.

138. Arch. Capitolare, Assisi, Co. S. Francesco, no. 3, 1340.——. For examples of paintings with wax images, depicted *ex voto*, see Volbach, *Pinacoteca vaticana Kataloge*, vol. 2, fig. 7.

139. "And I, the writer, have actually witnessed someone whose cat has strayed making a vow that if he recovered it, he would send a wax image [of the cat] to the Virgin at Orsanmichele. And he actually did this! Now while this may not be a violation of the faith, surely it is a mockery of God, the Virgin and all the Saints. For [God] desires our heart and our mind; he is not interested in our wax images, nor in such conceits and vanities" (translated by Brucker, *Renaissance Florence*, 211).

140. Warburg, *La rinascita del paganesimo*, 137–41. See also Masi, "La ceroplastica in Firenze," and von Schlosser, "Geschichte der Portratbildnerei in Wachs." On uses of wax molds, see Cennini, *Il libro dell'arte*, 129.

141. ASF, Not. antecos., no. 9592, n.p., 1374.vi.2.

142. ASPi, Osp. di S. Chiara, no. 2070, 343v–345r, 1285.v.5.

143. For an introduction to bas-reliefs, see Pope-Hennessy, *Italian Sculpture*. For notable examples of wooden sculpture during these centuries, see Pope-Hennessy, "Sienese Wooden Sculpture," 323–24; Carli, *La scultura lignea senese* and *La scultura lignea italiana;* more recently, the catalogue *Scultura Dipinta;* and a conference paper by Paoletti, *"Ars Orandi,"* which I thank the author for the opportunity of reading.

144. ASF, Not. antecos., no. 9982, 10r–11v, 1411.vii.2.

145. ASF, Dipl., S.M. Nuova, 1343.iv.25.

146. ASPr, Perg., Misericordia, 1315.vi.17.

147. ASF, Not. antecos., no. 3570, 1363.v.21.

148. ASPr, Not. Prot., no. 7, 28r–30v, 1387.vi.20.

149. ASF, Dipl., Misericordia di Arezzo, 1393.xi.19.

150. The church, located in the diocese of Lucca, was a dependency of the Benedictine abbey of S. Benedetto a Polirone sul Pò: Repetti, *Dizionario*, 1: 761.

151. ASF, Dipl., Arch. Gen., 1413.iv.12.

152. ASF, Not. antecos., no. 3702, 100v–101r, 1363.vi.18.

153. Ibid., no. 5881, n.p., 1372.i.1.

154. ASPr, Not. Prot., no. 22, 79r–80r, 1400.i.27.

155. ASF, Not. antecos., no. 8066, 121v–127v, 1409.vii.20.

156. Arch. dei Laici, reg. 726, 60r–61r, 1374.vi.2.

157. See citation at the beginning of Chapter 3.

7. Paintings

1. For general discussions of the commissioning of paintings, see Baxandall, *Painting and Experience,* and Hager, *Die Anfänge des italienischen Altarbildes.* On altarpieces, see van Os, *Sienese Altarpieces.*

2. Alberti, *Trattato della pittura,* bk. 2, par. 52). See also Hills, "Renaissance Altarpieces," 39.

3. Bibl. Com., Notarile, C.N. 21, 14r–15r, 1400.v.30.

4. ASF, Dipl., Arch. Gen., 1416.x.13.

5. ASF, Not. antecos., no. 7991, 14v–15v, 1401.viii.16.

6. ASF, Dipl., Olivetani d'Arezzo, 1348.———.

7. ASF, Not. antecos., no. 5880, 131r, 1371.viii.23.

8. Belting, *The Image and Its Public,* 14.

9. Wackernagel, *The Florentine Artist,* 40–41, and Baxandall, *Painting and Experience,* 5.

10. ASF, Dipl., S.M. Novella, 1348.vii.22; see Chapter 6, note 95. In a codicil to his will redacted on 8 October 1349, Torinus left an additional 270 florins for the construction of the Porta Maggiore of the church of Santa Maria Novella; see Orlandi, *"Necrologio,"* vol. 2, app. 2, doc. 24, 436–37. According to Lunardi, *Arte e storia,* 31, the commission for the Old Testament cycle was not carried out within one year as demanded in the testament but most likely awaited Paolo Uccello's execution of the same subject for the Chiostro Verde in the fifteenth century. Lunardi speculates that the fresco cycle was originally intended for the Chiostro but not executed because the vaults of the Chiostro were not securely finished by 1349.

11. ASPr, Perg., Mt. Morcino, no. 78, 1362.iii.23. Crispolti, *Perugia Augusta,* 133, mentions this chapel: "Le due Cappelle, o altari di S. Andrea e di S. Caterina, l'una all'incontro dell'altra, per due tavole di Errigo Fiammingo."

12. Bellosi, "La mostra di affreschi," 78. Others, such as the antiquarian Marchese Antonio Albergotti (*Notizie sugli uomini illustri aretini*) and Boskovits, *Pittura fiorentina,* 141, claim that Arezzo did possess a strong "local school" in the Trecento. See del Vita, "Notizie e documenti su antichi artisti aretini," 230; "Contributi per la storia dell'arte aretina"; Pasqui, "Pittori aretini"; Gamurrini, "Pittori aretini"; Salmi, *San Domenico and San Francesco;* Donati, "Per la pittura aretina del Trecento"; and Masseti, *Spinello Aretino.*

13. Of 47 paintings, 30 derive from public notarial protocols, and of 165 works of art, 98 come from these sources.

14. See Borsook, *The Mural Painters of Tuscany*, xxxii.

15. Belting, *The Image and Its Public;* van Os, *Sienese Altarpieces,* "Text and Image"; Hager, *Die Anfänge des italienischen Altarbildes;* Ringbom, *Icon to Narrative;* Trexler, "Florentine Religious Experience." For the importance of "thaumaturgic or other miraculous powers" of art in the fifteenth and early sixteenth centuries, see Burke, *Culture and Society,* 112–13.

16. While Trexler, in "Florentine Religious Experience," successfully dispels nineteenth-century romantic notions of the artist and the function of painting, he fails to examine religious art historically over the period of his analysis. Instead, he encapsulates the period from the thirteenth through the sixteenth centuries with general statements such as "the belief in power-laden natural objects was general in that age" (9).

17. Boskovits, *Pittura fiorentina:* "a costo di ripetermi . . . un aspetto assai importante nella produzione del pittore . . . il profitto prevedibile aveva il suo peso anche in decisioni che oggi diremmo strettamente artistiche" (171). Belting, in *The Image and Its Public,* suggests a similar transition in his historical schema of the icon: "The third turning point is summed up by the concept of the early Renaissance. This can be seen, for example, in the new control the artist had over his work, as a consequence of which the art of the image became its function" (7).

18. ASPi, Osp. di S. Chiara, no. 2071, 23r–25v, 1285.xii.10. The earliest appearance of a painting in these documents was also in the Pisan records. Another immigrant, Lazarus f.q. Talliapanis, from Borgo San Genesio, who was living in Pisa, left four lire in his 1264 testament for oil to illuminate "night and day" a lamp in front of the figure of the Virgin Mary and Jesus Christ and another lamp in front of the figure of the Holy Cross in his parish church of San Cristoforo Chinzica: ibid., no. 2065, 72r–74v, 1264.ii.9.

19. The altar of San Giovanni Evangelista was on the left arm of the transept in the lower church; it was later ceded to the duke of Athens. See Nessi, *La Basilica di S. Francesco,* 54, 341, 356, 388.

20. Sacro Convento, instr. V, 47, 1300.iv.14. For similar phrases in commission documents, though for a later period, the sixteenth century, see Glasser, *Artists' Contracts,* 31. This document has been cited by Fortini, *Nova vita di S. Francesco,* 3: 512; Zaccaria, "Diario storico," 290, n. 142; and Nessi, *La Basilica di S. Francesco.* For a general discussion of artists' contracts, see also Conti, "L'evolution dell'artista," 127–34; Burke, *Culture and Society,* 87–95; and Baxandall, *Painting and Experience,* 1–27.

21. These findings stand somewhat in variance with the conclusions drawn by Borsook, who argues in *The Mural Painters of Tuscany* that the great period of Tuscan wall paintings originated at the end of the Duecento. She does not distinguish between paintings of individual saints or altarpieces and fresco cycles. On the other hand, Ringbom, *Icon to Narrative,* finds the fundamental transition to the "close-up" half-length figure in narrative painting in the fifteenth

century. On the distinction between the narrative and the devotional image, see Panofsky's functional and formal distinctions in "Imagio Pietatis"; Ringbom's criticisms in *Icon to Narrative*, 56; and Belting's reassessment in *The Image and Its Public*, 48–52: "We now return to the question of whether devotional images should be distinguished from *historiae*. The answer may be given in the positive" (52).

22. Warburg, "Arte del ritratto e borghesia fiorentina," in *La rinascita del paganesimo antico*, 114–15.

23. Castelnuovo, "Il significato del ritratto."

24. Gilbert, "The Renaissance Portrait"; Pope-Hennessy, *The Portrait in the Renaissance*; Alazard, *The Florentine Portrait*; and Hughes, "Representing the Family."

25. ASPi, 72r–v, Osp. di S. Chiara, no. 18, 1315.ii.pridie.

26. ASF, Not. antecos., no. 7575, 246v, 1335.xii.6.

27. See Glasser, *Artists' Contracts*; Baxandall, *Giotto and the Orators*; and *Painting and Experience*, 1–27.

28. ASS, Not. antecos., no. 25, 97v, 1334.xii.4.

29. ASF, Dipl., Olivetani d'Arezzo, 1328.x.16.

30. ASF, Not. antecos., no. 13364, 3v, 1300.xi.8.

31. ASPr, Osp. di Misericordia, no. 3, 2v–3r, 1331.ii.27.

32. Ibid., no. 6, 20v–21v, 1345.iii.13.

33. ASF, Dipl., S.M. Nuova, 1327.iv.18.

34. Ibid., Arch. Gen., 1346.iii.16.

35. ASF, Not. antecos., no. 981, 108r–v, 1321.ix.21.

36. ASPi, Osp. di S. Chiara, no. 2078, 53r–v, 1311.viii.6.

37. ASPr, Osp. di Misericordia, no. 3, 19v–20r, 1332.iv.7.

38. Sacro Convento, instr. V, 47, 1300.iv.14.

39. ASF, Not. antecos., no. 981, 108r–v, 1321.ix.21.

40. ASS, Dipl., Arch. Gen., 1348.ix.22.

41. ASF, Not. antecos., no. 11050, 7r–9r, 1349.iv.1.

42. Sacro Convento, Instr. VIII, no. 51, 1348.vii.23.

43. ASF, Not. antecos., no. 5884, 49v–50v, 1348.ix.3.

44. ASF, Dipl., Olivetani d'Arezzo, 1348.————.

45. Arch. dei Laici, reg. 726, 19v–20v, 1348.vii.16.

46. Arch. Capitolare, Pace Puccii Notario, no. 57, 143r–, 1348.ix.21.

47. ASPr, Not. Bast., no. 39, 60v–67v, 1348.vii.1.

48. ASF, Dipl., Olivetani d'Arezzo, 1348.viii.27.

49. ASF, Not. antecos., no. 20833, n.p., 1348.viii.26.

50. Sacro Convento, Instr. IX, no. 44, 1360.viii.2.

51. The painting requested by the citizen and wool manufacturer of Arezzo Duccinus f.q. Andree would have included more than a single figure, but he failed to enumerate them in his will. At the outset, he left 100 lire to his heir and only son to have the image of the blessed Virgin Mary "with those figures which the testator said he had told his heir" painted in the church of San

Michele of Arezzo above the testator's sepulcher: ASF, Dipl., Misericordia d'Arezzo, 1362.v.28.

52. See Ringbom, *Icon to Narrative,* and Preiser, *Das Entstehen und die Entwicklung der Predella.*

53. ASF, Not. antecos., no. 3569, 91r, 1363.vii.5; cited in *La Chiesa fiorentina,* 215.

54. Previtali, "La periodizzazione," 27. Based on the small size of table paintings after 1350, Meiss, "Italian Primitives," 4, assumed that production for church altars had declined to a trickle, "due in part to the fact that many church altars had already received their retables in the preceding period of immense activity, both architectural and pictorial."

55. van Os, "The Black Death" and "Tradition and Innovation."

56. Boskovits, *Pittura fiorentina:* "che non si conoscono grandi cicli affrescati negli anni '70, e che dalla seconda metà del decennio forse diminuisce anche il numero delle tavole d'altare rispetto ai tempi precedenti. Tale caduta nella produzione non si limita del resto al campo della pittura, dato che rallenta pure il ritmo della costruzione e decorazione delle chiese . . . ora risultano quasi totalmente sospesi" (43).

Other art historians have assumed a strict relation between hard times and artistic production: when times were hard, artists did not work. See, for instance, Procacci, "Sulla cronologia," 31.

57. Meiss, *Painting in Florence and Siena,* 23, 32.

58. ASS, Dipl., Arch. Gen., 1374.viii.31.

59. To have some idea of how paltry this amount must have been for paintings in the late Trecento, compare it to the payment of 49 lire, 12 soldi, 2 denari made to the carpenter Paolo Bindi in 1339 for the wood and construction of only the predella for the *tavola* of San Crescenzo. It was followed by another payment of 42 lire, 9 soldi, 2 denari in 1340 "per la predella e per le colone de la tavola di San Cresciento la quale dipegnie el maestro Ambruogio Lorenzi." See Rowley, *Ambrogo Lorenzetti,* 131. For prices in the late Trecento, Datini's letters provide the largest number of examples: small portable triptychs could cost as little as 2 to 3.5 florins. See Boskovits, *Pittura fiorentina,* 169, and Corti, "Sul commercio dei quadri." For painters' wages in mid-Trecento workships, see Meiss, "Notable Disturbances," appendix, 186. For the fifteenth century, see Borsook, Review of Neri di Bicci, *Le Ricordanze,* 317; Wackernagel, *The Florentine Artist,* 339; and Lerner-Lehmkuhl, *Zur Struktur und Geschichte.* For the gilding alone of Filippo Lippi's Sant'Ambrogio altarpiece, Fra Diamante was paid eight lire in 1447. See Borsook, "Cults and Imagery," 195, n. 113.

60. ASPr, Not. Prot., no. 2, 64r–v, 1368.v.23. See also *Bibliotheca Sanctorum,* 3: 749.

61. Arch. S. Lorenzo, no. 899, 1371.ix.1. Meiss, in *Painting in Florence and Siena,* 157–58, argues that by embracing ascetic Christianity, painting in the second half of the Trecento turned completely away from "antique" subjects.

But pagan themes and figures did not hold a monopoly on antiquity, as the work of Rice, *Lefèvre d'Etaples*, Spitz, *The Religious Renaissance*, and others has shown. Indeed, the rector's choice of these obscure late third-century martyrs reflects a taste for ancient history and culture in the late Trecento.

Richa, *Chiese fiorentine*, 2: 53, was aware of this testament and claims that the rector was "an intimate friend of Petrarch," but mistakenly attributes the foundation to San Lorenzo instead of Santa Cecilia. The patrician rector's chapel was, however, erected in San Lorenzo. Amerigo Corsini, in *Visite Pastorali* (1422), lists this chapel among those of San Lorenzo: "SS. Tiburtii et valeriani dotata per olim dominum Niccolaum Bennucci" (13v).

62. ASPr, Perg., S.M. di Monte Luce, 1367.xi.12.

63. ASF, Dipl., Olivetani d'Arezzo, 1372.i.20. "In primis quia anima dignior est corpore et in omnibus merito corpori preferenda, voluit, iussit, reliquit et mandavit quod de bonis suis quedam capella per eum facta in ecclesia nova fratrum Sancti Augustini de Aretio et nondum perfecta compleatur et mictatur executa per infrascriptos heredes et fideicommissarios et ibidem pingatur figura beati Jacopi et sub eius titulo intituletur. Item reliquit et legavit dicte Capelle pro pictura ipsius et calice, planeta, missali, cero et aliis necessariis et opportunis fulcimentis dicte capelle florenos de auro quinquaginta qui spendantur et convertantur in fornimentis capelle predicte ex dicto die ad sex menses post mortem dicti testatoris."

64. Vasari, *Le Vite*, vol. 2, *Commento*, ed. Barocchi, 643–44.

65. Vasari, Ibid., *Testo*, 2, ed. Bettarini: "Da Cortona andato a Arezzo l'anno 1369, quando appunto i Tarlati, già stati signori di Pietramala, avevano in quella città fatto finire il convento e il corpo della chiesa di Sant'Agostino . . . , nelle minori navate, delle quali avevano molti cittadini fatto fare cappelle e sepolture per le famiglie loro—, il Berna vi dipinse a fresco, nella cappella di San Iacopo, alcune storiette della vita di quel Santo; e sopra tutto molto vivamente la storia di Marino barattiere; il quale avendo per cupidigia di danari dato, e fattone scritta di propria mano, l'anima al diavolo, si raccomanda a San Iacopo, perché lo liberi da quella promessa, mentre un diavolo col mostrargli lo scritto gli fa la maggior calca del mondo. Nelle quali tutte figure espresse il Berna con molta vivacità gli affetti dell'animo, e particolarmente nel viso di Marino da un canto la paura e dall'altro la fede e sicurezza, che gli fa sperare da San Iacopo la sua liberazione se bene prontamente dice e mostra le sue ragioni al Santo; che dopo avere indotto in Marino estremo pentimento del peccato e promessa fatto, lo libera e tornalo a Dio" (254).

66. Alpers, *"Ekphrasis."*

67. See Stubblebine, *Giotto*, 108–9.

68. ASF, Dipl., Olivetani d'Arezzo, 1372.i.20: "Item reliquit et dari voluit pro illicitis et male extortis per eum et incertis libras ducentas denarii aretii spendendas per fideicommissarios suos infrascriptos et primo illis a quibus extortos esse[n]t et habitos. Et si non reperirentur, concertantur ın maritando

puellas vel mictendo aliquas puellas in monesterium vel aliter prout visum
fuerit dictis fideicommissariis pro anima ipsius. Item cum non remictatur pec-
catus nec restituatur ablatum reliquit, iussit, voluit et mandavit restitui omnibus
ab eo debentibus legiptime recipere et habere quicquid apparet debere recipere
de bonis suis."

69. From merely reading the documents at their disposal, the executors,
or the friars, might have focused on another of the testator's sins. In a long
document redacted the same day as his will, Marianus pleaded to Count
Franceschinus Pucci de Arca to legitimate his bastard son, Cola, giving him
and his heirs the same rights as his other son, Luca. The major portion of
Marianus's will in fact dealt with the distribution of property between these
two sons. The division was not equal. While the legitimated Cola received a
house and several pieces of land, Luca was named as the universal heir. If
Luca were to die without legitimate heirs, then Cola would inherit only half
of the estate, and Marianus's *fideicommissarii* were to distribute the other half
to unspecified "pious causes." Evidently, Marianus did not perceive the sin of
fathering an illegitimate son as bearing the same weight for his future in
purgatory as he did the sin of usury. He resolved the former through secular
means without charitable gifts or pious phraseology. Perhaps he had com-
municated this anguish to either the Augustinian friars or his executors. Unfortunately, a separate commission document does not exist.

70. Arch. dei Laici, reg. 726, 51v–52r, 1374.v.23.

71. Ibid., 51v, 1374.viii.1.

72. Bibl. Com., Not., A. I. Ser Giovanni di Giacomo, 69v–71v, 1374.vii.24.

73. ASF, Not. antecos., no. 205, 32v, 1365.vii.1.

74. Arch. dei Laici, reg. 726, 52v–53v, 1374.v.18: "Et voluit quod in pede
dicti orti videlicet iuxta ecclesia sancte trinitatis fiat et fieri debeat maiestas beate
marie viriginis et figura beati urbani cum ymagine sua ad pedes eorum."

75. Ibid., 60r–v, 1374.vi.2.

76. Ibid., 52v–53v, 1374.v.18.

77. G. F. Gamurrini, "I pittori aretini," 92–94, has transcribed these documents.

78. ASF, Not. antecos., no. 5880, 131r–, 1371.viii.23.

79. The evidence from surviving paintings of the increase in the number
of chosen saints and the paucity of "histories" matches my conclusions drawn
from the testaments. See Meiss, "Italian Primitives": "In later Trecento altarpieces, however, historical scenes tend to be relegated to the predella or
eliminated altogether. The reduced importance of historical scenes in Trecento
altarpieces is the result of several factors. The growing cult of the saints
multiplied the images of them in the altarpiece and crowded histories from
the main fields" (11).

80. In the 1364–75 period, 8 paintings appear in 88 wills from Arezzo and
7 from 77 wills in Florence; for 1376–1425, there are 10 paintings from 194
wills in Arezzo and 4 from 176 wills in Florence.

81. ASPr, Perg., San Domenico, no. 90, 1383.viii.14.

82. ASPr, Mt. Morcino, no. 407, 1425.ix.12.

83. ASF, Not. antecos., no. 15219, 103r–v, 1382.xii.31.

84. ASPi, Dipl., Primaziale, 1393.viii.6.

85. Ibid., San Martino, 1391.viii.24.

86. *Bibliotheca Sanctorum,* 9: 923–47 (Nicola, vescovo di Mira).

87. ASF, Not. antecos., no. 10736, 73v–74v, 1391.ii.6. van Os, "Tradition and Innovation," 66, comments on the popularity of local saints at Montalcino in the latter part of the Trecento.

88. ASF, Dipl., Misericordia d'Arezzo, 1382.iv.16.

89. ASPr, Not. Bast., no. 11, 74v–77r, 1390.vii.13.

90. ASF, Not. antecos., no. 12064, 16r–v, 1393.vii.12.

91. ASPr, Not. Prot., no. 22, 110r–v, 1400.vi.26.

92. ASPr, Perg., Mt. Morcino, no. 228, 1389.iii.4.

93. Meiss, *Painting in Florence and Siena,* characterizes the period "from narrative to ritual" (16–26).

94. ASF, Not. antecos., no. 9982, 11v–13r, 1411.vii.6.

95. Borsook, *The Mural Painters of Tuscany,* 94, and Salmi, *San Domenico and San Francesco,* 38.

96. I can find no trace of this commission in Richa, *Notizie istoriche delle chiese fiorentine,* or in Paatz and Paatz, *Die Kirchen von Florenz.*

97. van Os, in "Tradition and Innovation," 55, maintains that a "democratization in patronage" characterized art commissions of the second half of the Trecento, in terms both of the individual patrons and of a new emphasis on local corporations and guilds. In "Italian Primitives," 5, 12, Meiss also connected changes in style to changes in the social class of patrons, which for unexplained reasons later vanished from his magnum opus of 1951.

98. ASF, Not. antecos., no. 8066, 121v–128r, 1409.vii.20.

99. ASPr, Perg., Mt. Morcino, no. 407, 1425.ix.12.

100. In a codicil not selected for these samples, this testator gave Santa Maria Novella a further 270 florins for the construction of the church's main portal: see Meiss, *Painting in Florence and Siena,* 79, and di Pierro, "Contributo alla biografia," 11–15.

101. See Becker, "Aspects of Lay Piety," 177, and Meiss, *Painting in Florence and Siena,* 78. According to Matteo Villani, the Company of Orsanmichele received 350,000 florins in the year of the Black Death; and according to Ghiberti's biography of Trecento painters, Orcagna received 86,000 florins for his marble tabernacle.

102. For equally low or even lower prices in the 1380s, see Corti, "Sul commercio dei quadri," 84–91, who finds commissions for bedroom Madonnas at 13½ florins; small rondels of painted figures called "i due dische da parto e la basetta" for one florin 18 soldi in a 1384 contract; and frieze decorations for as little as 5 soldi di piccioli. These art forms do not, however, appear in my samples of testaments.

103. Borsook, Review of Neri di Bicci, *Le Ricordanze,* 317. Similarly, Wack-

ernagel, *The Florentine Artist,* 339, and Lerner-Lehmkuhl make the same assessment. The other principal determinant of price was the size of the work, for which the testaments never provide measurements. Baxandall's analysis of the art market in *Painting and Experience,* 1–27, is far more simplistic, reducing the determination of price to "matter and skill."

104. Borsook, Review of Neri di Bicci, 313, 315.

105. Ibid., 317. Domestic tabernacles cost far less, from 5 lire 8 soldi to 43 lire; however, all of the commissions found in the samples of testaments were destined for church decoration and not for private devotion. Neri di Bicci's prices appear higher than those which Wackernagel, in *The Florentine Artist,* 339–40 (based largely on Lerner-Lehmkuhl, *Zur Struktur und Geschichte*), estimates from the same period: "Prices from one hundred and two hundred florins are the general rule for altarpieces of the high classical period, with the standard that only pictures very rich in figures approach the upper price limit named." For frescoes, Wackernagel's figures are considerably lower—between 15 and 30 florins.

106. Offner, *Corpus of the Florentine Painting,* ser. 3, vol. 1, xv; Meiss, "Italian Primitives," *Painting in Florence and Siena,* 6–7; Boskovits, *Pittura fiorentina,* 17, 52, 85.

107. Dunkerton et al., *Giotto to Dürer,* maintain that "many individuals, including those of relatively modest means, had small religious paintings at home" (60). Their only example to back this claim comes, however, from the records of possibly the wealthiest merchant in central Italy at the beginning of the fifteenth century—Francesco Datini.

108. In *Duccio,* despite its subtitle, *Tuscan Art and the Medieval Workshop,* White says little about workshop organization; see, instead, Procacci, "Di Jacopo di Antonio," and van Os, "Tradition and Innovation." For business partnerships among early Quattrocento painters, see Corti, "La Compagnia"; for the organization of workshops, mostly in the later Quattrocento, see Wackernagel, *The Florentine Artist,* 299–347. See also the illustrative materials in Neri di Bicci, *Le ricordanze,* and Dunkerton et al., *Giotto to Dürer,* 139ff.

109. Skaug is now completing a monograph that classifies over 7,000 punch marks, presenting the fruits of over 20 years of research. Among his earlier articles that point to the pivotal importance of 1363 in the dispersion of tools and changes in workshop practices, see "The St. Anthony Abbot," "The 'Rinuccini Tondo,' " and "Punch Marks." In addition, see Frinta, "The Quest for a Restorer's Shop," "An Investigation of the Punched Decoration," and "The Decoration of the Gilded Surfaces."

110. The plague carried off several of the most important painters of the period—Bernardo Daddi, his associate called by Offner the "Assistant of Daddi," most probably both Lorenzetti brothers, and, according to Meiss, "a great many minor painters" (*Painting in Florence and Siena,* 66).

111. van Os, "Tradition and Innovation," 50. The literature on proto-

industry has become extensive since Mendels's seminal essay, "Proto-industrialization: The First Phase of the Industrialization Process." In addition, see Kriedte, Medick, and Schlumbohm, *Industrialization before Industrialization*. For a thoroughgoing review and critique of this literature, see Mastboom, "The Role of Eastern Gelderland," 12–25.

112. Meiss, *Painting in Florence and Siena*, 165.

113. Ibid., 74.

114. Meiss had sketched the outlines of this cultural and stylistic picture of the late Trecento at least seven years before in "The Italian Primitives." In this formative article, Meiss's emphasis on class was stronger than what later emerged in *Painting in Florence and Siena*: "These qualities of later Trecento art express a state of mind that was influenced by several contemporary events: the economic crisis beginning in the forties, the Black Death of 1348, and the shift of power from the merchants and bankers to the lesser guilds and the lower middle classes, bearers of a more conservative culture" (12). He also saw patronage in class terms: "These little panels . . . constituted the first venture of a new social class in the domestic ownership of paintings" (4).

115. Meiss, *Painting in Florence and Siena*, 61.

116. Smart, *The Dawn of Italian Painting*, 107–8; Polzer, "Aristotle, Mohammed, and Nicholas V in Hell," "Fourteenth-Century Iconography of Death and the Plague"; Swarzenski, "Before and after Pisano." van Os, "Tradition and Innovation," mistakenly claims that Boskovits, in *Pittura fiorentina*, pushes back the dates of what Meiss considered "the Black Death style" in Florence to the 1320s. While Boskovits does argue that Orcagna's *Triumph of Death* predated the Black Death and was painted around 1345, his dates for the rejection of the Giottoesque and the origins of a new style in painting are consistent with Meiss's, around 1340. In "Notable Disturbances," Meiss revised his dates for several miniatures by the Pisan Francesco Triani but held fast to his earlier stylistic interpretations of Triani's frescoes in the Camposanto.

117. Paoletti, "The Strozzi Altarpiece," 282, argues that the iconography of this altarpiece is not "all retardataire or reflective of Dugento conventions," but instead reflects the ecclesiology of the Dominicans, who desired to enhance the hierarchical strength of the papacy. This emphasis, however, far from contradicting Meiss, supports his more general arguments concerning the renewed emphasis on ecclesiastical hierarchy and the severity of church power. Paoletti further attacks Meiss: "If the whole complex does not refer to the plague and if the conventions which Orcagna used in the altarpiece also have established meanings unrelated to the plague then we have good reason to challenge any connections of the altarpiece itself with the horrors of 1348" (283). But Meiss never makes any claim that painting after the Black Death incorporated specific plague iconography; nor does he argue for a simple one-to-one correspondence between the plague of 1348 and an immediate "cataclysmic reaction" (Paoletti's phrase, 299).

118. Fabbri and Rutenburg, "The Tabernacle of Orsanmichele," 389, 403–4.

119. Cole, *Italian Art,* 103.

120. Cole, "Orcagna and the Black Death Style," 36. Moreover, Gardner, in "Andrea di Bonaiuto," has considered the overall function of the frescoes in their architectual surroundings in the Dominican charterhouse. While rejecting the influence of Jacopo Passavanti and his *Specchio* for the iconographical programs of these frescoes, he nonetheless agrees with Meiss's stylistic interpretations: "The investigations of Millard Meiss . . . have greatly clarified our knowledge of the style of the painter" (121–22).

121. Cole, "Orcagna and the Black Death Style," 29.

122. Cole, *Italian Art,* 102. In "The Black Death," van Os concludes his survey of the literature around the Meiss thesis (which, curiously, does not confront Boskovits's bold reinterpretations) with a similarly nihilistic stance: "Above all, it is as if all hope has been abandoned of finding a convincing interpretation of artistic development in conjunction with historical change" (241).

123. See Maginnis's useful summary report, "The Literature of Sienese Trecento Painting": "Since the appearance of the book, over twenty years ago, the accepted dating for some of the works Meiss discussed has shifted to the pre-1348 period. These changes do not, however, substantially alter Meiss's characterization of the third quarter of the century, for his argument rests on the prevalence of attitudes, of certain stylistic characteristics and iconographic themes rather than upon their being unique to that period" (301). Curiously, Maginnis does not here analyze the revised chronology argued in Boskovits's mammoth reconstruction of artistic style and historical contexts, *Pittura fiorentina.* Since Maginnis's review, the most radical departure is van Os's overview, "The Black Death," 243, 244, 247, which attributes the sylistic changes after the Black Death to the breakdown of the large workshops of the previous generation along with changes in patronage from the city to the provinces and from the oligarchs to "the *vox populi*" (which, however, once again dovetails with Meiss's earlier analysis).

124. Based on the reviews of this impressive work, it is safe to say that few art historians have placed it in its proper context as a reinterpretation of culture in late Trecento Florence. Most do not even discuss Boskovits's findings in relation to Meiss's thesis.

125. Antal, *Florentine Painting.*

126. Boskovits, *Pittura fiorentina,* 9.

127. Ibid., 24, 36: "in perfetto parallelo col pittore, nel Trecentonovelle vengono presentate le storie in un linguaggio svagato sì, e a volte ruvido, ma schietto e libero da ogni ricercatezza: una parlata adatta a esprimere una gran varietà di situazioni e atteggiamenti umani, un idioma ricco e flessible." And

on page 38, "anni '60, l'interesse naturalistico costituisce una novità assoluta in quell'ambiente."

128. Fengler, "Bartolo di Fredi's Old Testament Frescoes."

129. Boskovits, *Pittura fiorentina*, 46.

130. Ibid., 54, 71.

131. Ibid., 62.

132. See Baron, *The Crisis of the Early Italian Renaissance*, 28–47; and, more recently, Banti, *D'Appiano*, 10–16, 90.

133. Banti, *D'Appiano*, 9, 59, 71–93.

134. Boskovits, *Pittura fiorentina*, 138. Eight years later, in *The Painters of the Miniaturist Tendency*, 12–79, Boskovits appears to have abandoned this complex historical schema for the second half of the Trecento. In this catalogue, it is as though the pestilence of 1340, the bankruptcies, and the Black Death did not figure: "From the early 1330s, Daddi's style developed the idiosyncrasies which were to characterize it throughout the rest of his career: a joyful and spontaneous narrative style, harmonious balance of colours, precision of detail and drawing" (71). "In the final phase of his development, Daddi's interests were directed towards a greater realism; his narratives became more detailed and the characterization of his figures more sympathetic and natural" (74). Moreover, instead of initiating a revival of naturalism and values associated with Giotto, the early sixties in this survey ended such a period: "So with Puccio's death, probably in 1362, the rich chapter of the "miniaturist tendency" comes to an end. . . . a figurative idiom capable of conveying deep human feeling though naturalistic expression and action, dies out with him . . . his figures never lose their joyous communicativeness and human warmth" (74).

135. Boskovits, *Pittura fiorentina*, 44.

136. See Trexler, *The Papal Interdict on Florence*.

137. In addition to the statistics presented here, see Boskovits's assumptions concerning his "decade of crisis," 1370–80, in *Pittura fiorentina*: "si decidevano a far esequire opere d'arte, si accontentavano di cose meno costose" (44).

138. Not only those commodities subject to factory production but a wide array of products, from Victorian locks and finished cabinets to tea, experienced adulteration and degradation: see Samuel, "The Workshop of the World." On art as an economic good, see Montias, "Cost and Value in Seventeenth-Century Dutch Art."

139. Meiss, "Italian Primitives," describes a triptych from the 1360s in Pienza: "The triptych was painted rapidly, and the layers of color were not always superimposed in the usual way. The brush stroke is visible in many places" (12).

140. Boskovits, in *Pittura fiorentina*, is one of the few in the recent historiography to discuss prices and workshop practices in the Trecento. Unfor-

tunately, he does not integrate these data into his analysis but tacks them onto the end as an epilogue, "L'artista alla fine del Trecento," 159–78, which in no way buttresses his earlier conclusions. The changes in prices do not match the "revolutions" he claims for style and content in the body of the text. Boskovits claims only that the prestige of the artist's profession began to ameliorate by the early Quattrocento (160), that is, in the period after his detailed analyses of changes in style and sentiment.

141. Meiss, *Painting in Florence and Siena,* 31; Boskovits, *Pittura fiorentina,* 46.

142. See Goldthwaite, *The Building of Renaissance Florence,* "The Empire of Things," 153–75, and "The Economy of Renaissance Italy"; and Previtali, "La periodizzazione." Wackernagel, *The Florentine Artist,* 369, posits a similar relation between demand and the extraordinary conditions of the Florentine art market in Renaissance. His argument, however, stresses the "supply" of artists as much as a widespread demand from patrons representing a wide array of Florentine society. For the obverse relationship, see, among others, Marx, *Capital,* vol. 1, chap. 14, 2, 459–60. Since Wackernagel and Lerner-Lehmkuhl, less work has been done on the art market and the organization of workshops than on other aspects of art history (see Borsook's remarks in the review of Neri di Bicci's *Ricordanze,* 313.) Some exceptions are Caplow, "Sculptors' Partnerships"; Camesasca, *Artisti in bottega;* Middeldorf's review of Wackernagel; and Corti, "Sul commercio dei quadri."

In contrast, new studies abound in the north of Europe, at least for the early modern period. Of these, the most important have come from the economist Montias: *Artists and Artisans in Delft,* and "Socio-Economic Aspects of Netherlandish Art." See also Benedict, "The Popular Market for Art"; Wilson, "Workshop Patterns and the Production of Painting in Sixteenth-Century Bruges"; and Jacobs, "The Marketing and Standardization of South Netherlandish Carved Altarpieces."

143. Borsook, *The Mural Painters of Tuscany:* "The new architectural style introduced by Brunelleschi took Classical Antiquity as its point of departure. . . . After the busy fullness of the fourteenth-century church interiors, those designed by Brunelleschi, Alberti and their followers appear bare. . . . What they seized upon [was] the essential structural definition of forms . . . For Alberti, the walls of the ideal church interior were predominantly white" (xli–xliii). In *De re aedificatoria* Alberti inveighs against crowding every place with altars, preferring the ancient rule of one altar in the middle of the temple. See Hills, "The Renaissance Altarpiece," 45.

144. Borsook, *The Mural Painters of Tuscany:* "A part of its legacy to future generations was the fashion of whitewashing muralled church interiors in order to give them a neat, clean look. This had already begun at Santa Croce during the early Quattrocento and was repeated for centuries thereafter" (xliii).

145. Similarly, van Os, "Tradition and Innovation," comments on the variety

of new patrons and new forms of altarpieces in the Sienese territory during the second half of the Trecento, which led to numerous short-term solutions: "In patronage democratization created confusion. . . . Only the aesthetic approach of Renaissance architects and painters would eventually generate new and widely accepted forms and compositions for the altarpiece" (66).

146. Trexler, "Florentine Religious Experience," 28.

147. On the appearance of churches before Vasari's "remorseless *sistema-zioni*," see Wackernagel's description of the old Santa Maria Novella in *The Florentine Artist:* "What we find today since the reorganization carried out by Vasari as well as the puristic neo-Gothic restoration around 1860 is a spacious, clearly comprehensible interior organization. . . . This, however, is the complete opposite of the former condition, which must probably have been regarded already in the High Renaissance as no longer quite satisfying and in the Mannerist period as downright intolerable. . . . Altars and tombs also appeared everywhere throughout the whole church space in planless asymmetrical distribution and variety of form. The church was thus a remarkably richly branching, multipartite organism, whose teeming abundance of forms was thoroughly entwined and interwoven with no less rich a variety of colors. . . . To this were added everywhere the coats of arms of donors and the banners or other memorial objects draped on many tombs. What an effect this lavishly orchestrated polyphony must have produced. . . . The appearance of its present condition, fragmentary and indistinct, gives only a dim suggestion of the original costly splendor of this space. And the jumble of forms and colors in the total picture of the church interior remains wholly inconceivable" (51–52).

148. According to Moisè, *Santa Croce,* 73, as early as 1429 the Commune of Florence imposed a tax on families who possessed chapels and tombs in churches for the purposes of ornamenting and whitewashing church walls. van Os, "Painting in a House of Glass," makes a similar argument for Sienese art, at least of the second half of the Quattrocento, maintaining that Pius II's dicta on chapel space stated in his commentaries were obeyed: "No one shall deface the whiteness of the walls and the columns. No one shall draw pictures. No one shall hang up pictures. No one shall erect more chapels and altars than there are at present." On Vasari's Cinquecento efforts, see Boas, *Giorgio Vasari;* Goldberg, *After Vasari;* and Hall, *Renovation and Counter-Reformation.* Wackernagel, *The Florentine Artist,* 39, 113, called them "remorseless," Vasari's "forcible Mannerist *sistemazioni.*"

149. Rodolico, *La democrazia fiorentina;* Rutenburg, *Popolo e movimenti popolari;* Cohn, *The Laboring Classes.*

150. Malavolti, *Dell'historie di Siena,* pt. 2, bk. 8, 152v–153r.

151. Because of his anti-oligarchic policies, D'Appiano was called "the Tyrant of Pisa": see Capponi, *Storia della Repubblica di Firenze,* bk. 4, 408–32, and Mallett, *The Florentine Galleys,* 8–9.

152. Despite his bourgeois origins, D'Appiano was also related to powerful noble ranchers in the region around Donoratico. Banti, *D'Appiano*, 78–79; Tangheroni, *Politica, commercio, agricoltura*, 71.

153. Cohn, *The Laboring Classes*, 179–210, "Criminality and the State"; Molho, "The Florentine Oligarchy," "Politics and the Ruling Class"; Trexler, *Public Life*.

154. Previtali, *La fortuna dei primitivi;* Meiss, "Italian Primitives."

8. Conclusion

1. This number does not include the formulaic bequests required by statutory laws.

2. Tabacco, *The Struggle for Power*, 136–43.

3. See Pertile, *Storia del Diritto Italiano*, 3: 323ff., and Drew, *The Lombard Laws*, 31–35.

4. Onory, "L'Umbria Bizantina," 55–77; Bognetti, "Il Ducato Longobardo di Spoleto," 79–102.

5. Bloch, *Apologie pour l'histoire*, 5.

6. Wieruszowski, "Arezzo as a Center of Learning"; Black, *Benedetto Accolti*, 5–12; Lazzeri, *Guglielmino Ubertini*, 110.

7. In addition to the statistics on pious giving presented here, see Antal, *Florentine Painting*, 74, and Lesnick, *Preaching in Medieval Florence*.

8. See Ermini, *Storia dell'Università di Perugia*, and "Fattori di successo dello studio perugino."

9. Denley, "Academic Rivalry and Interchange": "The thirteenth century saw the beginnings of two Tuscan *studi*, that of Arezzo, which dates almost from the beginning of the century, and that of Siena, whose origins can be traced back to documents of the 1240s, but which formally opened in 1275" (194).

10. Wieruszowski, "Arezzo as a Center of Learning"; Black, *Benedetto Accolti*, 17ff.; Lazzeri, *Guglielmino Ubertini*, 103–13. The 1255 statutes of the Aretine *studium* are the oldest of any university.

11. Fabroni, *Historia Academiae Pisanae*.

12. Brucker, "Florence and Its University," and "Renaissance Florence: Who Needs a University?" For the later period, see Verde, *Lo Studio Fiorentino*. The Signoria of Florence established the *studium generale* on 29 August 1348.

13. See, most recently, Black, "Humanism and Education."

14. See Baldelli, "La letteratura volgare": "Parallelamente al fiorire del volgare scritto, rilevante la presenza della cultura latina a Pisa. . . . I maggiori centri di produzione dei più antichi testi volgari sono anche fra i maggiori centri di letteratura, a tutti i livelli, in latino. . . . Nell'area toscana, la coincidenza fra presenza culturale latina e attività in volgare scritto è patente a Pisa. . . . La prima città in cui si coglie la novità della scrittura monumentale non isolata,

ma anzi come prassi difusa, è Pisa, la prima città in Italia e in Europa" (69–70). See also Petrucci, *La scrittura,* 3–15.

15. Grendler, *Schooling in Renaissance Italy.*

16. Black, "Humanism and Education"; and see Petrucci and Miglio, "Alfabetizzazione e organizzazione scolastica nella toscana," 476.

17. Greenblatt, *Renaissance Self-Fashioning,* 3.

18. Chabod, "The Concept of the Renaissance."

19. The inconsistencies in these patterns do not negate the broader patterns of change that psychoanalysts and psychohistorians like Rudolph Binion, *Hitler among the Germans,* 15, have found accompany relived trauma—the will "to control, to master" an experience "too painful to assimilate . . . after having been overcome by it the first time." The direction of change is neither predictable nor logical in the short run, as instead the patient or the society is jolted from an earlier mental posture: see Chapter 3, note 22.

Notes to Appendix A

1. See Catoni and Fineschi, *L'Archivio notarile,* 13–22, and *Statuti senese dell'arte dei giudici e notai,* 84–85.

2. For the scheme of triplicate redactions customary in Umbrian contracts, see Bartoli Langeli, "Nota introduttiva," xix.

3. Cenci, *Documentazione,* vol. 1.

4. Other ecclesiastical archives with testaments exist in the vast Diplomatico collections. So as not to overburden the Florentine sample with selections from the Diplomatico, I concentrated on those collections from Florence's major hospital, Santa Maria Nuova, the Dominican archives of Santa Maria Novella, the Franciscan ones of Santa Croce, and several other monastic houses.

5. On the character of fragmentary copies kept by cathedrals, hospitals, and monastic orders, see Bertram, "Mittelalterliche Testamente," 520; on the massive collection of fragmentary testaments and excerpted legacies kept by the hospital of Santa Maria della Scala in Siena, see Redon, "Autour de l'Hôpital."

6. The adjusted R-square for this model is .183; the archive variable (testaments from the parchment collections as opposed to the public notarial protocols and *bastardelli*) is significant at .0019; its beta coefficient is + .06.

7. Arch. dei Laici, reg. 726, 3r–v, 52v–54v, 55v.

8. See, for example, the exceptional testaments drafted by Pierozius quondam Ser Federigi, Arch. dei Laici, reg. 726, 60r–61r; and that of Landucius Ser Andree Giotti degli Acceptantibus, 62v–63r.

9. The adjusted R-square is .199, the number of cases is 534, and the beta coefficients for these periods are as follows: 1363, − .168; 1364–75, − .158; 1376–1400, − .312; 1401–25, .224. All of these time periods are significantly different from the periods before the Black Death at .0001 or less.

10. For Perugia, the last quartile of this analysis includes the years 1400 to 1425 instead of 1401 to 1425. I included the plague year 1400 so as to bring notarial records into this last period of analysis. From the notarial protocol of Cola Bartolini (Protocol no. 22) I drew 19 testaments. After this date and before 1426, I was not able to locate other notarial books that drew testaments together.

Bibliography

Archives

AREZZO
Archivio di Stato, Arezzo (ASA)
  Protocollo d'antichi notari aretini (Antichi notari)
  Pergamene e carte varie (Perg.)
  L'Archivio della Fraternità dei Laici di Arezzo (Arch. dei Laici)
  Testamenti
Archivio Capitolare di Arezzo (Arch. Capitolare, Arezzo)

ASSISI
Sacro Convento di Assisi; Fondo Antico di San Francesco (Sacro Convento)
  Instrumenta I–X
  Archivi amministrativi
  Buste Z: Testamenti (1363–1543)
Biblioteca Comunale (Bibl. Com.)
  Notarile
Archivio Capitolare di Assisi (Arch. Capitolare, Assisi)
  Archivium Assisium ecclesie S. Rufini
  Compagnia di San Francesco (Co. S. Francesco)
  Compagnia di Santo Stefano (Co. S. Stefano)

FLORENCE
Archivio di Stato, Firenze (ASF)
  Notarile antecosimiano (Not. antecos.) [including notarial protocols from Florence, Arezzo, and Pisa]
  Diplomatico (Dipl.)
    Archivio Generale, Florence (Arch. Gen.)
    Domenicani d'Arezzo
    Misericordia d'Arezzo
    Olivetani d'Arezzo

Olivetani di Firenze
Santa Maria in Gradibus, Arezzo
Santa Maria Nuova
Santa Maria Novella
Santa Croce
Santa Felicità
Santissima Annuziata
Santa Maria di Badia
Cistercensi, Florence
Catasto
Statuti
Archivio Arcivescovile, Firenze
Visite
Biblioteca Medicea Laurenziana, Archivio San Lorenzo (Arch. S. Lorenzo)

PERUGIA
Archivio di Stato, Perugia (ASPr)
Notarile Bastardelli (Not. Bast.)
Notarile Protocolli (Not. Prot.)
Pergamene (Perg.)
San Domenico
San Francesco al Prato
San Maria di Monte Luce
Monte Morcino
Misericordia
Ospedale di Santa Maria della Misericordia, Contratti (Osp. di Misericordia)
Archivio di San Pietro
Liber contractuum

PISA
Archivio di Stato, Pisa (ASPi)
Ospedale di Santa Chiara (Osp. di S. Chiara)
Protocolli
Contratti e testamenti
Diplomatico (Dipl.)
Acquisto Cappelli
Misericordia
Olivetani di Pisa
Opera di Primaziale
Sant'Anna

San Benedetto
San Domenico
San Lorenzo alle Rivolte
Santa Marta
San Martino
San Michele in Borgo
San Paolo all'Orto

SIENA

Archivio di Stato, Siena (ASS)
    Notarile antecosimiano (Not. antecos.)
    Diplomatico (Dipl.)
        Archivio Generale (Arch. Gen.)

Printed Sources

Agazzari, Fra Filippo degli. *Gli "Assempi."* Edited by Piero Misciatelli. Siena, 1922.

Alberti, Leon Battista. *Trattato della pittura.* In *Opera volgari,* vol. 3, edited by Cecil Grayson. Bari, 1973.

Alighieri, Dante. *La Divina Commedia.* Edited by C. H. Grandgent, revised by Charles S. Singleton. Cambridge, Mass., 1972.

Angiolieri, Cecco. *Il canzoniere.* Edited by Sebastione Blancato. Milan, 1946.

Antoniella, Augusto, ed. *L'Archivio della Fraternità dei Laici di Arezzo.* Inventari e Cataloghi Toscani 17. Florence, 1985.

Barsotti, Riccardo. *Gli antichi inventari della cattedrale di Pisa.* Pisa, 1959.

Barsotti, Riccardo, Lucia Bertolini, Franco Russoli, and Emilio Tolaini, eds. *Mostra della sculptura pisana del Trecento: Pisa—Museo do S. Matteo.* Pisa, 1946.

Biscioni, Antonio Maria. *Lettere di Santi e Beati fiorentini: Raccolte ed illustrate.* Florence, 1736.

Boccaccio, Giovanni. *Epistle.* Edited by Pier Giorgio Ricci. *La letteratura italiana,* Storia e testi, vol. 9. Milan, 1965.

Catherine of Siena. *Epistolario di Santa Caterina da Siena.* Edited by Eugenio Dupré Theseider. Rome, 1940.

———. *I, Catherine: Selected Writings of St. Catherine of Siena.* Edited and translated by Kenelm Foster and Mary J. Ronayne. London, 1980.

———. *The Letters of Saint Catherine of Siena.* Vol. 3. Translated by Suzanne Noffke. Binghamton, N.Y., 1988.

Cavalca, Domenico. *Medicina del Cuore, ovvero Trattato della Pazienza.* Rome, 1756. Also in *Prosatori minori del Trecento.* Vol. 1, *Scritti di religione,* edited by Don Giuseppe de Luca, 39–47. Milan, 1954.

Cenci, Cesare. *Documentazione di vita assisana, 1300–1530*. Vol. 1, *1300–1448*. Spicilegium Bonaventurianum, vol. 10. Grottaferrata, 1974.

Cennini, Cennino. *Il libro dell'arte: The Craftsman's Handbook*. Translated by Daniel V. Thompson, Jr. New Haven, 1933.

Chronica Antiqua Conventus Sanctae Catharinae de Pisis. In *Archivio storico italiano (ASI)*, vol. 6, pt. 2. 1845.

Compagni, Dino. *Dino Compagni's Chronicle of Florence*. Edited by Daniel Bornstein. Philadelphia, 1986.

Il constituto del commune di Siena dell'anno 1262. Edited by Lodovico Zdekauer. Milan, 1897.

Il costituto del comune di Siena volgarizzato nel MCCCIX–MCCCX. 2 vols. Edited by Alessandro Lisini. Siena, 1903.

Crispolti, Cesare. *Perugia Augusta*. Perugia, 1648.

Cronaca della città di Perugia dal 1309 al 1491 nota col nome di Diario del Graziani. Edited by Ariodante Fabretti. *ASI*, vol. 16, pt. 1. Florence, 1850.

Cronaca fiorentina di Marchionne di Coppo Stefani. Edited by Niccolò Rodolico. *Rerum Italicarum Scriptores (RIS)*, vol. 30, pt. 1. Città di Castello, 1903.

Cronaca Pisana di Ranieri Sardo dell'anno 962 sino al 1400. Edited by Francesco Bonaini. *ASI*, vol. 6, pt. 2, 2d ser. Florence, 1845.

Cronaca senese attributa ad Agnolo di Tura del Grasso detta la Cronaca maggiore. Edited by Alessandro Lisini and Fabio Iacometti. In *Cronache Senesi, RIS*, n.s. vol. 15, pt. 6, 253–564. Bologna, 1931–39.

Cronaca senese di Donato di Neri e di suo figlio Neri. In *Chronache Senesi*, 567–685.

Cronica di Matteo Villani. Edited by Francesco Gherardi Dragomanni. 2 vols. Florence, 1846–47.

Le Croniche di Giovanni Sercambi Lucchese. 2 vols. Edited by Salvatore Bongi. Rome, 1892.

de Lat, Jan. *Reis-en handatlas van Vlaanderen, Brabanden aanleggende landschappen*. Amsterdam, 1740.

Fiorilli, C. *I dipinti a Firenze nell'arte dei medici, speziale e merciai*. Florence, 1921.

Formularium Florentinum Artis Notariae (1220–1242). Edited by Gino Masi. Milan, 1943.

Friex, Eugene H. *Tables des cartes des Pays Bas et des frontières de France*. Brussels, 1712.

Giovannini, Prisca, and Sergio Vitolo, eds. *Il Convento del Carmine di Firenze: Carratteri e documenti*. Florence, 1981.

Liber Contractuum (1331–32) dell'Abbazia Benedettina di San Piero in Perugia. Edited by Don Costanzo Tabarelli, O.S.B. Fonti per la storia dell'Umbria. Vol. 3. Perugia, 1967.

Malavolti, Orlando. *Dell'historie di Siena*. Venice, 1599.

Molti e facezie del Piovano Arlotto. Edited by Gianfranco Folena. Milan and Naples, 1953.

Museo di San Marco. *Mostra del Tesoro di Firenze Sacra.* Florence, 1933.

Neri di Bicci. *Le ricordanze (10 marzo 1453−24 aprile 1475).* Edited by Bruno Santi. Pisa, 1976.

Il notaio nella civiltà fiorentina: Secoli XIII−XIV. Florence, 1988.

Orlandi, Stefano, ed. *"Necrologio" di S. Maria Novella: Testo integrale dall'inizio al MDIV corredato di note biografiche tratte da documenti coevi.* 2 vols. Florence, 1955.

Pasqui, Ubaldo. *Documenti per la storia della città di Arezzo.* 3 vols. Florence, 1899.

Passavanti, Jacopo. *Lo Specchio di vera penitenzia.* Edited by Maria Lenardon. Florence, 1925.

Pellini, Pompeo. *Dell'historia di Perugia.* Venice, 1664.

Petrarca, Francesco. *Rime, Trionfi, Poesie latine.* Edited by F. Neri, G. Martellotti, E. Bianchi, and N. Sapegno. *La letteratura italiana,* Storia e testi, vol. 6. Milan and Naples, 1952.

Petrarch's Testament. Edited by Theodore Mommsen. Ithaca, N.Y., 1957.

Prosatori minori del Trecento. La letteratura italiana, Storia e testi, vol. 12. Milan, 1955.

Raniero da Perugia. *Ars notaria.* Edited by Augusto Gaudentio. In *Scripta Anecdote Glossatorum vel Glossatorum aetate composita,* 2: 25−75. Bologna, 1892.

Rationes Decimarum Italiae nei secoli XIII e XIV, Tuscia, I. La decima degli anni 1274−1280. Edited by Pietro Guidi, Studi e testi, vol. 58. Vatican City, 1932. *Tuscia, II. La decima degli anni 1295−1304.* Edited by Martino Giusti. Studi e testi, vol. 98. Vatican City, 1942. *Umbria.* Edited by Pietro Sella. Studi e testi, vols. 161, 162. Vatican City, 1952.

Richa, Giuseppe. *Notizie istoriche delle chiese fiorentine: Divise ne' suoi quartieri.* 10 vols. Florence, 1754−62.

Rodulphi, Rolandi. *Summa totius artis notariae.* Venice, 1574.

Roncioni, Raffaello. *Delle istorie pisane: Libra XVI.* Edited by Francesco Bonaini. *ASI,* vol. 6, pt. 1 (bks. 1−10). Florence, 1844.

Sacchetti, Franco. *Il Trecentonovelle.* Edited by Antonio Lanza. Florence, 1984.

La SS. Annunziata di Firenze: Studi e documenti sulla chiesa e il convento. Edited by Eugenio Casalini. Florence, 1971.

Scultura dipinta: Maestri di Legname e Pittori a Siena, 1250−1450. Florence, 1987.

Statuta populi e communis Florentiae (a. 1415). Freiburg, 1778−81.

Statuti di Perugia dell'anno MCCCXLII. Edited by Giustiniano Degli Azzi. Corpus Statutorum Italicarum, vols. 4, 9. Rome, 1913−16.

Statuti della Republica Fiorentina. Vol. 2, *Statuto del Podestà dell'anno 1325.* Edited by Romolo Caggese. Florence, 1921.

Statuti inediti della Città di Pisa dal XII al XIV secolo. Edited by Francesco Bonaini. Vol. 1, *Breve Pisani Communis, An. MCCLXXXVI.* Vol. 2, *Constituta legis et usus MCCXXIIII.* Florence, 1854–70.

Statuti senesi dell'arte dei giudici e notai dal XIV secolo. Fonti e studi del Corpus membranarum italicarum, 7. Edited by Giuliano Catoni. Rome, 1972.

Statuto di Arezzo (1327). Edited by Giulia Marri Camerani. Fonti di Storia Aretina, vol. 1. Florence, 1946.

Storie Pistoresi (1300–1348). Edited by S. A. Barbi. *RIS,* new ed., vol. 11, pt. 5. Città di Castello, 1907–27.

Summa notariae Aretii composita annis MCCXL–MCCCIII. Edited by Carlo Cicognario. In *Bibliotheca Iuridica Medii Avei,* 3: 283–335. Bologna, 1901.

Tavole di Ragguaglio per la riduzione dei pesi e misure . . . del granducato di Toscana. Florence, 1782.

Tavole di Riduzione delle misure e pesi toscani alle misure e pesi analoghi. Florence, 1809.

Tavole di Ragguaglio delle diverse misure locali di capacità e di peso dei singoli territori dello Stato Pontifico. Edited by Giuseppi Bofondi. Rome, 1855.

Vasari, Giorgio. *Le Vite de' più eccellenti pittori, scultori, e archettori nelle redazioni del 1550 e 1568. Testo,* edited by Rosanna Bettarini. *Commento,* edited by Paolo Barocchi. 6 vols. + Florence, 1966–.

Volbach, Wolfgang. *Pinacoteca vaticana Kataloge.* Vol. 2, *Il Trecento: Firenze e Siena.* Vatican City, 1987.

Zaccaria, Giuseppe. *Diario storico della basilica e sacro convento di S. Francesco.* In *Miscellanea Franciscana,* vol. 63, 290–361, 1963.

Secondary Sources

Alazard, Jean. *The Florentine Portrait.* Translated by Barbara Whelpton. London, 1948.

Aldinucci, Angiolo. "Economia aretina nei secoli XIV e XV." In *Contributi allo studio della storia di Arezzo,* 2d ser., edited by the Rotary Club di Arezzo. Arezzo, 1981. (Hereafter *Contributi.*)

Alpers, Svetlana Leontief. *"Ekphrasis* and Aesthetic Attitudes in Vasari's *Lives." Journal of the Courtauld and Warburg Institutes* 23 (1960): 190–215.

Antal, Frederick. *Florentine Painting and Its Social Background: The Bourgeois Republic before Cosimo de' Medici's Advent to Power: XIV and Early XV Centuries.* London, 1947.

Antoniella, Augusto. *L'Archivio della Fraternità dei Laici di Arezzo.* Inventari e Cataloghi Toscani 17. Florence, 1985.

Ardito, Felice. *Nobiltà, popolo, e signoria del Conte Fazio di Donoratico in Pisa nella Ia metà del secolo XIV.* Cuneo, 1920.

Arias, Emilio, Emilio Cristiani, and Paolo E. Gabba, eds. *Camposanto monumentale di Pisa: Le Antichità.* 2 vols. Pisa, 1977.

Ariès, Philippe. *Western Attitudes toward Death: From the Middle Ages to the Present.* Translated by P. Ranum. Baltimore, 1974.

————. *The Hour of Our Death.* Translated by Helen Weaver. New York, 1981.

Ashtor, Eliyahn. *Levant Trade in the Later Middle Ages.* Princeton, 1983.

Aston, Trevor H., and C.H.E. Philpin, eds. *The Brenner Debate: Agrarian Class Structure and Economic Development in Pre-Industrial Europe.* Cambridge, 1985.

Bagliani, Agostino Paravicini. *I Testamenti dei Cardinali del Duecento.* Miscellanea della Società Romana di Storia Patria, vol. 25. Rome, 1980.

Baldelli, Ignazio. "La letteratura volgare in Toscana dalle Origini ai primi decenni del secolo XIII." In *Letteratura italiana: Storia e geografia*, Vol. 1, *L'età medievale*, 65–78. Turin, 1987.

Balestracci, Duccio. *La zappa e la retorica: Memorie familiari di un contadino toscano del Quattrocento.* Florence, 1984.

————. "Per una storia degli ospedale di contado nella Toscana tra XIV e XVI secolo: Strutture, arredi, personale, assistenze." In *La società del bisogno: Poverità e assistenza nella Toscana medievale*, edited by Giuliano Pinto, 37–59. Florence, 1990.

Banker, James R. *Death in the Community: Memorialization and Confraternities in an Italian Commune in the Late Middle Ages.* Athens, Ga., 1988.

————. Review of Samuel K. Cohn, *Death and Property in Siena, 1205–1800: Strategies for the Afterlife. Journal of Interdisciplinary History* 20 (1990): 672–75.

Banti, Ottavio. *Iacopo D'Appiano: Economia, società, e politica del comune di Pisa al suo tramonto (1392–1399).* Pubblicazioni dell'Università Istituto di Storia, vol. 4. Pisa, 1971.

————. *Breve storia di Pisa.* Pisa, 1989.

Baron, Hans. "Franciscan Poverty and Civic Wealth." *Speculum* 13 (1938): 1–37.

————. *The Crisis of the Early Italian Renaissance: Civic Humanism and Republican Liberty in an Age of Classicism and Tyranny.* 2 vols. Princeton, 1955.

Bartolotti, Lando. *La città nella storia d'Italia: Siena.* Bari, 1975.

Bartoli Langeli, Attilio. "La realtà sociale assisana e il patto del 1210." In *Assisi al tempo di San Francesco. Società internazionale di studi francescani: Atti del V Convegno internazionale, Assisi, 13–16 ottobre 1977*, 271–336. Assisi, 1978.

————. "Nota introduttiva." In *Chiese e conventi degli ordini mendicanti in Umbria nei secoli XIII e XIV: I Protocolli di Perugia*, edited by M. Immacolata Bossi. Archivi dell'Umbria: Inventari e ricerche, no. 12. Perugia, 1987.

Baxandall, Michael. *Giotto and the Orators: Humanist Observers of the Painting in Italy and the Discovery of Pictorial Composition, 1350–1450.* Oxford, 1971.

————. *Painting and Experience in Fifteenth-Century Italy.* London, 1980.

Becker, Marvin. *Florence in Transition.* 2 vols. Baltimore, 1967–68.

————. "Individualism in the Early Italian Renaissance: Burden and Blessing." *Studies in the Renaissance* 19 (1972): 273–97.

————. "Aspects of Lay Piety in Early Renaissance Florence." In *The Pursuit of Holiness in Late Medieval and Renaissance Religion: Papers from the University of Michigan Conference,* edited by Heiko Oberman and Charles Trinkaus, 177–200. Leiden, 1974.

————. *Medieval Italy: Constraints and Creativity.* Bloomington, Ind., 1981.

Bellomo, Manlio. *Ricerche sui rapporti patrimoniali fra coniugi: Contributo alla storia della famiglia medievale.* Varese, 1961.

————. *La condizione giuridica della donna in Italia: Vicende antiche e moderne.* Turin, 1970.

Bellosi, Luciano. "La mostra di affreschi staccati al Forte Belvedere." *Paragone* 201 (1966): 73–79.

Bellosi, Luciano, Alessandro Angelini, and Giovanna Ragionieri. "Le arti figurative." In *Prato: Storia di una città.* Vol. 1, *Ascesa e declino del centro medievale (dal mille al 1494),* edited by Giovanni Cherubini, 907–62. Florence, 1991.

Beloch, Julius. *Bevölkerungsgeschichte Italiens.* Vol. 1. Berlin and Leipzig, 1937.

Bellucci, M. "Notizie storiche sugli antichi ospedali perugini." *Bollettino del Rotary Club di Perugia* (April 1965): 6–16.

Belting, Hans. *The Image and Its Public in the Middle Ages: Form and Function of Early Paintings of the Passion.* Translated by Mark Bartusis and Raymond Meyer. New Rochelle, N.Y., 1990. [Berlin, 1981.]

Benedict, Philip. "Towards the Comparative Study of the Popular Market for Art: The Ownership of Paintings in Seventeenth-Century Metz." *Past and Present* 109 (1985): 100–117.

Berenson, Bernard. *Italian Painters of the Renaissance.* London, 1952.

Bertram, Martin. "Mittelalterliche Testamente: Zur Entdeckung einer Quellengattung in Italien." *Quellen und Forschungen aus italienischen Archiven und Bibliotheken (QFIAB)* 68 (1988): 507–45.

————. "Hundert Bologneser Testamente aus einer Novemberwoche des Jahres 1265." *QFIAB* 69 (1989): 80–110.

————. "Bologneser Testamente. Erster Teil: Die urkundliche Überlieferung." *QFIAB* 70 (1990): 151–233.

Bibliotheca Sanctorum. Istituto Giovanni XXIII. 12 vols. Rome, 1961.

Binion, Rudolph. *Hitler among the Germans.* 2d ed. DeKalb, Ill., 1984.

————. *Soundings: Psychohistorical and Psycholiterary.* New York, 1981.

————. *Introduction à la psychohistoire*. Paris, 1982.

————. "Corrigenda." *Psychohistory Review* (1986): 69–79.

Biraben, Jean-Noel. *Les hommes e la peste en France et dans les pays européens*. 2 vols. Paris, 1975–76.

Bizzocchi, Roberto. *Chiesa e potere nella Toscana del Quattrocento*. Bologna, 1987.

Black, Robert. *Benedetto Accolti and the Florentine Renaissance*. Cambridge, 1985.

————. "Humanism and Education in Renaissance Arezzo." In *I Tatti Studies: Essays in the Renaissance*, 3: 171–237. Florence, 1989.

Bloch, Marc. *Apologie pour l'histoire, ou métier d'historien*. Paris, 1949.

Bloch, Maurice, and Jonathan Parry, eds. *Death and the Regeneration of Life*. Cambridge, 1982.

Boas, T.S.R. *Giorgio Vasari: The Man and the Book*. Princeton, 1979.

Bognetti, Gian Piero. "Il Ducato Longobardo di Spoleto." In *L'Umbria nella storia, nella letteratura, nell'arte*, 79–102. Bologna, 1954.

Bois, Guy. *Crise du féodalisme: Economie rurale et démographie en Normandie orientale du début du 14e siècle au milieu du 16e siècle*. Paris, 1976.

Bonanno, Claudio, Metello Bonanno, and Luciana Pellegrini, "I Legati *pro anima* ed il problema della salvezza nei testamenti fiorentini della seconda metà del Trecento." *Ricerche storiche* 15 (1985): 183–220.

Borsook, Eve. *The Mural Painters of Tuscany from Cimabue to Andrea del Sarto*. 2d ed. Oxford, 1980.

————. "Cults and Imagery at Sant'Ambrogio in Florence." *Mitteilungen des Kunsthistorischen Institutes* 25 (1981): 158–64.

————. Review of Neri di Bicci's *Le Ricordanze*. *Art Bulletin* (1979): 313–18.

Borsook, Eve, and Johannes Offerhaus. *Francesco Sassetti and Ghirlandaio at Santa Trinità: History and Legend in a Renaissance Chapel*. Doornspijk, 1981.

Boskovits, Miklós. *Pittura fiorentina alla viglia del Rinascimento, 1370–1400*. Florence, 1975.

————. *The Fourteenth Century: The Painters of the Miniaturist Tendency. A Critical and Historical Corpus of Florentine Painting*, Edited by Richard Offner with Klara Steinweg. Continued by Boskovits and Mina Gregori. Florence, 1984.

Bowsky, William. "The Impact of the Black Death upon Sienese Government and Society." *Speculum* 39 (1964): 368–81.

————. *A Medieval Italian Commune: Siena under the Nine, 1287–1355*. Berkeley, 1981.

————. *Piety and Property in Medieval Florence: A House in San Lorenzo*. In *Quaderni di "Studi Senesi,"* no. 69. Milan, 1990.

Brentano, Robert. "Death in Gualdo Tadino and in Rome." *Studia gratiana* 19 (1976): 79–100.

Bresc, Henri. *Un monde méditerranéen: Economie et société en Sicile, 1300–1450*. 2 vols. Rome, 1986.

Bridbury, A. R. *Economic Growth in England in the Later Middle Ages*. London, 1962.

Brooke, Rosalind B. "La prima espansione francescana in Europa." In *Espansione del Francescanesimo tra Occidente e Oriente nel secolo XIII: Atti del VI convegno internazionale, Assisi, 12–14 ottobre 1978*. Assisi, 1979.

Brown, J. W. *The Dominican Church of Santa Maria Novella*. Edinburgh, 1902.

Brown, Judith. *In the Shadow of Florence: Provincial Society in Renaissance Pescia*. Oxford, 1982.

———. "Prosperity or Hard Times in Renaissance Italy?" *Renaissance Quarterly* 42 (1989): 761–80.

Brown, Peter. *The Cult of the Saints: Its Rise and Function in Latin Christianity*. Chicago, 1981.

Brucker, Gene A. "Florence and Its University, 1348–1434." In *Action and Conviction in Early Modern Europe*, edited by T. Rabb and J. Seigel, 220–36. Princeton, 1969.

———. *Renaissance Florence*. 2d ed. Berkeley, 1983.

———. *Giovanni and Lusanna: Love and Marriage in Renaissance Florence*. Berkeley, 1986.

———. "Renaissance Florence: Who Needs a University?" In *The University and the City: From Medieval Origins to the Present*, edited by T. Bender, 47–58. New York, 1988.

———. "Monasteries, Friaries, and Nunneries in Quattrocento Florence." In *Christianity and the Renaissance: Image and Religious Imagination in the Quattrocento*, edited by Timothy Verdon and John Henderson, 41–62. Syracuse, N.Y., 1990.

Bucci, Mario. *Campo Santo Monumentale di Pisa*. Pisa, 1960.

Burckhardt, Jacob. *The Civilization of the Renaissance in Italy*. Translated by S.G.C. Middlemore. New York, 1958.

Burke, Peter. *Culture and Society in Renaissance Italy, 1420–1540*. New York, 1972

———. *Historical Anthropology of Early Modern Italy*. Cambridge, 1987.

Burresi, Mariagiulia. *Andrea, Nino, e Tommaso, scultori pisani*. Milan, 1983.

Bynum, Caroline W. *Holy Feast and Holy Fast: The Religious Significance of Food to Medieval Women*. Berkeley, 1987.

Caleca, Antonino. "Un profilo dell'arte pisana del Trecento." In *Andrea, Nino, e Tommaso, scultori pisani*, edited by Mariagiulia Burresi. Milan, 1983.

Camesasca, Ettore. *Artisti in bottega*. Milan, 1966.

Campbell, J. K. *Honour, Family, and Patronage*. Oxford, 1964.

Camporeale, Salvatore. "Senso della morte e amore della vita nel Rinascimento: Susone, Valla, Erasmo, e il 'problema della salvezza.'" *Memorie Domenicane,* n.s. 8–9 (1977–78): 439–50.

――――. "Giovanni Caroli e la 'Vitae fratrum S.M. Novellai': Umanesimo e crisi religiosa (1460–1480)." *Memorie Domenicane,* n.s. 12 (1981): 141–267.

――――. "Giovanni Caroli: Dal 'Liber dierum' alle 'Vitae fratrum.'" *Memorie Domenicane,* n.s. 16 (1985): 199–233.

――――. "Giovanni Caroli, 1460–1480: Death, Memory, and Transformation." In Tetel, Witt, and Goffen, *Life and Death in Fifteenth-Century Florence,* 16–27.

――――. "Humanism and the Religious Crisis of the Late Quattrocento: Giovanni Caroli, O.P., and the 'Liber dierum lucensium.'" In *Christianity and the Renaissance,* 445–66.

Capelli, Adriano. *Cronologia, cronografia, e calendario perpetuo, dal principio dell'èra cronologico-sincrone e quadri sinottici per verificare le date storiche.* 4th ed. Milan, 1978.

Capitani, Ovidio. "Città e comuni." In *Storia d'Italia.* Vol. 4, *Comuni e Signorie: Istituzioni, società, e lotte per l'egemonia,* edited by Ovidio Capitani, Raoul Manselli, Giovanni Cherubini, Antonio Ivan Pini, and Giorgio Chittolini, 5–57. Turin, 1981.

Caplow, Harriet McNeal. "Sculptors' Partnerships in Michelozzo's Florence." *Studies in the Renaissance* 21 (1974): 145–73.

Caponeri, Marilena Rossi. "Nota su alcuni testamenti della fine del secolo XIV relativi alla zona di Orvieto." In *Chiese e conventi degli ordini mendicanti in Umbria nei secoli XII–XIV,* edited by M. R. Caponeri and L. Riccetti. Archivi dell'Umbria: Inventari e Ricerche, vol. 9. Bari, 1988.

Capponi, Gino. *Storia della Repubblica di Firenze.* Florence, 1875.

Carli, Enzo. *Il Camposanto di Pisa.* Rome, 1937.

――――. *La scultura lignea senese.* Milan and Florence, 1951.

――――. *La scultura lignea italiana dal XII al XVI.* Milan, 1961.

Carmichael, Ann. *Plague and the Poor in Renaissance Florence.* Cambridge, 1986.

Carpentier, Elisabeth. *Une ville devant la peste: Orvieto et la Peste Noire de 1348.* Paris, 1962.

Carta d'Italia all scala di 1:25,000. 4th ed. Istituto geografico militare. Florence, 1962.

Casagrande, Giovanna. "La recente storiografia umbra sulle confraternite: Prospetti di ricerca." *Ricerche di storia sociale e religiosa* 15–16 (1979): 135–44.

Casini, Bruno. *Il fondo degli ospedali riunite di S. Chiara di Pisa.* Pisa, 1961.

Cassandro, Michele. "Commercio, manifatture, e industrie." In *Prato: Storia di una città,* 1: 395–477.

Castelnuovo, Enrico. "Il significato del ritratto pittorico nella società." In *Storia d'Italia*. Vol. 5, *Documenti*, edited by Ruggiero Romano and Corrado Vivanti, 1035–94. Turin, 1973.

Castelnuovo, Enrico, and Carlo Ginzburg. "Centro e periferia." In *Storia dell'arte italiana*, vol. 1, edited by Giovanni Previtali, 285–352. Turin, 1979.

Catoni, Giuliano. "Gli oblati della Misericordia: Poveri e benefattori a Siena nella prima metà del Trecento." In *La società del bisogno*, 1–17.

————, ed. *Le pergamene dell'università di Siena e la "Domus Misericordiae": Seminario di Archivistia*. Siena, 1975–76.

Catoni, Giuliano, and Sonia Fineschi. *L'Archivio notarile (1221–1862): Inventario*. Pubblicazioni degli archivi di Stato, no. 87. Rome, 1975.

Chabod, Federico. "The Concept of the Renaissance." In *Machiavelli and the Renaissance*, translated by David Moore, 149–200. New York, 1958.

Chartier, Roger, et al., eds. *A History of Private Life*. Vol. 3, *Passions of the Renaissance*. Translated by Arthur Goldhammer. Cambridge, Mass., 1989.

Chaunu, Pierre. *La mort à Paris: 16, 17, et 18e siècles*. Paris, 1978.

Cherubini, Giovanni. *Signori, Contadini, Borghesi: Ricerche sulla società italiana del basso medioevo*. Florence, 1974.

————. "Schede per uno studio della società aretina alla fine del Trecento." Publications of the Rotary Club of Arezzo, no. 867, 1 May 1977.

La chiesa fiorentina. Edited by Carlo Calzolai. Florence, 1970.

Chiffoleau, Jacques. *La comptabilité de l'au-delà: Les hommes, la mort, et la religion dans la région d'Avignon à la fin du moyen âge (vers 1320–vers 1480)*. In Collection de l'Ecole français de Rome, vol. 47. Rome, 1980.

————. "Perchè cambia la morte nella regione di Avignon alla fine del Medioevo." *Quaderni storici* 17 (1982): 449–65.

Cipolla, Carlo M. *Studi di storia della moneta: Il movimento dei cambi in Italia dal secolo XII al XV*. In *Studi nelle scienze-giuridiche e sociali*, no. 101. Pavia, 1948.

Cohn, Samuel Kline, Jr. "Criminality and the State in Renaissance Florence, 1344–1466." *Journal of Social History* 13 (1980): 211–33.

————. *The Laboring Classes in Renaissance Florence*. New York, 1980.

————. "Florentine Insurrections, 1342–1385." In *The English Uprising of 1381*, edited by R. H. Hilton and T. H. Aston, 143–64. Cambridge, 1984.

————. "La 'nuova storia sociale' di Firenze." *Studi storici* 26 (1985): 353–71.

————. *Death and Property in Siena, 1205–1800: Strategies for the Afterlife*. Baltimore, 1988.

————. Review of Peter Burke, *Historical Anthropology of Early Modern Italy*. *American Historical Review* 93 (1988): 1359–60.

Cole, Bruce. "Some Thoughts on Orcagna and the Black Death Style." *Antichità viva* 22 (1983): 27–37.

————. *Italian Art, 1250–1550: The Relation of Renaissance Art to Life and Society.* New York, 1987.

Contadini e proprietari nella Toscana moderna: Atti del Convegno di studi in onore di Giorgio Gorgetti. 2 vols. Florence, 1979.

Conti, Alessandro. "L'evolution dell'artista." In *Storia dell'arte italiana,* vol. 2, *L'artista e il pubblico,* 127–34. Turin, 1979.

Conti, Elio. *La formazione della struttura agraria moderna nel contado fiorentino.* 2 vols. Rome, 1965.

Conti, Piero Ginori. *La Basilica di S. Lorenzo di Firenze e la famiglia Ginori.* Florence, 1940.

Cortese, Ennio. "Per la storia del munio in Italia." *Rivista italiana per le scienze giuridiche* 8 (1955–56): 323–474.

Corti, Gino. "Sul commercio dei quadri a Firenze verso la fine del secolo." *Commentari* 22 (1971): 84–91.

————. "La Compagnia di Taddeo e di Bartolo e Gregorio di Cecco, con altri documenti inediti." *Mitteilungen des Kunsthistorischen Institutes in Florenz* 25 (1981): 373–77.

Coturri, E. "L'Ospedale così detto 'di Bonifazio' in Firenze." *Pagine di storia della medicina* 3 (1959): 15–33.

Coulton, George G. *The Black Death.* New York, 1930.

Cresi, Domenico. "Statistica dell'ordine minoritico dell'anno 1282." *Archivium Franciscanum Historicum* 66 (1963): 157–62.

Cristiani, Emilio. *Nobiltà e popolo del comune di Pisa: Dalle origini del podestariato alla Signoria dei Donoratico.* Naples, 1962.

————. "Sul valore politico del cavaliere nella Firenze dei secoli XIII e XIV." *Studi medievali,* 3d ser., 3 (1962): 365–71.

————. "Un inventario delle Pergamene dell'archivio Capitolare di Pisa ridatto da Raffaello Roncioni nel 1610." *Bollettino Storia di Pisa* 33–35 (1964–66): 617–67.

————. "Il ceto dirigente." In *La Toscana nel secolo XIV: Caratteri di una civiltà regionale,* edited by Sergio Gensini, 27–40. Centro di studi sulla civiltà del tardo medieovo, San Miniato, 2. Pisa, 1988.

Cristofani, Antonio. *Delle storie di Assisi: Libri sei.* 3d ed. Assisi, 1902.

Croix, Alain. *La Bretagne aux 16e et 17e siècles: La vie, la mort, la foi.* Paris, 1961.

da Caprese, P. Saturino, O.F.M. *Guida Illustrata della Verna.* Prato, 1902.

D'Ajano, R. B. "Lotte sociali a Perugia nel secolo XIV." *Vierteljahrschrift für Sozial-und Wirtschaftsgeschichte* 8 (1916): 337–49.

D'Angiolini, Piero, and Claudio Pavone, eds. *Guida generale degli Archivi di Stato italiani.* 3 vols. Rome, 1981–86.

Davidsohn, Robert. *Geschichte von Florenz.* 4 vols. Osnabruck, 1896–1927. [*Storia di Firenze.* 8 vols. Translated by Giovanni Battista Klein. Florence, 1972.]

Davis, Charles T. "Ubertino da Casale and His Conception of 'Altissima Paupertas.'" *Studi Medioevali,* 3d ser., 22 (1981): 2–56.

Davis, John. *Land and Family in Pisticci.* London, 1973.

————. *People of the Mediterranean.* London, 1977.

degli Azzi Vitelleschi, Giustiniano. *Le Relazioni tra la Republica di Firenze e l'Umbria.* 2 vols. Perugia, 1904–9.

Delcorno, Carlo. *Giordano da Pisa e l'antica predicazione volgare.* Florence, 1975.

del Guerre, G. *L'Ospedale pisano di papa Alessandro.* Pisa, 1931.

Della Pina, M. "Andamento e distribuzione della popolazione." In *Livorno e Pisa: Due città e un territorio nella politica dei Medici,* 25–30. Pisa, 1980.

del Panta, Lorenzo. "Cronologia e diffusione delle crisi di mortalità in Toscana dalla fine del XIV agli inizi del XIX secolo." *Ricerche storiche* 7 (1977): 293–343.

————. *Le epidemie nelle storia demografica (secoli XIV–XIX).* Turin, 1980.

————. "Dalla mortalità epidemica alla mortalità controllata." In *Vita morte e Miracoli di gente comune: Appunti per una storia della popolazione della Toscana fra XIV e XX secolo,* edited by Carlo Corsini, 66–94. Florence, 1988.

Delumeau, Jean. *Le peur en Occident (XIVe–XVIIIe siècles): Une cité assiégée.* Paris, 1983.

————. *Le pèché et la peur: La culpabilisation en Occident (XIIIe–XVIIIe siècles).* Paris, 1983.

del Vita, Alessandro. "Contributi per la storia dell'arte aretina." *Rassegna d'arte* 13 (1913): 185–88.

————. "Notizie e documenti su antichi artisti aretini." *L'Arte* 16 (1913): 228–32.

Denley, Peter. "Academic Rivalry and Interchange: The Universities of Siena and Florence." In *Florence and Italy: Renaissance Studies in Honour of Nicolai Rubinstein,* edited by Peter Denley and Caroline Elam, 193–208. London, 1988.

Desplanques, Henri. *Campagnes ombriennes—Contribution à l'étude des paysages ruraux en Italie centrale.* Paris, 1969.

Dickson, Gary. "The Flagellants of 1260 and the Crusades." *Journal of Medieval History* 15 (1989): 227–67.

Dini, Bruno. "Lineamenti per la storia dell'arte della Lana in Arezzo nei secoli XIV–XV." In *Contributi.*

————. *Arezzo intorno al 1400: Produzioni e Mercato.* Arezzo, 1984.

————, ed. *Tracce di una storia economica di Firenze e della Toscana in generale dal 1252–1550.* Arezzo, 1974.

————, ed. *Industria e commercio nella Toscana medievale*. Florence, 1989.

di Pierro, Carmine. "Contributo alla biografia di fra Iacopo Passavanti fiorentino." *Giornale storico della letterature italiana* 47 (1906): 1–24.

Donati, Pier Paolo. "Per la pittura aretina del Trecento." *Paragone* 215 (1968): 22–39.

Douglas, Langton. *A History of Siena*. London, 1902.

Drew, Katherine. *The Lombard Laws*. Philadelphia, 1976.

Du Fresne Du Cange, Carolo. *Glossarium Mediae et Infimae Latinitatis*. 10 vols. Graz, 1954.

Dunkerton, Jill, Susan Foister, Dillian Gordon, and Nicholas Penny. *Giotto to Dürer: Early Renaissance Painting in the National Gallery*. New Haven, 1991.

Emery, Richard W. *The Friars in Medieval France*. New York, 1962.

Epstein, Stephan. *Alle origini della fattoria toscana: L'ospedale della Scala di Siena e le sue terre (metà-'200–metà-'400)*. Florence, 1987.

Era, Antonio. *Ricerche sul Formularium Florentinum diversorum contractuum*. Sassari, 1924.

Ercole, Francesco. "L'istituto dotale nella pratica e nella legislazione statutaria dell'Italia superiore." *Rivista italiana per le scienze giuridiche* 45 (1908): 191–302; 46 (1910): 167–257.

Ermini, Giuseppe. "Fattori di successo dello studio perugino delle origini." In *Storia e arte in Umbria nell'età comunale: Atti del VI Convegno di Studi Umbria, Gubbio, 26–30 maggio 1968*, pt. 2, 289–309. Perugia, 1971.

————. *Storia dell'Università di Perugia*. 4 vols. Florence, 1971–75.

Eubel, Conrad. *Hierarchia Catholica Medii Aevi sive Summorum Pontificum, S.R.E. Cardinalinum Ecclesiarum Antistitum Series ad anno 1198 usque ad annum 1431 Perducta*. Vol. 1. Regensberg, 1913.

Fabbri, Nancy Rash, and Nina Rutenburg. "The Tabernacle of Orsanmichele in Context." *Art Bulletin* 63 (1981): 385–405.

Fabroni, Angelo. *Historia Academiae Pisanae*. 3 vols. Pisa, 1791–95.

Fanfani, Amintore. *Un mercante del Trecento (Giubileo Carsidoni)*. Milan, 1935.

Fasoli, Gino. "Ricerche sulla legislazione antimagnatizia nei communi dell'alta e media Italia." *Rivista di storia del diritto italiano* 12 (1939): 116–17.

Fengler, Christie Knapp. "Bartolo di Fredi's Old Testament Frescoes in San Gimignano." *Art Bulletin* 63 (1981): 374–84.

Fiumi, Enrico. *Storia economica e sociale di San Gimignano*. Florence, 1961.

Fortini, Arnaldo. *Nova vita di S. Francesco*. 4 vols. Assisi, 1959.

Fourquin, Guy. *Histoire économique de l'occident médiéval*. Paris, 1969.

Friedman, David. "The Burial Chapel of Filippo Strozzi in Santa Maria Novella in Florence." *L'Arte* 9 (1970): 109–32.

Frinta, Mojmîr, S. "An Investigation of the Punched Decoration of Medieval Italian and Non-Italian Panel Paintings." *Art Bulletin* 47 (1965): 261–65.

————. "The Quest for a Restorer's Shop of Beguiling Invention: Restoration and Forgeries in Italian Panel Painting." *Art Bulletin* 60 (1978): 7–23.

————. "The Decoration of the Gilded Surfaces in Panel Painting around 1300." In *Akten des XXV internationalen Kongresses für Kunstgeschichte Wien, 1983*. Vol. 6, *Europäische Kunst um 1300*, 69–75. Vienna, Cologne, and Graz, 1986.

Frugoni, Arsenio. "Sui flagellanti del 1260." *Bullettino dell'Istituto storico italiano* 75 (1963): 214–15.

Fumi, Luigi. *Eretici e ribelli nell'Umbria: Studio storico di un decennio, 1320–1330*. Todi, 1916.

Fustel de Coulanges, N.D. *La Cité antique: Etude sur le culte, le droit, les institutions de la Grèce et de Rome*. Paris, 1864.

Gamurrini, G. F. "I pittori aretini dall'anno 1150 al 1527." *Rivista d'arte* 10 (1917–18): 88–97.

Gardner, Julian. "Arnolfo di Cambio and Roman Tomb Design." *Burlington Magazine* 115 (1973): 420–39.

————. "Andrea Di Bonaiuto and the Chapterhouse Frescoes in Santa Maria Novella." *Art History* 2 (1979): 107–38.

Garin, Eugenio. *L'Umanesimo italiano*. Bari, 1952.

————. *Portraits from the Quattrocento*. Translated by Victor and Elizabeth Velen. New York, 1972.

Gaston, Robert. "Liturgy and Patronage in San Lorenzo, Florence, 1350–1650." In *Patronage, Art, and Society in Renaissance Italy*, edited by F. W. Kent and Patricia Simon, 111–33. Oxford, 1987.

Gatti, Gerardo. "Antonomia privata e volontà di testare nei secoli XIII e XIV." In *Nolens Intestatus Decedere: Il testamento come fonte della storia religiosa e sociale*. Archivi dell'Umbria, Inventari e Ricerche 7, 17–26. Perugia, 1983.

Gavitt, Philip. *Charity and Children in Renaissance Florence: The Ospedale degli Innocenti, 1410–1536*. Ann Arbor, Mich., 1990.

Genicot, Léopold. "Crisis: From the Middle Ages to Modern Times." In *The Cambridge Economic History of Europe*, vol. 1, edited by M. M. Postan, 660–742. Cambridge, 1966.

Giardina, Camillo. " 'Advocatus' e 'mundualdus' nel Lazio e nell'Italia meridionale." *Rivista di storia del diritto italiano* 9 (1936): 291–310.

Gilbert, Creighton. "The Renaissance Portrait." *Burlington Magazine* 110 (1968): 278–85.

Gilmore, Myron. *The World of Italian Humanism, 1453–1517*. New York, 1952.

Ginatempo, Maria. *Crisi di un territorio: Il popolamento della toscana senese alla fine del Medioevo*. Florence, 1988.

Glasser, Hannelore. *Artists' Contracts of the Early Renaissance.* New York, 1977.

Goitein, S. D. *A Mediterranean Society: The Jewish Communities of the Arab World as Portrayed in the Documents of the Cairo Geniza.* 5 vols. Berkeley, 1967–88.

Goldberg, Edward. *Patterns in Late Medieval Art Patronage.* Princeton, 1983.

————. *After Vasari: History, Art, and Patronage in Late Medici Florence.* Princeton, 1988.

Goldthwaite, Richard. *Private Wealth in Renaissance Florence: A Study of Four Families.* Princeton, 1968.

————. "I prezzi del grano a Firenze dal XIV al XVI secolo." *Quaderni storici* 28 (1975): 5–36.

————. *The Building of Renaissance Florence: An Economic and Social History.* Baltimore, 1980.

————. "The Empire of Things: Consumer Demand in Renaissance Italy." In Kent and Simons, *Patronage, Art, and Society in Renaissance Italy,* 153–75.

————. "The Economy of Renaissance Italy: The Preconditions for Luxury Consumption." *I Tatti Studies: Essays in the Renaissance,* 2: 15–39. Florence, 1987.

————. "The Medici Bank and the World of Capitalism." *Past & Present* 114 (1987): 3–31.

Goldthwaite, Richard, and W. R. Rearick. "Michelozzo and the Ospedale di San Paolo in Florence." *Mitteilungen des kunsthistorischen Institutes in Florenz* 21 (1977): 221–306.

Goody, Jack. *Death, Property, and the Ancestors: A Study of the Mortuary Customs of the Lodagaa of West Africa.* Stanford, Calif., 1962.

————. "Inheritance, Property, and Women: Some Comparative Considerations." In *Family and Inheritance,* 10–36.

————. *The Development of the Family and Kinship in Europe.* Cambridge, 1983.

Goody, Jack, Joan Thirsk, and E. P. Thompson, eds. *Family and Inheritance: Rural Society in Western Europe, 1200–1800.* Cambridge, 1976.

Gottfried, Robert S. *The Black Death: Natural and Human Disaster in Medieval Europe.* London, 1983.

————. *Doctors and Medicine in Medieval England, 1340–1530.* Princeton, 1986.

Graesse, Johann Georg Theodor, Friedrich Benedict, and Helmut Plechl. *Orbis Latinus: Lexikon lateinischer geographischer Namen des Mittelalters und der Neuzeit.* Braunschweig, 1972.

Grande dizionario della lingua italiana. Edited by Salvatore Battaglia. 15 vols. Turin, 1961–.

Greenblatt, Stephen J. *Renaissance Self-fashioning from More to Shakespeare.* Chicago, 1980.

Grendler, Paul F. *Schooling in Renaissance Italy: Literacy and Learning, 1300–1600.* Baltimore, 1989.

Grohmann, Alberto. *Città e territorio tra medioevo ed moderna.* 2 vols. Perugia, 1981.

————. *Le città nella storia d'Italia: Perugia.* 2d ed. Bari, 1985.

————. *Le città nella storia d'Italia: Assisi.* Bari, 1989.

Guêze, R. "Le origini dell'ospedale di Santa Maria della Misericordia in Perugia." *Bollettino della deputazione di storia patria per l'Umbria (BDSPU)* 60 (1963): 83–87.

Guichard, Pierre. *Structures sociales "orientales" et "occidentales" dans l'Espagne musulmane.* Paris, 1977.

Hager, Helmut. *Die Anfänge des italienischen Altarbildes: Untersuchungen zur Entstehungsgeschichte des toskanischen Hochaltarretabels.* Römische Forschungen der Bibliotheca Hertziana, vol. 17. Munich, 1962.

Haines, Margaret. "Brunelleschi and Bureaucracy: The Tradition of Public Patronage at the Florentine Cathedral." In *I Tatti Studies: Essays in the Renaissance,* 3: 89–125. Florence, 1989.

Hall, Marica. *Renovation and Counter-Reformation: Vasari and Duke Cosimo in Santa Maria Novella and Santa Croce, 1565–1577.* Oxford, 1979.

Heers, Jacques. *Esclaves et domestiques au Moyen Age dans le monde méditerranéen.* Paris, 1981.

Henderson, John. "Le Confraternite religiose nella Firenze del tardo medioevo: Patroni spirituali e anche politici?" *Ricerche storiche* 15 (1985): 77–94.

————. "Charity in Late-Medieval Florence: The Role of Religious Confraternities." In *Florence and Milan: Acts of Two Conferences at Villa I Tatti in Florence,* 2: 147–63. Florence, 1988.

————. "The Parish and the Poor in Florence at the Time of the Black Death: The Case of S. Frediano." *Continuity and Change* 3, pt. 2 (1988): 247–72.

————. "Religious Confraternities and Death in Early Renaissance Florence." In *Florence and Italy,* 383–94.

————. "The Hospitals of Late-Medieval and Renaissance Florence: A Preliminary Survey." In *The Hospital in History,* edited by L. Granshaw and R. Porter, 63–92. New York and London, 1989.

————. *Piety and Charity.* Forthcoming.

Herlihy, David. *Pisa in the Early Renaissance.* New Haven, 1958.

————. *Medieval and Renaissance Pistoia: The Social History of an Italian Town, 1200–1430.* New Haven, 1967.

————. "The Distribution of Wealth in a Renaissance Community: Florence, 1427." In *Towns and Societies,* edited by P. Abrams and E. Wrigley, 131–57. Cambridge, 1978.

————. *Opera Muliebria: Women and Work in Medieval Europe.* New York, 1990.

Herlihy, David, and Christiane Klapisch-Zuber. *Les Toscans et leur familles: Une étude du catasto florentin de 1427.* Paris, 1978.

Herklotz, Ingo. *"Sepulcro" e "Monumenta" del Medioevo.* Rome, 1985.

Hertz, Robert. *Death and the Right Hand.* Translanted by R. Needham and C. Needham. London, 1960.

Heywood, William. *Palio and Ponte: An Account of the Sports of Central Italy from the Age of Dante to the Twentieth Century.* London, 1904.

————. *A History of Perugia.* New York, 1910.

Hicks, David L. "Sources of Wealth in Renaissance Siena: Businessmen and Landowners." *Bullettino Senese di storia patria (BSSP)* 93 (1986): 9–42.

Hills, Paul. "The Renaissance Altarpiece: A Valid Category?" In *The Altarpiece in the Renaissance,* edited by P. Humfrey and M. Kemp, 34–48. Cambridge, 1990.

Hinnebusch, William A. *The History of the Dominican Order.* 2 vols. Staten Island, N.Y., 1966–73.

Hoffman, Philip T. *Church and Community in the Diocese of Lyon, 1500–1789.* New Haven, 1984.

Hoger, Annegret. "Studien zur Entstehung der Familienkapelle und zu Familien-Kapellen und-Altaren des Trecento in Florintiner Kirchen." Ph.D. diss., Bonn, 1976.

Holmes, George. *Florence, Rome, and the Origins of the Renaissance.* Oxford, 1986.

Hood, William. "Fra Angelico at San Marco: Art and Liturgy of Cloistered Life." In *Christianity and the Renaissance,* 108–31.

Hook, Judith. *Siena, a City and Its History.* London, 1979.

Hughes, Diane Owen. "Struttura familiare e sistemi di successione ereditaria nei testamenti dell'Europa medievale." *Quaderni Storici* 33 (1976): 929–52.

————. "Representing the Family: Portraits and Purposes in Early Modern Italy." *Journal of Interdisciplinary History* 17 (1986): 7–38.

Huizinga, Johan. *The Waning of the Middle Ages: A Study of the Forms of Life, Thought, and Art in France and the Netherlands in the XIVth and XVth Centuries.* Translated by F. Hopman. London, 1924.

Imberciadori, Ildebrando. *Mezzadria classica toscana con documentazione inedita del sec. 9 al sec. 14.* Florence, 1951.

Izbicki, Thomas M. "'Ista questio est antiqua': Two *Consilia* on Widows' Rights." *Bulletin of Medieval Canon Law* 8 (1978): 47–50.

Jacobs, L. F. "The Marketing and Standardization of South Netherlandish Carved Altarpieces: Limits on the Role of the Patron." *Art Bulletin* 81 (1989): 203–29.

Kent, Dale. *The Rise of the Medici: Faction in Florence, 1426–1434.* Oxford, 1978.

Kent, Dale, and Francis W. Kent. *Neighbours and Neighbourhood in Renaissance Florence: The District of the Red Lion in the Fifteenth Century.* Locust Valley, N.Y., 1982.

Kent, Francis W. *Household and Lineage in Renaissance Florence.* Princeton, 1977.

Kirshner, Julius. *Pursuing Honor While Avoiding Sin: The Monte delle doti of Florence.* In *Quaderni di "Studi Senesi,"* 71. Milan, 1978.

———. "Wives' Claims against Insolvent Husbands in Late Medieval Italy." In *Women of the Medieval World: Essays in Honor of John H. Mundy,* edited by J. Kirshner and S. Wemple, 256–303. Oxford, 1985.

———. "Materials for a Gilded Cage: Non-Dotal Assets in Fourteenth- and Fifteenth-Century Florence, 1300–1500." In *The Family in Italy from Antiquity to the Present,* edited by David Kertzer and Richard Saller, 184–207. New Haven, 1991.

Kirshner, Julius, and Jacques Pluss. "Two Fourteenth-Century Opinions on Dowries: Paraphernalia and Non-dotal Goods." *Bulletin of Medieval Canon Law* 9 (1979): 65–77.

Klapisch-Zuber, Christiane. *Les Maîtres du marbre (Carrare 1300–1600).* Paris, 1969.

———. "Déclin démographique et structure du ménage: L'exemple de Prato, fin XIVe–fin XVe." In *Famille et parenté dans l'occident médiéval: Actes du Colloque de Paris (6–8 juin 1974),* edited by Georges Duby and Jacques Le Goff, 255–73. Rome, 1977.

———. *Women, Family, and Ritual in Renaissance Italy.* Translated by Lydia G. Cochrane. Chicago, 1985.

———. *La famiglia e le donne nel Rinascimento a Firenze.* Bari, 1988.

Kreytenberg, Gert. *Andrea Pisano und die toskanische Skulptur des 14 Jahrhunderts.* In Italienische Forshungen herausgegben vom Kunsthistorischen Institut in Florenz, vol. 14. Munich, 1984.

Kriedte, Peter, Hans Medick, and Jurgen Schlumbohm. *Industrialization before Industrialization: Rural Industry in the Genesis of Capitalism.* Translated by Beate Schempp. Cambridge, 1981.

Kristeller, Paul. "The Immortality of the Soul." In *Renaissance Thought and Its Sources,* edited by Michael Mooney, 181–96. New York, 1979.

Kuehn, Thomas. "Women, Marriage, and *Patria Potestas* in Late Medieval Florence." *Revue d'histoire du droit* 49 (1981): 127–47.

———. "'Cum Consensu mundualdi': Legal Guardianship of Women in Quattrocento Florence." *Viator* 13 (1982): 309–33.

———. *Emancipation in Late Medieval Florence.* New Brunswick, N.J., 1982.

———. Review of Cohn, *Death and Property. Journal of Modern History* 62 (1990): 624–26.

Lane, Arthur. "Florentine Painted Glass and the Practice of Design." *Burlington Magazine* 91 (1949): 43–48.

Lane, Frederic C., and Reinhold C. Mueller. *Money and Banking in Medieval and Renaissance Venice.* Vol. 1, *Coins and Moneys of Account.* Baltimore, 1985.

Langer, William L. "The Next Assignment." *American Historical Review* 63 (1958): 283–304.

Lanzi, Luigi Antonio. *Storia pittorica della Italia.* 2 vols. Bassano, 1795–96.

la Roncière, Charles de. "L'influence des franciscains dans la campagne de Florence au XIVe siècle (1280–1360)." *Mélanges de l'école française de Rome: Moyen âge, temps modernes (MEFRM)* 87 (1975): 27–103.

————. *Florence: Centre économique régional au XIVe siècle.* 5 vols. Aix-en-Provence, 1977.

————. "Aspects de la religiosité populaire en toscane: Le contado florentin des années 1300." In *La Toscana nel secolo XIV,* 337–84.

La Sorsa, Saverio. *La compagnia d'Or S. Michele ovvero una pagina della beneficenza in Toscana nel secolo XIV.* Trani, 1902.

Lazzeri, Corrado. *Guglielmino Ubertini: Vescovo di Arezzo (1248–1289) e i suoi tempi.* Florence, 1920.

————. *Aspetti e figure di vita medievale in Arezzo.* Arezzo, 1937.

Le Bras, Gabriel. "Un programme: La géografie religieuse." *Annales d'histoire sociale.* Vol. 1, *Hommages à Marc Bloch,* 87–112. 1945.

Lebrun, François. *Les hommes et la mort en Anjou aux 17e et 18e siècles: Essai de démographie et de psychologie historiques.* Paris, 1971.

Le Goff, Jacques. "Ordres mendicants et urbanisation dans la France médiévale." *Annales, E.S.C.* 25 (1970): 924–46.

Le Goff, Jacques, and Pierre Toubert. "Une histoire totale du moyen âge, est-elle possible?" In *Actes du 100e Congrès national des Société savants.* Paris, 1975.

Lensi, Alfredo. *La Verna.* Florence, 1934.

Leo, Heinrich. *Entwicklung der Verfassung der lombardischen Städt bis zu der ankunft Kaiser Friedrich I.* Hamburg, 1824.

Leonij, L. "La peste e la compagnia del Cappelletto a Todi nel 1363." *ASI,* 4th ser., 2 (1878): 3–11.

Lerner, Robert. "The Black Death and Western Eschatological Mentalities." In Williman, *The Black Death,* 77–105.

Lerner-Lehmkuhl, Hanna. *Zur Struktur und Geschichte des Florentinischen Kunstmarketes.* Wattenscheid, 1936.

Le Roy Ladurie, Emmanuel. *Les paysans du Languedoc.* 2 vols. Paris, 1966.

————. "Chaunu, Lebrun, Vovelle: The New History of Death." In *The Territory of the Historian,* vol 1, 273–84. Translated by Ben Reynolds and Siân Reynolds. Chicago, 1979.

Lesnick, Daniel. *Preaching in Medieval Florence: The Social World of Franciscan and Dominican Spirituality*. Atlanta, 1989.

Lightbown, Ronald W. *Donatello and Michelozzo: An Artistic Partnership and Its Patrons in the Early Renaissance*. 2 vols. London, 1980.

Little, Lester. *Religious Poverty and the Profit Economy in Medieval Europe*. Ithaca, 1978.

————. *Liberty, Charity, Fraternity: Lay Religious Confraternities at Bergamo in the Age of the Commune*. Bergamo and Northampton, Mass., 1989.

Lopez, Robert. "Hard Times and Investment in Culture." In *The Renaissance: A Symposium*, 19–32. New York, 1953.

Lopez, Robert, and Harry A. Miskimin. "The Economic Depression of the Renaissance." *Economic History Review* 14 (1962): 408–27.

L'Oreficeria nella Firenze del Quattrocento. Florence, 1977.

Luchs, Alison. "Stained Glass above Renaissance Altars: Figure Windows in Italian Church Architecture from Brunelleschi to Bramante." *Zeitschrift für Kunstgeschichte* 48 (1985): 177–225.

Lunardi, Roberto. *Arte e storia in Santa Maria Novella*. Florence, 1983.

Luzzati, Michele. "Le origini di una famiglia nobile pisana: I Roncioni nei secoli XII al XIII." *BSSP* 73–75 (1966–68): 60–118.

————. "I registri notarili pisani dal XIII al XV secolo." In *Sources of Social History: Private Acts of the Late Middle Ages*, edited by Paolo Brezzi and Egmont Lee, 7–22. Toronto, 1984.

————. *Firenze e la Toscana nel Medioevo: Seicento anni per la costruzione di uno stato*. Turin, 1986.

McNeill, William. *Plagues and Peoples*. New York, 1976.

Maginnis, Hayden B. J. "The Literature of Sienese Trecento Painting, 1945–1975." *Zeitschrift für Kunstgeschichte* 40 (1977): 276–309.

Maine, Sir Henry. *Dissertations on Early Law and Custom*. London, 1883.

Maier, Charles S. "La storia comparata." In *Il mondo contemporaneo*, vol. 10, *Gli strumenti della ricerca*, pt. 2, *Questioni di metodo*, 1395–1410. Florence, 1983.

Maire-Vigueur, J.-C. "Les institutions communales de Pisa aux XIIe et XIIIe siècles." *Le Moyen Age* 79 (1973): 519–27.

Malanima, Paolo. "L'attività industriali." In *Prato: Storia di una città*. Vol. 2, *Un microcosmo in movimento (1494–1815)*, edited by Elena Fasano Guarini, 217–80. Florence, 1986.

Mallett, Michael. *The Florentine Galleys in the Fifteenth Century*. Oxford, 1967.

————. "Pisa and Florence in the Fifteenth Century." In *Florentine Studies*, edited by Nicolai Rubinstein. London, 1968.

Martines, Lauro. *Power and Imagination: City-States in Renaissance Italy*. New York, 1979.

————. "The Uses of Mortality." *Times Literary Supplement,* 1–7 Sept. 1989, 956.

Marx, Karl. *Capital,* vol. 1. Edited by Ernest Mandel and translated by Ben Fowles. London, 1976.

Masi, Gino. "La ceroplastica in Firenze nei secoli XV–XVIe e la famiglia Benintendi." *Rivista d'arte* 9 (1916): 134–43.

Massari, Cesare. *Saggio sulle pestilenze di Perugia e sul governo sanitario: di esse dal secolo XIV.* Perugia, 1838.

Masseti, Anna Rosa Calderoni. *Spinello aretino giovane.* Pisa, 1973.

Mastboom, Joyce. "The Role of Eastern Gelderland in Dutch Economic Development, 1650–1850." Ph.D. diss., Brandeis University, 1990.

Mazzatinti, Giuseppe, ed. *Gli Archivi della storia d'Italia.* 9 vols. Rocco di S. Casciano, 1897–1915.

Mazzatinti, Giuseppe, M. F. Pulignani, and M. Santoni, eds. *Archivio storico per le Marche e per l'Umbria.* 4 vols. Foligno, 1884–89.

Mazzi, Maria Serena, and Sergio Raveggi. *Gli uomini e le cose nelle campagne fiorentine del Quattrocento.* Florence, 1983.

Meersseman, Giles Gerard. *Ordo Fraternitatis: Confraternite e pietà dei laici nel mondo medioevo.* 3 vols. Rome, 1977.

Meiss, Millard. "Italian Primitives at Konopištĕ." *Art Bulletin* 28 (1946): 1–16.

————. *Painting in Florence and Siena after the Black Death: The Arts, Religion, and Society in the Mid-Fourteenth Century.* Princeton, 1951.

————. "An Illuminated *Inferno* and Trecento Painting in Pisa." *Art Bulletin* 47 (1965): 21–34.

————. "Notable Disturbances in the Classification of Tuscan Trecento Paintings." *Burlington Magazine* 113 (1971): 178–88.

Melis, Federigo. "Lazzaro Bracci: La funzione di Arezzo nell'economia dei secoli XIV–XV." *Atti e memorie dell'academia Petrarca,* n.s. 38 (1965–67): 1–18.

————. "L'economia delle città minori della Toscana." In *Le zecche minori toscane al XIV secolo: Atti del 3° Convegno Internazionale di Studi (Pistoia, 1967),* 13–40. Bologna, 1975.

————. *Industria e commercio nella Toscana medievale.* Edited by Bruno Dini. Florence, 1989.

————. "Momenti dell'economia del Casentino nei secoli XIV e XV." In *Industria e commercio,* 192–211.

Meloni, Piero L. "Per la storia delle confraternite disciplinate in Umbria nel secolo XIV." In *Storia e arte in Umbria nell'età communale: Atti del VI Convegno di Studi Umbria, Gubbia,* pt. 2, 533–87. Perugia, 1971.

Mendels, Franklin F. "Proto-industrialization: The First Phase of the Industrialization Process." *Journal of Economic History* 32 (1972): 241–61.

Mengozzi, Niccolò. *Il monte dei Paschi e le aziende in esso riunite: Note e storiche.* 6 vols. Siena, 1891–1902.

Mercantini, Maria. *La pieve di S. Maria ad Arezzo: Tumultose vicende di un restauro ottocentesco.* Arezzo, 1982.

Middeldorf, Ulrich. Review of M. Wackernagel, *World of the Florentine Renaissance Artist. Art Bulletin* 21 (1939): 298–300.

Mira, Giuseppe. "L'estimo di Perugia dell'anno 1285." In *Annali della facoltà di scienze politiche ed economia e commercio dell'Università degli studi di Perugia,* 397–400. Milan, 1956.

————. "Il fabbisogno dei cereali in Perugia e nel suo contado nei secoli XII e XIV." In *Studi in onore di Armando Sapori,* 1: 505–17. Milan, 1957.

————. "Aspetti dell'organizzazione corporativa in Perugia nel XIV secolo." *Economia e storia* 6 (1959): 366–98.

————. "Aspetti di vita economica nell'Assisi di San Francesco." In *Assisi al tempo di San Francesco. Società internazionale di studi francescani: Atti del V Convegno internazionale Assisi, 13–16 October 1977,* 123–79. Assisi, 1978.

Moisé, Filippo. *Santa Croce di Firenze: Illustrazione storico-artistica.* Florence, 1845.

Molho, Anthony. "The Florentine Oligarchy and the Balìa of the Late Trecento." *Speculum* 43 (1968): 25–51.

————. "Politics and the Ruling Class in Early Renaissance France." *Nuova rivista storica* 52 (1968): 401–20.

————. *Florentine Public Finances in the Early Renaissance, 1400–1433.* Cambridge, Mass., 1971.

————. "Visions of the Florentine Family in the Renaissance." *Journal of Modern History* 50 (1978): 304–11.

Molho, Anthony, and Julius Kirshner. "The Dowry Fund and the Marriage Market in Early Quattrocento Florence." *Journal of Modern History* 50 (1978): 403–38.

Mollat, Michel. "Le sentiment de la mort e de la vie et la pratique religieuse à la fin du Moyen Age." *La vie spirituelle,* suppl., 77 (1966): 218–29.

Monfasani, John. "The Fraticelli and Clerical Wealth in Quattrocento Rome." In *Renaissance Society and Culture: Essays in Honor of Eugene F. Rice, Jr.,* edited by John Monfasani and Ronald G. Musto, 177–95. New York, 1991.

Monti, Gennaro. *Le confraternite medievali dell'alta e media Italia.* 2 vols. Venice, 1927.

Montias, John Michael. *Artists and Artisans in Delft: A Socio-Economic Study of the Seventeenth Century.* Princeton, 1982.

————. "Cost and Value in Seventeenth-Century Dutch Art." *Art History* 10 (1987): 455–66.

————. "Socio-Economic Aspects of Netherlandish Art from the Fifteenth to the Seventeenth Century: A Survey." *Art Bulletin* 72 (1990): 358–73.

Moorman, John R. H. *The History of the Franciscan Order, from Its Origin to the Year 1517*. Oxford, 1968.

Morandi, Ubaldo. *Cattedrale di Siena: Ottavo centanario della consacrazione, 1179–1979*. Siena, 1979.

Moreni, Domenico. *Notizie istoriche dei Contorni di Firenze*. 4 vols. Florence, 1791–95.

Moriani, Antonella. "Assistenza e beneficenza ad Arezzo nel XIV secolo: La Fraternità di Santa Maria della Misericordia." In *La società del bisogno*, 19–35.

Mosiici, Luciana. "Note sul più antico protocollo notarile del territorio fiorentino e su altri registri di imbreviature del secolo XIII." In *Il Notariato nella civiltà toscana: Atti di un Convegno (Maggio 1981)*, 171–238. Rome, 1985.

Moskowitz, Anita Fiderer. *The Sculpture of Andrea and Nino Pisano*. Cambridge, 1986.

Mundy, John H. "Charity and Social Work in Toulouse, 1100–1250." *Traditio* 22 (1966): 203–87.

Murray, Alexander. "Piety and Impiety in Thirteenth-Century Italy." In *Studies in Church History*. Vol. 8, *Popular Belief and Practice*, edited by G. J. Cuming and Derek Baker, 83–106. Cambridge, 1972.

————. "Religion among the Poor in Thirteenth-Century France: The Testimony of Humbert de Romans." *Traditio* 30 (1974): 285–324.

Neretti, Luigi. *Fra Benedetto da Foiano della chiana*. Collana di storia locale, 8. Foiano, 1988.

Nessi, Silvestro. *La Basilica di S. Francesco in Assisi e la sua documentazione*. Assisi, 1972.

Nicolaj [Petronio], Giovanna. "Notariato aretino tra medioevo ed età moderno: Collegio, statuti, e matricole dal 1339 al 1739." In *Studi in onore di Leopoldo Sandri*, 633–60. Pubblicazioni degli Archivi di Stato 98. Rome, 1983.

————. "Storia di vescovi e di notai ad Arezzo fra XI e XII secolo." In *Il Notariato nella civiltà toscana: Atti di un Convegno (Maggio 1981)*, 147–70. Rome, 1985.

Nicolini, Ugolino. "Nuove testimonianze su fra Raniero Fasani e i suoi disciplinati." *BDSPU* 60 (1963): 331–46.

————. "Ricerche sulla sede di Fra Raniero Fasani fuori di Porta Sole a Perugia." *BDSPU* 63 (1966): 189–204.

Norberg, Kathryn. *Rich and Poor in Grenoble, 1600–1814*. Berkeley, 1984.

Offner, Richard. *A Critical and Historical Corpus of the Florentine Painting*, ser. 3, vol. 1. New York, 1931.

Onory, Sergio Mochi. "L'Umbria Bizantina." In *L'umbria nella storia, nella letteratura, nell'arte,* 55–77. Bologna, 1954.

Origo, Iris. "The Domestic Enemy: The Eastern Slave in Tuscany in the Fourteenth and Fifteenth Centuries." *Speculum* 30 (1955): 521–66.

————. *The Merchant of Prato: Francesco do Marco Datini.* London, 1957.

————. *The World of San Bernardino.* New York, 1962.

Orlandelli, Gianfranco. "Genesi dell' 'ars notariae' nel secolo XIII." *Studi medievali,* 3d ser., 6 (1965): 329–66.

Orlandi, Stefano. "Il VII centanario della predicazione di S. Pietro Martire a Firenze: I ricordi di S. Pietro Martire." *Memorie Domenicane* 63 (1946): 26–41, 59–87; 64 (1947): 31–48, 109–36, 170–211.

Ottokar, Nicola. *Il Comune di Firenze alla fine del Dugento.* Florence, 1926.

Ottolenghi, D. "Studi demografici sulla popolazione di Siena dal secolo XVI al XIX." *BSSP* 10 (1903): 297–358.

Paatz, Walter, and Elisabeth Paatz. *Die Kirchen von Florenz: Ein kunstgeschichtliches Handbuch.* 7 vols. Frankfurt am Main, 1940–54.

Pampaloni, Guido. *L'ospedale di Santa Maria Nuova.* Florence, 1961.

————. "Popolazione e società nel centro e nei sobborghi." In *Prato: Storia di una città,* 1: 361–93.

Panofsky, Erwin. "Imagio Pietatis." In *Festschrift für M. J. Friedländer zum 60. Geburtstag,* 261–308. Leipzig, 1927.

————. *Tomb Sculpture: Four Lectures on Its Changing Aspects from Ancient Egypt to Bernini.* Edited by H. W. Janson. New York, 1964.

Paoletti, John. "The Strozzi Altarpiece Reconsidered." *Memorie Domenicane,* n.s. 20 (1989): 279–300.

————. "*Ars Orandi:* Wooden Sculpture in Italy as Sacral Presence." Typescript. N.d.

Papi, Massimo D. "Confraternite ed ordine mendicanti a Firenze: Aspetti di una ricerca quantitative." *Mélanges de l'école française de Rome* 89 (1977): 723–32.

————. "Le Confraternite fiorentine fra medioevo e rinascimento: Stato della questione e prospettiva d'indagine." *Ricerche di storia sociale e religiosa* 15–16 (1979): 121–33.

Pardi, Giuseppe. "La popolazione di Siena e del Senese attraverso i secoli." *La Città: Estratta dal BSSP* 1 (1924): 1–48.

Pardo, Vittorio Franchetti. *Le città nella storia d'Italia: Arezzo.* Bari, 1986.

Park, Katherine. *Doctors and Medicine in Early Renaissance Florence.* Princeton, 1985.

Pasqui, Ubaldo. "La biblioteca di Ser Simone figlio di ser Benvenuto di Bonaventura della Tenca." *ASI,* 5th ser., 4 (1889): 250–55.

————. "Pittori aretini vissuti dalla metà del sec. XII al 1527." *Rivista d'arte* 10 (1917–18): 32–87.

Passerini, Luigi. *Storia degli stabilmenti de beneficenza ed'istruzione elementare gratuita della città di Firenze.* Florence, 1853.

Pastore, Alessandro. *Crimine e giustizia in tempo di peste nell'Europa moderna.* Bari, 1991.

Pellegrini, L. "Mendicanti e parroci: Coesistenza e conflitti di due strutture organizzative della 'cura animarum.'" In *Francescanesimo e vita religiosa dei laici nel '200: Atti del VIII Convegno internazionale (Assisi, 16 ottobre 1980).* Rimini, 1982.

Pertile, Antonio. *Storia del diritto italiano.* Vol. 3, *Storia del diritto privato.* Padua, 1871.

Peterson, David. "Conciliarism, Republicanism, and Corporatism: The 1415–1420 Constitution of the Florentine Clergy." *Renaissance Quarterly* 42 (1989): 183–226.

————. "An Episcopal Election in Quattrocento Florence." In *Popes, Teachers, and Canon Law in the Middle Ages,* edited by James Ross Sweeney and Stanley Chodorow. Ithaca, 1989.

Petralia, Giuseppe. "Per la storia dell'emigrazione quattrocentesca da Pisa e della migrazione Toscana-Sicilia nel Basso Medieoevo." In *Strutture familiari, epidemie, migrazioni nell'Italia medievale,* edited by Rinaldo Comba, Gabriella Piccinni, and Guiliano Pinto, 373–88. Naples, 1984.

Petrucci, Armando. *La scrittura: Ideologia e rappresentazione.* Turin, 1986.

Petrucci, Armando, and Luisa Miglio. "Alfabetizzazione e organizzazione scolastica nella toscana del XIV secolo." In *La Toscana nel secolo XIV,* 465–84.

Pevsner, Nikolaus. "The Term Architect in the Middle Ages." *Speculum* 17 (1942): 549–62.

Piccini, Gabriela. *"Seminare, fruttare, raccogliere": Mezzadri e salariati sulle terre di Monte Oliveto Maggiore (1374–1430).* Milan, 1982.

Pierotti, Romano. "Aspetti del mercato e della produzione a Perugia fra la fine del secolo XIV e la prima metà del XV: La bottega di Cuoiame di Niccolò di Martino di Pietro." *BSPU* 72 (1975): 79–185, 1395–1442; 73 (1976): 1–131.

Pinto, Giuliano. *La Toscana nel tardo medioevo: Ambiente, economia rurale, società.* Florence, 1982.

————, ed. *La società del bisogno: Poverità e assistenza nella Toscana medievale.* Florence, 1990.

Pinto, Giuliano, and Paolo Pirillo, eds. *Il contratto di mezzadria nella Toscana medievale.* 2 vols. Florence, 1987.

Pitt-Rivers, Julian. "Honour and Social Status: The Concept of Honour." In

Honour and Shame: The Values of Mediterranean Society, edited by J. Peristiany, 19–77. London, 1965.

Polzer, Joseph. "Aristotle, Mohammed, and Nicholas V in Hell." *Art Bulletin* 46 (1964): 457–69.

————. "Aspects of the Fourteenth-Century Iconography of Death and the Plague." In Williman, *The Black Death,* 108–30.

Pope-Hennessy, John. "An Exhibition of Sienese Wooden Sculpture." *Burlington Magazine* 91 (1949): 323–24.

————. *Introduction to Italian Sculpture.* London, 1955.

————. *The Portrait in the Renaissance.* Bollingen Series, 35. New York, 1966.

Postan, M. M. *The Medieval Economy and Society: An Economic History of Britain in the Middle Ages.* London, 1972.

Preiser, Arno. *Das Entstehen und die Entwicklung der Predella in der italienischen Malerie.* Hildesheim, 1973.

Previtali, Giovanni. *La fortuna dei primitivi dal Vasari ai neoclassici.* Turin, 1964.

————. "La periodizzazione della storia dell'arte italiana." In *Storia dell'arte italiana,* vol. 1, edited by Giovanni Previtale, 5–95. Turin, 1979.

Procacci, Ugo. "Sulla cronologia delle opere di Masaccio e di Masolino tra il 1425 e il 1428." *Rivista d'arte,* 3d ser., 28 (1953): 3–55.

————. "Di Jacopo di Antonio e delle compagnie di pittori del Corso degli Adimari nel XV secolo." *Rivista d'arte,* 3d ser., 35 (1960–61): 3–70.

Pullan, Brian. *Rich and Poor in Renaissance Venice: The Social Institutions of a Catholic State, to 1620.* Oxford, 1971.

————. "Poveri, mendicanti, e vagabondi (secoli XIV–XVII)." In *Storia d'Italia: Annali.* Vol. 1, *Dal feudalesimo al capitalismo,* edited by Ruggiero Romano and Corrado Vivanti, 981–1048. Turin, 1978.

————. "Support and Redeem: Charity and Poor Relief in Italian Cities from the Fourteenth to the Seventeenth Century." *Continuity and Change* 3 (1988): 177–208.

Rearick, Janet Cox. *Dynasty and Destiny in Medici Art.* Princeton, 1984.

Redon, Odile. "Autour de l'Hôpital Santa Maria della Scala à Sienne au XIIIe siècle." *Ricerche storiche* 15 (1985): 17–34.

Repetti, Emmanuel. *Dizionario geografico fiscio e storico della Toscana.* 6 vols. Florence, 1833–44.

Riccetti, Lucio. "Orvieto: Testamenti del 'Liber donationem' (1221–1281)." In *Nolens Intestatus Decedere.*

————, ed. *Il duomo di Orvieto.* Bari, 1988.

Ricci, Paola Romizi. "Il notaio perugino Pietro di Lippolo e le sue 'imbreviature' del 1348." *Annali della Facoltà di lettere e filosofia* 7 (1969–70): 347–500.

Rice, Eugene. *Prefatory Epistles of Jacques Lefèvre d'Etaples and Related Texts.* New York, 1972.

Riemer, Eleanor. "Women, Dowries, and Capital Investment in Thirteenth-Century Siena." In *The Marriage Bargain: Women and Dowries in European History*, edited by Marion A. Kaplan, 59–79. New York, 1985.

Rigon, Antonio. "Influssi francescani nei testamenti padovani del due e trecento." *Le Venezie francescane*, n.s. 2 (1985): 105–19.

Ringbom, Sixten. *Icon to Narrative: The Rise of the Dramatic Close-up in the Fifteenth-Century Devotional Painting*. Acta Academiae Aboensis, vol. 331, no. 2. Albo, 1965.

Rodolico, Niccolò. *La democrazia fiorentina nel suo tramonto 1378–1382*. Bologna, 1905.

Romano, Ruggiero. *Tra due crisi: l'Italia del Rinascimento*. Turin, 1971.

Ronzani, Mauro. "Gli ordini mendicanti e le istituzioni ecclesiastiche preesistenti a Pisa nel Duecento." In *Les ordres mendicants et la ville en Italie Centrale (v. 1220–v. 1350): Actes de la table ronde*. Rome, 27–28 April 1977. *MEFRM* 89 (1977).

————. "Penitenti e ordini mendicanti a Pisa sino all'inizio del Trecento." *MEFRM* 89 (1977): 733–41.

————. "Il francescanismo a Pisa fino alla metà del Trecento." *Bolletino storico Pisano* 14 (1985): 1–56.

Rosenthal, Elaine G. "The Position of Women in Renaissance Florence: Neither Autonomy nor Subjection." In *Florence and Italy*, 369–81.

Ross, Janet, and Nelly Erichsen. *The Story of Pisa*. London, 1909.

Rossi, A. "Lo sviluppo demografico di Pisa dal XII al XV secolo." *BSSP* 14–16 (1945–47): 7–61.

Rossi Sabatini, G. *L'espansione di Pisa nel Mediterraneo fino alla Meloria*. Florence, 1935.

Rowley, George. *Ambrogio Lorenzetti*. Princeton, 1958.

Rubinstein, Nicolai. "La lotta contro i magnati a Firenze: La prima legge sul 'sodamento' e la pace del Card. Latino." *ASI* 93 (1935): 161–72.

Rutenberg, Victor. *Popolo e movimenti popolari nell'Italia del '300 e '400*. Translated by G. Borghini. Bologna, 1971.

Saalman, Howard. *The Bigallo*. New York, 1969.

Salmi, Mario. "I Bacci di Arezzo nel sec. XV e loro cappella nella chiesa di S. Francesco." *Rivista d'Arte* 9 (1916): 224–37.

————. *San Domenico e San Francesco di Arezzo*. Rome, 1951.

————. *San Domenico and San Francesco in Arezzo*. Translated by Althea Loshak. Rome, 1954.

Saltmarsh, John. "Plague and Economic Decline in England in the Later Middle Ages." *Cambridge Historical Journal* 7 (1941–43): 23–41.

Salvatorelli, Luigi. "La politica interna di Perugia in un poemetto volgare della metà del Trecento." *BDSPU* 50 (1953): 5–110.

————. "Spiritualità umbra." In *L'umbria nella storia, nella letteratura, nell'arte,* 1–26.

Salvemini, Gaetano. *Magnati e popolani in Firenze dal 1280 al 1295.* Florence, 1899.

Samuel, Raphael. "The Workshop of the World: Steam Power and Hand Technology in Mid-Victorian Britain." *History Workshop* 3 (1973): 6–72.

Sandri, Lucia. "Ospedali e utenti dell'assistenze nella Firenze del Quattrocento." In *La società del bisogno,* 61–100.

Sapori, Armando. "La beneficenza delle compagnie mercantili del trecento." *ASI,* 7th ser., vol. 4 (1925): 251–72.

————. *Le marchand italien au moyen âge: Conférences et bibliographie.* Paris, 1952.

Schevill, Ferdinand. *Siena: The Story of a Medieval Commune.* New York, 1909.

Schlosser, Julius von. "Geschichte der Portratbildnerei in Wachs." *Jahrbuch der Kunsthistorischen Sammlungen des Allerhochsten Kaiserhauses* 29 (1911): 171–258.

Schneider, Jane. "Of Vigilance and Virgins: Honor, Shame, and Access to Resources in Mediterranean Societies." *Ethnology* 10 (1971): 1–24.

Sereni, Emilio. *Storia del paesaggio agrario italiano.* Bari, 1961.

Shrewsbury, John F. D. *A History of Bubonic Plague in the British Isles.* Cambridge, 1970.

Silva, Pietro. *Pisa sotto Firenze dal 1406 al 1433.* Pisa, 1910.

Skaug, Erling. "The St. Anthony Abbot Ascribed to Nardo di Cione at the Villa I Tatti, Florence." *Burlington Magazine* 117 (1975): 540–43.

————. "The 'Rinuccini Tondo'—An Eighteenth-Century Copy or a Four-teenth-Century Original?" In *Atti del convegno di studi delle opere d'arte a dieci anni dell'alluvione in Firenze, 1976,* 333–39, 571–75. Florence, 1981.

————. "Punch Marks—What Are They Worth? Problems of Tuscan Work-shop Interrelationships in the Mid-Fourteenth Century: The Ovile Master and Giovanni da Milano." In *Proceedings of the 24th International Congress of the History of Art/CIHA.* Vol. 3, *La pittura nel XIV e XV secolo: Il contributo dell'analisi tecnica alla storia dell'arte,* 253–82. Bologna, 1983.

Smart, Alastair. *The Dawn of Italian Painting, 1250–1400.* Ithaca, 1978.

Spitz, Lewis. *The Religious Renaissance of the German Humanists.* Cambridge, Mass., 1963.

Strocchia, Sharon. "Burials in Renaissance Florence, 1300–1500." Ph.D. diss., University of California, Berkeley, 1981.

————. "Death Rites and the Ritual Family." In Tetel, Witt, and Goffen, *Life and Death in Fifteenth-Century Florence,* 120–45.

Stubblebine, James H. *Giotto: The Arena Chapel Frescoes: Illustrations, Introductory Essay, Backgrounds, Sources, and Criticism.* New York, 1969.

Swarzenski, Hanns. "Before and after Pisano." *Boston Museum Bulletin* 68 (1970): 178–96.

Sznura, Franek. "Edilizia privata e urbanistica in tempo di crisi." In *Prato: Storia di una città,* 1: 301–58.

Tabacco, Giovanni. "Interpretazioni e ricerche sull'aristocrazia comunale di Pisa." *Studi medievali,* 3d ser., 3 (1962): 707–27.

———. "Nobiltà e potere ad Arezzo in età communale." *Studi medievali* 15 (1974): 1–24.

———. "Nobili e cavalieri a Bologna e a Firenze tra XII e XIII secolo." *Studi medievali,* 3d ser., 17 (1976): 41–79.

———. *The Struggle for Power in Medieval Italy.* Translated by Rosalind B. Jensen. Cambridge, 1989.

Tangheroni, Marco. *Politica, commercio, agricoltura a Pisa nel Trecento.* Pubblicazioni dell'Istituto di Storia: Facoltà di lettere dell'Università di Pisa, no. 5. Pisa, 1973.

———. "Il sistema economico della toscana nel Trecento." In *La Toscana nel secolo XIV,* 41–66.

Tateo, Francesco. "I Toscani e gli altri." In *La Toscana nel secolo XIV,* 5–26.

Tenenti, Alberto. *Il Senso della morte e l'amore della vita nel Rinascimento (Francia et Italia).* 2 ed. Turin, 1977.

———. "Processi formativi e condizionamenti del senso della morte e delle sue espressioni (secoli XII–XVIII)." *Ricerche di storia sociale e religiosa* 8 (1979): 5–22.

Tetel, Marcel, Ronald Witt, and Rona Goffen, eds. *Life and Death in Fifteenth-Century Florence.* Durham, N.C., 1989.

Todini, Filippo. *La pittura umbra: Dal Duecento al primo Cinquecento.* 2 vols. Milan, 1989.

Topografische kaart van België / Carte topographique de Belgique (1:100,000). Brussels, 1986.

Trexler, Richard. *Economic, Political, and Religious Effects of the Papal Interdict on Florence, 1376–1378.* Frankfurt am Main, 1964.

———. "Death and Testament in the Episcopal Constitutions of Florence (1327)." In *Renaissance Studies in Honor of Hans Baron,* edited by Anthony Molho and John Tedeschi, 29–74. De Kalb, Ill., 1971.

———. *Synodal Law in Florence and Fiesole, 1306–1518.* Studi e testi, vol. 286. Vatican City, 1971.

———. "The Bishop's Portion: Generic Pious Legacies in the Late Middle Ages in Italy." *Traditio* 28 (1972): 397–450.

———. "Le célibat à la fin du Moyen Age: Les religieuses de Florence." *Annales, E.S.C.* 27 (1972): 1329–50.

———. "Florentine Religious Experience: The Sacred Image." *Studies in the Renaissance* 19 (1972): 8–41.

———. "The Foundlings of Florence, 1395–1455." *Journal of Psychohistory* 1 (1973–74): 259–84.

———. *Public Life in Renaissance Florence.* New York, 1980.

Tripet, Arnaud. *Pétrarque ou la connaissance de soi.* Geneva, 1967.

Valeri, Elpidio. *La fraternità dell'Ospedale di Santa Maria della Misericordia in Perugia nei secoli XIII–XIV.* Perugia, 1972.

van Os, Henk. "The Black Death and Sienese Painting." *Art History* 4 (1981): 237–49.

———. *Sienese Altarpieces, 1215–1460—Form, Content, Function.* 2 vols. Gröningen, 1984–90.

———. "Text and Image: The Case of a Jewish Prophet in Carmelite Disguise." In *Non Nova, sed Nove: Mélanges de civilisation médiévale, dédiés à Willem Noomen,* edited by Martin Gosman and Jaap Van Os, 163–68. Gröningen, 1984.

———. "Tradition and Innovation in Some Altarpieces by Bartolo di Fredi." *Art Bulletin* 67 (1985): 50–66.

———. "Painting in a House of Glass: The Altarpieces of Pienza." *Simiolus* 17, no. 1 (1987): 23–38.

Varese, Prospero. "Condizioni economiche e demografiche di Arezzo nel secolo XV." In *Annali del R. Istituto Magistrale di Arezzo,* 39–67. Arezzo, 1924–25.

Vauchez, André, and Raoul Manselli. "'Ordo fraternitatis': Confraternite e pietà dei laici nel medioevo." *Rivista di storia della chiesa in Italia* 32 (1978): 186–202.

Verde, Armando F., O.P. *Lo Studio fiorentino 1473–1503: Ricerche e documenti.* 4 vols. Florence, 1973–85.

Verlinden, Charles. *L'esclavage dans l'Europe médiévale.* 2 vols. Bruges, 1955.

Volpe, Giocchino. *Studi sulle istituzioni comunali a Pisa (Città e contado, Consoli e Podestà) Secoli XII–XIII.* Pisa, 1902.

Vovelle, Michel. *Piété baroque et déchristianisation en Provence au XVIIIe siècle: Les attitudes devant la mort d'après les clauses des testaments.* Paris, 1973.

———. *La mort et l'occident, de 1300 à nos jours.* Paris, 1983.

Wackernagel, Martin. *The World of the Florentine Renaissance Artist: Projects and Patrons, Workshop and Art Market.* Translated by Alison Luchs. Princeton, 1980.

Wainwright, Valerie. "Conflict and Popular Government in Fourteenth-Century Siena: Il Monte dei Dodici." In *Atti del III Convegno di studi sulla storia dei ceti dirigenti in Toscana,* 57–80. Florence, 1981.

———. "The Testing of a Popular Sienese Regime: The 'Riformatori' and the Insurrection of 1371." In *I Tatti Studies: Essays in the Renaissance,* 2: 107–70. Florence, 1987.

Waley, Daniel. *The Papal States in the Thirteenth Century.* London, 1961.

———. "Le istituzioni communali di Assisi nel passaggio dal XII al XIII secolo." In *Assisi al tempo di San Francesco. Società internazionale di studi francescani: Atti del V Convegno internazionale Assisi, 13–16 ottobre 1977*, 53–70. Assisi, 1978.

———. *The Italian City-Republics.* 3d ed. London, 1988.

Warburg, Aby. *La rinascita del paganesimo antico.* [*Gesammelte Schriften*, 1932.] Florence, 1966.

Watkins, Renée Neu. "Petrarch and the Black Death: From Fear to Monuments." *Studies in the Renaissance* 19 (1972): 196–223.

Weissman, Ronald. *Ritual Brotherhood in Renaissance Florence.* New York, 1982.

———. "Taking Patronage Seriously: Mediterranean Values and Renaissance Society." In *Patronage, Art, and Society*, 25–45.

White, John. *Duccio: Tuscan Art and the Medieval Workshop.* London, 1979.

Wickham, Chris J. *The Mountains and the City: The Tuscan Appennines in the Early Middle Ages.* Oxford, 1988.

Wieruszowski, Helen. "Arezzo as a Center of Learning and Letters in the Thirteenth Century." *Traditio* 9 (1953): 321–91.

Williman, Daniel, ed. *The Black Death: The Impact of the Fourteenth-Century Plague. Papers of the Eleventh Annual Conference of the Center for Medieval and Early Renaissance Studies.* New York, 1982.

Wilson, Jean C. "Workshop Patterns and the Production of Painting in Sixteenth-Century Bruges." *Burlington Magazine* 132 (1990): 523–27.

Wolbach, Wolfgang F. *Guide del Museo Sacro Vaticano.* Vol. 2, *La Croce: Lo sviluppo dell'Oreficeria sacra.* Vatican City, 1938.

Woolf, Stuart J. "Plebi urbane e plebi rurali: Da poveri a proletari." *Storia d'Italia: Annali*, 1: 1049–78. Turin, 1978.

Zaccaria, Giuseppe. "L'Arte de Guarnellari e dei Bambagiari di Assisi." *BDSPU* 70 (1973): 1–92.

Zervas, Diane Finiello. *The Parte Guelfa: Brunelleschi and Donatello.* Locust Valley, N.Y., 1988.

Index

Assisi (*continued*)

lineage, 135, 168–71

paintings, 85, 246, 247, 248, 252, 253, 254

perpetual masses, 206, 207, 208, 211

plaques, 136

politics, 9, 10, 11

poor relief, 66, 133

population, 5, 6

property, 136, 168–71, 196, 197, 198, 200

religious orders

Augustinians of Santo Spirito, 33

Franciscans, 6, 39, 40, 41, 85, 135, 137, 248

of San Giovanni, 136

hermits (*carcerati* at Monte Subàsio), 40

San Corradi de Insula, 40

San Damiano, 40

San Francesco, 40

Santa Maria de Rochezola, 40

Santa Maria degli Angeli (the Porziuncola), 40, 322n. 19

nunneries, 43, 44

Poor Clares, 40

Olivetani, 339n. 98

Sacro Convento of San Francesco (Basilica of Assisi), 40, 84, 85, 86, 171, 252

restoration, 240

sculpture, 239

testaments, 11, 12, 13, 14, 290, 291, 293–94

tombs, 133, 136, 137

wax figures, 239

Baglioni family, 352n. 117

Baldelli, Ignazio, 379n. 14

Balestracci, Duccio, 307n. 1

Banker, James, 64, 307n. 1, 323n. 29, 328n. 107, 329n. 120, 330nn. 125, 127, 333n. 14, 363n. 123

Banti, Ottavio, 275

Barbolani family, 215

Bardi family, 179

Baron, Hans, 33, 275, 348n. 134

"civic humanism," 32, 275

Bartoli Langeli, Attilio, 16, 314n. 95

Baxandall, Michael, 372n. 103

Becker, Marvin, 32, 52, 266, 326n. 63, 329n. 121

Bellucci, M., 326n. 74

Belting, Hans, 245, 248, 366n. 17

Benedictines. *See under individual city-states, religious orders*

Benucci family, 207

Bertram, Martin, 16

Bibbiena, 21, 111, 299

Bicci, Neri di, 268

Binion, Rudolph, 379n. 19

Bizzocchi, Roberto, 340n. 113

Black, Robert, 312n. 74

Black Death, 4, 5, 6, 7, 8, 17, 18, 21, 32–33, 50–51, 52, 53, 54, 56, 57, 58, 59, 60, 63, 67, 69, 70, 72, 73, 74, 77, 78, 80, 84, 87, 88, 89, 90, 93, 98, 102, 108, 112, 116, 117, 135, 137, 140, 142, 143, 148, 149, 150, 153, 154, 155, 160, 161, 163, 169, 173, 174, 182, 186, 187, 189, 191, 195, 197, 198, 199, 206, 207, 212, 214, 216, 217, 218, 219, 220, 223, 227, 231, 232, 234, 236, 241, 243, 248, 249, 250, 251, 252, 253, 254, 256, 258, 259, 261, 262, 264–65, 266, 269, 271, 272, 273, 274, 276, 279, 287, 291, 292, 317n. 129, 337n. 65

Black Death studies, 25–26

Bloch, Marc, 281, 283

Boccaccio, Giovanni, 18, 140, 162, 344n. 48

Borgo San Sepolcro, 4, 61, 64, 89, 112, 323n. 29, 328n. 107, 329n. 120, 330nn. 125, 127

Borsook, Eve, 342n. 37, 358n. 53, 367n. 21, 377nn. 143, 144

Boskovits, Miklós, 248, 269, 271, 272, 273, 274, 275, 276, 277, 366n. 17, 368n. 56, 375n. 134, 376nn. 137, 140

Bowsky, William, 10

Bracci, Lazzaro, 8, 151, 312n. 75